Dry Eye Disease

Dry Eye Disease

Edited by

ANAT GALOR, MD, MSPH
Associate Professor of Ophthalmology
Bascom Palmer Eye Institute
University of Miami
Miami, Florida

ELSEVIER

Publisher: Sarah Barth
Acquisitions Editor: Kayla Wolfe
Editorial Project Manager: Sam W. Young
Project Manager: Sreejith Viswanathan
Cover Designer: Matthew Limbert

3251 Riverport Lane
St. Louis, Missouri 63043

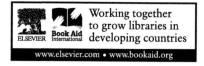

Working together
to grow libraries in
developing countries

www.elsevier.com • www.bookaid.org

List of Contributors

Penny A. Asbell, MD, FACS, MBA, FARVO
Professor
Department of Ophthalmology
University of Tennessee Health Science Center
Memphis, TN
United States

Christophe Baudouin, MD, PhD
Department of Ophthalmology
Quinze-Vingts National Ophthalmology Hospital &
    Vision Institute
Paris, France

Jose Benitez-del-Castillo, MD
Department of Ophthalmology
University Complutense
Hospital Clinic San Carlos
Madrid, Spain

William W. Binotti, MD
Cornea Service
Department of Ophthalmology
Tufts Medical Center
Tufts University School of Medicine
Boston, MA
United States

Vatinee Y. Bunya, MD, MSCE
Department of Ophthalmology
Scheie Eye Institute
Philadelphia, PA
United States

Yihe Chen, MD
Schepens Eye Research Institute of Massachusetts
    Eye and Ear
Department of Ophthalmology
Harvard Medical School
Boston, MA
United States

Stephanie M. Cox, OD
Cornea Service
Department of Ophthalmology
Tufts Medical Center
Tufts University School of Medicine
Boston, MA
United States

**Jennifer P. Craig, PhD, FCOptom, FAAO,
    FBCLA, FCLS**
Professor
Department of Ophthalmology
New Zealand National Eye Centre
The University of Auckland
Auckland, New Zealand

Reza Dana, MD, MSc, MPH
Schepens Eye Research Institute of
    Massachusetts Eye and Ear
Department of Ophthalmology
Harvard Medical School
Boston, MA
United States

Murat Dogru, MD, PhD
Department of Ophthalmology
Keio University School of Medicine
Tokyo, Japan

John A. Gonzales, MD
Francis I. Proctor Foundation
Department of Ophthalmology
University of California
San Francisco, CA
United States

Christopher John Hammond, MD, FRCOphth
Academic Section of Ophthalmology
Department of Twin Research & Genetic
    Epidemiology
King's College London, St Thomas' Hospital
London, United Kingdom

Pedram Hamrah, MD
Cornea Service
Department of Ophthalmology
Tufts Medical Center
Tufts University School of Medicine
Boston, MA
United States

Sandeep Jain, MD
Department of Ophthalmology and Visual Sciences
University of Illinois at Chicago
Chicago, IL
United States

Jerry Kalangara, MD
Department of Anesthesiology
Division of Pain Medicine
Emory University School of Medicine
Atlanta, GA
United States

Takashi Kojima, MD, PhD
Department of Ophthalmology
Keio University School of Medicine
Tokyo, Japan

Merin Kuruvilla, MD
Division of Pulmonary, Allergy, Critical Care, and Sleep
Emory University School of Medicine
Atlanta, GA
United States

Zuguo Liu, MD, PhD
Eye Institute of Xiamen University
China

Ilaria Macchi, MD
Ophthalmology Unit
Fabia Mater
Rome, Italy

Mina Massaro-Giordano, MD
Department of Ophthalmology
Scheie Eye Institute
Philadelphia, PA
United States

Elisabeth M. Messmer, MD, FEBO
Department of Ophthalmology
Ludwig-Maximilians-University
Munich, Germany

Maryam Mousavi, MOptom, PhD
Dean and Professor
School of Optometry
University of Alabama at Birmingham
Birmingham, AL
United States

Jessica Mun, BA
Clinical Research Coordinator
Department of Ophthalmology and Visual Sciences
University of Illinois at Chicago
Chicago, IL
United States

Jennifer B. Nadelmann, MD
Department of Ophthalmology
Scheie Eye Institute
Philadelphia, PA
United States

Kelly K. Nichols, OD, MPH, PhD
Dean and Professor
School of Optometry
University of Alabama at Birmingham
Birmingham, AL
United States

Jeremy N. Nortey, BS
Research Fellow
University of North Carolina School of Medicine
Chapel Hill, NC
United States

Francis I. Proctor Foundation
University of California
San Francisco, CA
United States

Sneh Patel, MS
University of Miami Miller School of Medicine
Miami, FL
United States

Bascom Palmer Eye Institute
University of Miami Miller School of Medicine
Miami, FL
United States

Vilavun Puangsricharern, MD
Excellence Center for Cornea and Limbal Stem Cell
    Transplantation
Department of Ophthalmology
King Chulalongkorn Memorial Hospital
Faculty of Medicine
Chulalongkorn University
Bangkok, Thailand

Daniela Roca, MD
Department of Ophthalmology and Visual Sciences
University of Illinois at Chicago
Chicago, IL
United States

Konstantinos D. Sarantopoulos, MD, PhD
Department of Anesthesiology
Perioperative Medicine, and Pain Management
University of Miami Miller School of Medicine
Miami, FL
United States

Chi Chin Sun, MD, PhD
Department of Ophthalmology
Chang Gung Memorial Hospital
Keelung, Taiwan

School of Medicine
College of Medicine
Chang Gung University
Taoyuan, Taiwan

Bayasgalan Surenkhuu, MD, MS
Research Specialist
Department of Ophthalmology and Visual Sciences
University of Illinois at Chicago
Chicago, IL
United States

Joseph Tauber, MD
Owner Tauber Eye Center
Kansas City, MO
United States

Louis Tong, MBBS, FRCS, MD, PhD
Ocular Surface Research Group
Singapore Eye Research Institute
Duke-NUS Graduate Medical School
Singapore National Eye Center
Yong Loo Lin School of Medicine
National University of Singapore
Singapore

Kazuo Tsubota, MD, PhD
Department of Ophthalmology
Keio University School of Medicine
Tsubota Laboratory, Inc.
Toyko, Japan

Ömür Ö. Uçakhan, MD
Professor
Department of Ophthalmology
Ankara University School of Medicine
Ankara, Turkey

Murugesan Vanathi, MD
Dr. Rajendra Prasad Centre for Ophthalmic Sciences
All India Institute of Medical Sciences (AIIMS)
New Delhi, India

Jelle Vehof, MD, PhD, FEBO
Departments of Ophthalmology and Epidemiology
University of Groningen
University Medical Center Groningen
Groningen
the Netherlands

Academic Section of Ophthalmology
King's College London
St Thomas' Hospital
London, United Kingdom

Chi Hoang Viet Vu, MD, PhD
Cornea Department
Vietnam National Eye Hospital
Hanoi
Vietnam

Michael T.M. Wang, MBChB
Ophthalmology Fellow
Department of Ophthalmology
New Zealand National Eye Centre
The University of Auckland
Auckland, New Zealand

Sarah R. Wellik, MD
Professor of Ophthalmology
University of Miami
Bascom Palmer Eye Institute
Miami, FL
United States

James S. Wolffsohn, BSc, MBA, PhD
School of Optometry
Aston University
Birmingham
United Kingdom

Norihiko Yokoi, MD, PhD
Department of Ophthalmology
Kyoto Prefectural University of Medicine
Kyoto, Japan

Kyung Chul Yoon, MD, PhD
Department of Ophthalmology
Chonnam National University Medical School and
    Hospital
Gwangju
Korea

Contents

CHAPTER 1

Questionnaire Design and Use to Assess Dry Eye Disease

JAMES S. WOLFFSOHN, BSC, MBA, PHD

The accepted TFOS DEWS II definition (2017)[1] of dry eye includes symptoms as a required element of a diagnosis of dry eye disease and this was also the case with the 2007 definition.[2] However, symptoms alone cannot make a diagnosis of dry eye disease.[3] Standardization is important for a diagnosis and hence in the 2017 TFOS DEWS II diagnostic methodology report[4] reviewed the many available questionnaires and recommended the use of the Ocular Surface Disease Index (OSDI) or the Dry Eye Questionnaire (DEQ-5). "The consensus view of the committee was to use the OSDI due to its strong establishment in the field or the DEQ-5 due to its short length and discriminative ability".[4] In addition, they noted the continuous nature of visual analogue scales makes them attractive for clinical trials compared to discrete Likert-based question rating.

DESIGN CONSIDERATIONS

The Food and Drug Administration (FDA) of the United States published a report in 2009[5] highlighting the critical features for the development of Patient Reported Outcome (PRO) measures. Many dry eye questionnaires were developed before this report was available, but it still gives a useful benchmark as to how robust these questionnaires are.

The conceptual framework explicitly defines the concepts measured by the instrument and how the items (questions) interrelate to give the scores produced by a PRO instrument. The instrument may contain several subconcepts that contribute to the overall measurement. Hence, for dry eye it is common to assess severity and frequency of several dry eye type symptoms that combine (usually just summed, with none attributed a greater weight than others if they are presumed to independently contribute) to an overall score.

Content validity is evidence that the instrument measures what it is intended to measure, i.e., it has been validated to differentiate different severities of a certain medical condition in a population of interest.

Other considerations include
- Number of items/respondent burden
  - The longer the questionnaire, the more the burden on respondents and the more likely questions will be missed or due attention will not be paid, affecting the responses.[6,7]
- Administration mode
  - Contact with a clinician when completing a questionnaire (such as asking the questions by telephone or face to face) can artificially reduce the symptoms/reported difficulty of a patient.[8] However, completing it independently could be more burdensome if vision is impaired or the eyes are uncomfortable.
- Response options
  - Free text is useful to collect additional information or for respondents to clarify their approach in scoring a question, but this is more qualitative.
  - Likert/rating scales allow respondents to identify their intensity of feeling by selecting a number from a range between two or more "anchor" descriptors. They rely on the separation between each number being equal, but the scale is not continuous. A larger range allows more sensitive increments, but may not improve the accurate recording by respondents.[9] There should be a wide enough range and suitable "anchor" descriptors to ensure that ceiling/floor effects do not occur (when a normal distribution is skewed as too many responses fall at the top or bottom of the scale respectively). An even range of numbers

Dry Eye Disease. https://doi.org/10.1016/B978-0-323-82753-9.00006-0

Rating Scale – How comfortable have your eyes been over the last month

No discomfort   0   1   2   3   4   5   Extreme discomfort

Likert Scale – I have not experienced any discomfort due to my eyes over the last month

Strongly agree (1)   Agree (2)   Neither agree or disagree (3)   Disagree (4)   Strongly Disagree (5)

Visual Analog Scale - How comfortable have your eyes been over the last month

No discomfort ———————————————————————————— Extreme discomfort

FIG. 1.1 Questionnaire response option types.

forces the respondent from a neutral response if using an agree/disagreement style question.

- Visual analogue scales are a line with anchor descriptors at each end, on which respondents identify their intensity of feeling by placing a mark which can then be measured as a proportion of the complete line length (Fig. 1.1). It has the advantage of being a continuous scale (no limited number options) and this approach has been shown in rating contact lens handling to be more repeatable and responsive than a Likert scale.[10]

- Instructions
  - The instructions to the respondent on how to complete the questionnaire, including what to do when a question is not relevant to their situation, must be clear. Of particular importance is the period over which they are reflecting, when generally ranges from the past month to their feelings at the time of completion. A short recall period is susceptible to variability due to environmental conditions and disease fluctuations, whereas a long recall period is susceptible to memory limitations.

- Format
  - There is limited research on whether the formatting (layout) of the questions impacts completion.[11] While a comparison of digital versus paper base questionnaires has not yet been conducted in eye care, a metaanalysis of electronic pain-related data capture methods demonstrated digitally completed PRO questionnaires are comparable with conventional paper methods in terms of score equivalence, data completeness, ease, efficiency, and acceptability.[12]

- Language
  - The language should be generally be about a 11- to 12-year-old reading level (grade 6 USA)[13]
- Translation or cultural adaptation availability
  - It is important that a respondent can understand the language in the questions and the intended meaning. Translation to another language should be done by a native dual-language speaker. The questionnaire should then be back translated by a second native speaker and rechecked to ensure the question meaning has been maintained.[14]

HOW SHOULD THE QUESTIONS BE SELECTED?

The initial PRO questions are usually generated from a literature review of previously reported symptoms/difficulties and the items used by previous questionnaires. Focus groups or interviews with patients, clinicians, and family members can also be used.[5] These should continue until no new relevant on important information emerges (saturation). It is debatable whether a dry eye questionnaire should include items on health-related quality of life, as while the impact on the patient is important, it is difficult to differentiate activities affected by dry eye compared to other health issues.[15] Another relevant issue that is generally not covered is the burden of treatment strategies. These elements are best covered, if relevant, by separate questionnaires, so each one remains unidimensional. The selected questions should be reviewed for relevance (do they reflect the experience of someone with the disease/condition) and coverage (does the questionnaire cover all the likely related experiences) by the target population (including a broad demographic and range of severity) and experts in the field. These individuals perform the initial assessment of clarity (cognitive interviews to check their understanding of what the questions mean) and readability. The questions should be relevant to most patients as "non-applicable" options cause problems for scoring.[5]

HOW SHOULD THE QUESTIONNAIRE BE VALIDATED?

Following question selection and refinement the questionnaire prototype should be trialled in a target population with a wide range of the "condition" being tested. Additional tests should be performed which are hypothesized to assess the same relationship to stratify this population by the severity of the "condition" should be conducted to test the construct validity of the questionnaire prototype (either as an association/correlation (discriminant and convergent validity) or the ability to statistically separate the identified severity levels (group validity)). This might include an overall single question about how a patient feels. If there is an accepted gold standard for the same concept, the extent to which this correlates with the questionnaire is the "criterion validity."

The choice of population induces a level of bias as the inclusion and exclusion criteria used to choose the test participants will affect the apparent effectiveness of the questionnaire. The questionnaire prototype is also tested a second time in a subgroup to assess its repeatability. If this is too soon after the initial testing, then it is likely to be influenced by patient recall. If the repeat completion is too long after the initial testing, variation in the "condition" with factors such as the environment can make the questionnaire seem unreliable.[8]

STATISTICAL ANALYSIS

Item Reduction and Scale Optimization

One the data have been collected, statistical analysis is applied to assess whether the questionnaire assesses a single trait, the items it uses are relevant to the majority of the population, that the items discriminate between individuals and that the items are reliable. Classical Test Theory was based upon the assumption that the amount of an attribute is characterized by the "raw" questionnaire score. It has been shown that raw scores derived from ordinal data cannot be used as an accurate measurement of an attribute,[16] while it also cannot be assumed that an attribute is normally distributed within a population. In addition, it cannot be assumed that all tasks in question are of equal difficulty. The more recent

Item Response Theory compares individuals to an independent standard rather than each other.[17] It uses a mathematical model that describes the relationship between the level of a latent trait for a particular person and the probability of that person selecting a particular response to an item. Rasch Analysis is a form of Item response Theory that is based on Poisson models and principals of the score indicating the severity (order), the raw score of a questionnaire can be used for the measurement of an attribute (additivity), and only a single attribute is measured by the questionnaire (unidimensionality). Questionnaires that have been developed using Rasch Analysis will therefore be independent of the sample used to obtain the initial responses allowing subsequent use to measure the attribute on any population without variation of the psychometric properties. It should be noted a variety of statistical information is produced in Rasch Analysis, but it is up to the developers to select the most appropriate outputs for item reduction.

All response scales must be scored in the same direction, i.e., a larger number should reflect an increasing amount of the condition, or vice versa. The statistics indicate whether items are too predictable or too random. Unused or rarely used response options are removed from the scale or combined with adjacent response options. Once the response-scale function has been optimized, the procedure for item reduction involves item fit statistics, item targeting, frequency of endorsement, and tests of normality (skew and kurtosis) which have specific requirements that need to be met in order to indicate conformance with the Rasch model. If the questionnaire does not meet all of the criteria, the item that fails the most criteria is eliminated from the questionnaire, and all of the statistics and criteria are recalculated and reassessed. This is repeated in an iterative process until all of the remaining items meet all of the criteria or until the removal of an item causes the separation index to fall below a value of 2, which indicates a loss in questionnaire precision.[18]

Psychometric Properties of the Final Questionnaire

Once the questionnaire has been finalized through statistical refinement of the questions and the response options, its ability to detect change (equally sensitive to gains and losses in the measurement concept and to change across the entire range expected for the population of interest) should be determined. This would typically involve use prior to and after a treatment strategy known to be effective. The ability of an instrument to detect change in a certain population demographic influences the sample size for evaluating the effectiveness of treatments in clinical trials.

The psychometric properties of a questionnaire refer to its reliability and validity[18]:

- reliability is defined as the extent to which measurements are repeatable, stable and free from error; usually expressed as a ratio of the variability in observed questionnaire scores to the total variability including error, generating a coefficient between 0 (unreliable) and 1 (indicating higher reliability).
  - internal consistency—a measure of the interrelationship between items in a questionnaire. Options include the item-total correlations (the observed scores for each item to be correlated in turn to the total questionnaire score excluding that particular item) or "Cronbach's alpha" (splitting all items of a questionnaire into two halves and then determining correlation between the two). Acceptable values are typically considered to be >0.70 (lower values suggest the PRO is not measuring a single trait/multidimensionality) and <0.90 (greater values suggest items are redundant).
  - test—retest reliability—the ability of the questionnaire to produce repeatable responses, when complete after a time interval. Intraclass Correlation Coefficient measures concordance (agreement) rather than just correlation (association) which can be strong even if the scores are systematically raised or depressed on the retest. A value of ≥0.8 is typically desired for good questionnaire test—retest reliability, although a value of at least 0.6 is considered acceptable.
- validity is a measure of how well the questionnaire is able to measure what it is supposed to measure, although a perfect correlation is not expected as this would indicate the questionnaire is redundant. There are five specific areas that together encompass the meaning of validity. Two are relevant to the development stage:
  - face validity is whether the questionnaire seems to a person with the condition/disease or expert, to be asking appropriate questions.
  - content validity requires a judgment on whether the coverage and content of the items is appropriate, in terms of being applicable to all people within the intended target population.

The other three assessments of validity are typically made after the questionnaire has been statistically analyzed.

  - construct validity is an assessment of whether questionnaire scores are related to other variables or attributes as would be expected to in theory.

The process typically consists of a two-phased approach:

- Representational validity requires comparison and correlation between the questionnaire scores and other similar measures of the attribute of interest (convergent validity) or by comparison to measures that are known not to tap the attribute of interest (divergent or discriminant validity), confirming that the questionnaire doesn't measure what it isn't supposed to measure.
- Elaborative validity confirms the need for the existence of the questionnaire, by showing that it can be used in some way, most often to monitor change ("discriminative validity").
- *Criterion validity* is similar to elaborative validity, but is a demonstration that the questionnaire can discriminate people between groups. This usually involves the use of a Receiver Operating Characteristic (ROC) curve (a plot of the sensitivity of the questionnaire against 100 minus the specificity of the questionnaire; Fig. 1.2). Sensitivity is the true-positive rate, i.e., the proportion of people correctly categorized by the questionnaire, while specificity is the true-negative rate, i.e., the proportion of "normal" people correctly identified as being "normal." The area under the ROC curve is an index of discriminative ability, where an area of 0.5 (diagonal line) indicates that a test has no discriminative ability and the closer the curve is to the top left corner of the plot, the greater the area and therefore discriminative ability (an area of 1.0 indicating perfect discriminative ability). This relies on there being an independent gold standard for comparison which is usually not the case.
- factorial validity confirms the number of attributes (subscales) the questionnaire measures. Factor analysis or principal component analysis allows the number of variables or factors in a questionnaire to be identified, as well as concurrently describing the proportion of the variation that each accounts for.

DRY EYE QUESTIONNAIRES

The development of the common dry eye questionnaires are presented in Table 1.1 along with the design elements and analysis applied to refine the questionnaire. Only those questionnaires that have been well established with attempts at detailed psychometric evaluation have been summarized. For example, questionnaires such as the Women's Health Study

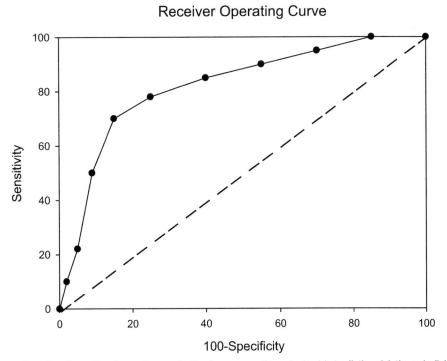

FIG. 1.2 Receiver Operating Curve demonstrating how a questionnaire is able to distinguish those individuals in an imagery dry eye group (sensitivity) without falsely selecting those from the nondry eye group (specificity) for different cut-off criteria.

questionnaire, which has a single question on dry eye symptom frequency, along with checking whether the individual has ever been diagnosed with dry eye, but no psychometric design evaluation, were excluded.[19]

The Ocular Surface Disease Index

Since the introduction of the OSDI by Schiffman and colleagues[20] (commissioned and copyrighted by by Allergan, Inc) in 2000, it has become the most widely used symptomology questionnaire in the dry eye community. However, it doesn't assess the severity of the symptoms, just their frequency, and as well as general ocular-related symptoms (sensitivity to light, grittiness, pain/soreness, blurred vision, and poor vision) it includes quality of life questions on limitation to activities (reading, driving at night, working with a computer or bank machine, and watching television) and whether the discomfort has environmental triggers (wind, humidity, and air conditioning). These responses are scored on a 5 point Likert scale (between all of the time (4) and none of the time (0)) and the results of the 3 subsections summed, multiplied by 25

and divided by the number of questions answered to reach the final OSDI score (on a 0–100 scale). This approach is to overcome the issue of patients noting questions as not being applicable (such as driving at night), but is not ideal. While the questionnaire was developed based on the comments of patients from previous clinical trials and comments from over 400 patients and 2 health professionals, the refinement from the initial 40 questions to the final 12 is just described as based on two small groups of patients with dry eye and one phase II clinical trial group. Internal consistency between the items was high, suggesting possible redundancy, factor analysis identified 3 subscales and repeatability was good (intraclass correlation of 0.82 overall, but less for the subscales), but Rasch modeling was not conducted.[20] The OSDI was able of differentiate dry eye patients from normal based on physician rating (sensitivity 0.60, specificity 0.83) or a composite dry eye score (combining Schirmers I, lissamine green and patient perception of ocular symptoms with no further details stated; sensitivity 0.80, specificity 0.79) and correlated well with other eye-specific health status measures.

TABLE 1.1
The Development of the Common Dry Eye Questionnaires with Psychometric Evaluation with the Design Elements and Analysis Applied to Refine the Questionnaire.

QUESTIONNAIRE		DESIGN ELEMENTS						REFINEMENT ANALYSIS			
Name/Authors	Items	Recall Period	Dry Eye Sufferers	Literature Review	Saturation of Questions	Scale Type	Participants	Robust Psychometric Testing	Repeatability Period	Sensitivity Testing	Scoring
McMonnies and Ho 1986[47]	12	Not stated	x	x	x	Variable Likerts	68	x	x	Rheumatological dry eye patients	Arbitrary weight of question items 0–33 or 0–45
SANDE Schaumberg et al. 2007[66]	2	2 months	x	x	x	VAS	26–52	x	ICC 1–2 days ~0.6–0.8 2 months ~0.40	None at time	Multiplication of VAS, rooted 0–100
Ocular Comfort Index[56]	12	1 week	Unknown number	Stated but no details	x	7 rating	150–452	✓	14 ± 7 days N = 100	OSDI n = 337 Ocular lubricants N = 150	Rasch scaled 0–100
Subjective Evaluation of Symptom of Dryness[21]	3	Not stated	x	x	x	5 point Likert	97	x	x	x	Categorization or added 0–12
Standard Patient Evaluation of Eye Dryness Questionnaire (SPEED)[30]	8	Present, 72 h and 3 weeks	x	x	x	4–5 point Likert	100	x	x	Lid wiper presence	Summed for 4 frequency (0–4) and severity (0–5) symptoms; 0–28
Dry Eye Questionnaire (5 Item)[50]	5	Typical day	x	x	x	5 (frequency) or 6 (severity) Likert	50	x	x	Control versus dry eye Non-Sjögren's versus Sjögren's patients	Added; 0–22
Ocular Surface Disease Index (OSDI)[20]	12	Last week	Over 400	x	x	5 point Likert	139	x Internal consistency calculated	2 weeks N = 76	109 dry eye versus 30 normals	Added, multiplied by 25 and divided by number of questions answered; 0–100
Revised Ocular Surface Disease Index (OSDI-6)[28]	6	Past month	Based on original	x	x	5 point Likert	264	✓	1 day N = 50	264 dry eye versus normals	Added 0–24

Questionnaire								Internal consistency calculated			
Texas Eye Research and Technology Center Dry Eye Questionnaire (TERTC-DEQ)[59]	28	Past week and past month	"Extensive focus groups"	Stated but no details	x	5 point rating	89	x	8–12 weeks N = 13	37 dry eye versus 52 normals	Scored 0–94
University of North Carolina Dry Eye Management Scale (UNC DEMS)[60]	1	Past week	Stated, but not accessible	Stated, but not accessible	x	10 point Likert	66	x	1 week N = 56	46 dry eye versus 20 normals	Measured 0–100
Impact of Dry Eye in Everyday Life (IDEEL)[62]	57	Past 2 weeks	6 focus groups N = 45	x	✓	Mainly 4 or 5 point Likert	210	✓	2 weeks N = 210	162 dry eye versus 48 normals	0–100 for each of three dimensions
Dry Eye-Related Quality-of-Life Score (DEQS)[65]	15	Past week	20	From 3 previous questionnaires	x	5 point (frequency) or 4 point (severity) Likert	142	✓ Although only on 24 of original 45 items	2 weeks	203 dry eye versus 21 normals + punctal plug treatment N = 10	Added, multiplied by 25 and divided by number of questions answered; 0–100

Subsequent Rasch analysis has suggested unidimensionality and discriminative ability,[21] but unidimensionality was equivocal,[22,23] it did not confirm to the Rasch model,[22] categories of "half of the time" and "most of the time" should be collapsed into one response option and the subscales were not valid.[23] Comparison of its predictive ability of dry eye patients compared to other questionnaires has been mixed.[24,25] Clinicians and participants consider a minimally clinically important change for mild to moderate dry eye symptoms to be 4.5–7.3 units and 7.3–13.4 units for severe dry eye.[26]

Pult and Wolffsohn have since used item response theory to create a short form of the OSDI known as the OSDI-6 (Fig. 1.3), with better psychometric properties and discriminative ability.[28] It contains two items from each of the three OSDI categories (with no "non-applicable" options) and is simply scored by adding the values of each response (0–24 range, with >4 the cut-off for dry eye). The OSDI has been accepted in the United States for use in FDA clinical trials and translated into other languages such as Japanese.[29]

Standardized Patient Evaluation of Eye Dryness

The Standardized Patient Evaluation of Eye Dryness (SPEED) questionnaire was introduced by Korb and colleagues in 2005 while differentiating the prevalence of lid wiper epitheliopathy in patients who had dry eye symptoms.[30] No design considerations or psychometric testing was reported. The symptoms investigated are dryness, grittiness or scratchiness, soreness or irritation, and burning or watering. The initial question (not scored) asks whether the symptoms are present at the present time, in the past 72 h or the past 3 months. The frequency or the symptoms are assessed on a 4 point Likert scale (never, sometimes, often and constant) and severity on a 5 point Likert scale (no problems, tolerable, uncomfortable, bothersome, and intolerable). The psychometric properties of the questionnaire were not assessed until 2013 when using Rasch analysis on the results of 50 patients (30 with dry eye disease) it was found to have unidimensions with 3 subscales (dryness, burning, and fatigue/soreness) be unidimensional, sensitive to dry eye patients as "diagnosed" by the OSDI, and repeatable (over 1 week),[31] although the concordant correlation coefficient of 0.923 suggests some question redundancy. A further analysis with 127 patients showed that while the questionnaire was largely robust, there was substantial mis-targeting of the items, with the author suggesting the questionnaire was improved if a fatigue item was removed (which was not part of the original questionnaire, but seems to have been introduced by 2012[32] and used in subsequent studies) and dryness seems to have been combined with grittiness and scratchiness, to make a six question version.[24] The SPEED psychometric properties were also tested in 150 contact lens wearers and 134 noncontact lens wearers. This identified that the initial question on timescales caused multidimensions, while the eight questions on frequency and severity had acceptable response category functioning, fitted well to the Rasch model and measurement precision. Analysis of these eight items still showed evidence of slight multidimensionality.[33] Cut-offs have been proposed with no symptoms (SPEED = 0), mild to moderate symptoms (SPEED = 1–9), and severe symptoms (SPEED ≥10).[34]

Symptom Assessment in Dry Eye

The SANDE, developed by Deborah Schaumberg and colleagues in 2007, consists of two visual analogue scale

	Constantly	Mostly	Often	Sometimes	Never
Have you experienced any of the following *during a typical day of the last month?*					
1. Eyes that are sensitive to light?	4	3	2	1	0
2. Blurred vision?	4	3	2	1	0
Have problems with your eyes limited you in performing any of the following *during a typical day of the last month?*					
3. Driving or being driven at night?	4	3	2	1	0
4. Watching TV, or a similar task?	4	3	2	1	0
Have your eyes felt uncomfortable in any of the following situations *during a typical day of the last month?*					
5. Windy conditions?	4	3	2	1	0
6. Places or areas with low humidity?	4	3	2	1	0

FIG. 1.3 Ocular Surface Disease Index—six item.[27] (Reprinted with permission from Elsevier.)

questions on frequency (between "rarely" and "all of the time") and severity (between "very mild" and "very severe") of dry eye and/or ocular irritation symptoms. The mark placed on the visual analogue scale is measured and scaled on a 0 to 100 scale with 100 being the worst; a global score is obtained by multiplying the result from both questions and then taking the square root of their product. SANDE scores have been shown in a number of subsequent studies to correlate with the OSDI r = 0.58−0.67,[35−37] but this only accounts for 34%−45% of the variance. This is probably as the OSDI is a frequency only questionnaire and more about environments than specific symptoms in general. Sensitivity of the SANDE has been shown in intraductal probing,[38] intense-pulsed light therapy,[39] Cyclosporine,[40] Manuka honey,[41] human nerve growth factor,[42] autologous serum,[43] graft versus host disease,[44] eye cleaning treatment for blepharitis,[45] and artificial tear use.[46]

A score of ≥30 in combination with a noninvasive breakup time <10s[25] has been shown to be diagnostic of dry eye disease as defined by TFOS DEWS II with a 86% sensitivity and 94% specificity.[4]

McMonnies Dry Eye Questionnaire

McMonnies Dry Eye Questionnaire[47] consists of 12 questions, together with the respondents demographics (age and sex). A weighted assignment of points were arbitrarily attributed to risk factors such as ocular sensitivity to irritants/environment/alcohol drinking, taking certain medications, arthritis, dryness of other tissues, and other thyroid abnormalities, together with having had dry eye treatment and the frequency of symptoms. Retrospective Rasch analysis has been applied, with some studies suggesting the questionnaire is unidimensional and able to distinguish dry eye patients,[21] while other found it to not conform with the requirements for a valid questionnaire.[22,48] However, it remains well used.

Dry Eye Questionnaire-5

Begley and colleagues developed a questionnaire in 1999 using visual analogue scales examining the frequency, severity and impact of dryness, soreness, burning, blur, light sensitivity, and itch[49] and another to assess contact lens wearers examining the presence, frequency, severity, and intrusiveness of common ocular symptoms, including dryness, scratchiness and irritation, soreness, light sensitivity, and blurry, changeable vision (Fig. 1.4).[51] However, no psychometric process was used to refine these questionnaires and the source of the items was not identified. A revised version

of the DEQ was used by the authors in 2003.[52] Rasch analysis was retrospectively applied and it met the Rasch analysis criterion of unidimensionality, was able to differentiate symptomatic and asymptomatic groups and correlated well to other dry eye questionnaires.[21]

A subset of the Dry Eye Questionnaire were selected by correlation with a self-reported question on the severity of dry eye (from "I don't have dry eye" (0) to "Extremely Severe" (5)) in 2010. These questions on the frequency and severity of dryness and discomfort and the frequency of eye watering were able to differentiate control versus dry eye (cut-off ≥6 out of 22) and non-Sjögren's versus Sjögren's patients (cut-off ≥12).[50]

The initial CLDEQ consisted of 36 questions (9 subscales: discomfort, dryness, visual changes, soreness and irritation, grittiness and scratchiness, foreign body sensation, burning, photophobia, and itching) and was derived from the literature and clinical knowledge of dry eye symptoms among contact lens wearer and patients with dry eye. Each subscale assessed the symptom frequency and intensity of the symptom over the first 2 h after contact lens insertion, midday and at the end of the day, to examine diurnal fluctuations in symptoms. This version was able to discriminate clinician diagnosed contact lens dry eye.[53] Similarly to the DEQ-5, the eight questions of the shorter form were selected as those most strongly correlated with a self-reported opinion on ocular comfort when wearing contact lenses (Poor, Fair, Good, Very Good, and Excellent) and was able to reflect changes in opinion after lens refitting.[54] The CLDEQ-8 has the same eye discomfort and dryness (frequency over a typical day and severity at the end of your wearing time) questions, together with changeable, blurry vision (on the same scales) and closing your eyes (rated as never (0), rarely (1) or sometimes (2)) giving a summed score from 0 to 37.[54] It did not fit the Rasch model unless it was reduced to a 4-item scale on eye discomfort and dryness frequency (5 point: "never" to "constantly" Likert scale) and intensity (6 point: "never have it" to "very intense" rating scale).[33]

Subjective Evaluation of Symptom of Dryness

Authors from the University of Waterloo, Canada, utilized a 3 question screening tool to differentiate "dry" from "nondry eye" patients. The questions were frequency of symptoms, presence of discomfort and interference with activity on 5 option Likert scales.[21] While it differentiated patients in a similar manner to McMonnies questionnaire, Dry Eye Questionnaire and OSDI,

DEQ 5

1. Questions about **EYE DISCOMFORT**:

   a. During a typical day in the past month, **how often** did your eyes feel discomfort?

   - **0** Never
   - **1** Rarely
   - **2** Sometimes
   - **3** Frequently
   - **4** Constantly

   b. When your eyes felt discomfort, **how intense was this feeling of discomfort** at the end of the day, within two hours of going to bed?

Never have it	Not at All Intense				Very Intense
0	**1**	**2**	**3**	**4**	**5**

2. Questions about **EYE DRYNESS**:

   a. During a typical day in the past month, **how often** did your eyes feel dry?

   - **0** Never
   - **1** Rarely
   - **2** Sometimes
   - **3** Frequently
   - **4** Constantly

   b. When your eyes felt dry, **how intense was this feeling of dryness** at the end of the day, within two hours of going to bed?

Never have it	Not at All Intense				Very Intense
0	**1**	**2**	**3**	**4**	**5**

3. Question about **WATERY EYES:**

   During a typical day in the past month, **how often** did your eyes look or feel excessively watery?

   - **0** Never
   - **1** Rarely
   - **2** Sometimes
   - **3** Frequently
   - **4** Constantly

   Score: 1a + 1b + 2a + 2b + 3 = Total

   ___ + ___ + ___ + ___ + ___ = _____

FIG. 1.4 Dry Eye Questionnaire 5-item.[50] (Reprinted with permission of the authors.)

no further psychometric analysis was performed. It has only been shown to detect improvement with application of a lipid-based artificial tear formulation taken for 3 month.[55]

Ocular Comfort Index

The ocular comfort index was developed by Paul Murphy and Michael Johnson in 2007[56] and consists of 12 items scored on a 7 point response rating. The items assess the frequency ("never" to "always") and intensity ("never had it" to "severe") of dryness, grittiness, stinging, tiredness, pain, and itch. The initial items were developed by patients and a literature review (although the details are not given) and questions on comfort, clarity/bothersomeness of vision changes were excluded by Rasch analysis. The initial study included assessing the sensitivity to detect the treatment effect of an ocular lubricant in 100 dry eye patients (-5.5 to -8.0 units) and correlation with the OSDI (r = 0.73). McMonnies questionnaire was found to better identify contact lens induced dry eye than the ocular comfort index, but the latter was not designed to diagnose.[57] The validity of the Rasch conformity has been confirmed, although the analysis suggested that more than one trait might be contributing to the final score.[22] One of the initial authors published an abstract in 2011 suggesting that patient interviews had identified that the original questionnaire did not capture the scope of dry eye disease symptoms and hence a modified version would be validated,[58] but this has never been published. Instead the original version has been used in multiple treatment studies.

Texas Eye Research and Technology Center Dry Eye Questionnaire

The Texas Eye Research and Technology Center Dry Eye Questionnaire (TERTC-DEQ) questionnaire has 28 items examining the frequency, and intensity in the morning and late evening of comfort, soreness/irritation/grittiness/scratchiness/burning/stinging, dryness, and itch, together with how bothersome symptoms are and the contribution of discomfort, dryness, soreness/grittiness/burning, the taking of certain medications, dryness of mucosal tissues, the effectiveness of certain dry eye treatments (if used), and the frequency of use of artificial tears.[59] It mainly uses 5 point rating and Likert scales, with symptoms assessed during a typical day over the last week and treatments over the past month. It can differentiate dry eye patients (cut-off 32.3 points), was correlated with McMonnies questionnaire (r = 0.51), but the high internal consistency (Cronbach's alpha = 0.95)[59] suggests question redundancy.

University of North Carolina Dry Eye Management Scale

This single item severity of symptoms that "may include: pain, burning, tearing, grittiness, feeling like something is in your eye" is scored on a 10 point Likert scale. The paper suggests it was developed through literature search and dry eye patient/expert consultation,

but the link is not accessible and not published. Hence, the robustness of the item reduction is not possible to assess, but the single item was shown to be correlated to the OSDI (r = 0.80), repeatable (ICC = 0.90), and able to discriminate dry eye patients.[60] The minimal clinical important difference is 1 point.[61]

Impact of Dry Eye in Everyday Life

The Impact of Dry Eye in Everyday Life (IDEEL) questionnaire developed in 2003[62] is a well-designed questionnaire with robust psychometric testing. The initial 116 items were refined to a 57-item instrument, organized into 3 different modules; the Dry Eye Symptom-Bother (20 items on 1 dimension); the Dry Eye Impact on Daily Life (27 items covering 3 dimensions); and the Dry Eye Treatment Satisfaction (10 items covering two dimensions). The items are mainly scored on 4 or 5 point Likert scales although some questions require a dichotomous "Yes" or "No" response, with each module scored on a 0–100 scale. The Minimal Clinically Important Difference is 12 points.[63] A Chinese version has now been validated.[64] While the IDEEL questionnaire has good psychometric properties, it takes about 30 min to complete, is not unidimensional, and needs users to purchase it.

Dry Eye–Related Quality-of-Life Score

The DEQS is a Japanese questionnaire developed in 2013 with two subscales[65]: bothersome ocular symptoms (foreign body sensation, dry sensation in eyes, painful or sore eyes, ocular fatigue, heavy sensation in eyelids, redness in eyes); and impact on daily life (difficulty opening eyes, blurred vision when watching something), sensitivity to bright lights, problems with eyes when reading, problems with eyes when watching television or looking at a computer or cell phone, feeling distracted because of eye symptoms, eye symptoms affect work, not feeling like going out because of eye symptoms, and feeling depressed because of eye symptoms. The 15 items each has a frequency component (5 point Likert scale) and severity component (4 point Likert scale) so up to 30 responses are required. The average of the severity responses (discounting those not applicable) is multiplied by 25 to create a 0–100 scale.

There were 45 items in the initial pool which were refined down to 24 for testing from the opinion of 20 patients with dry eye. Only these items were part of the larger psychometric testing which identified good test–retest reliability (ICC = 0.81 to 0.93) and high internal consistency (Cronbach's alpha = 0.83–0.93) between questions in each subscale (suggesting redundancy). The DEQS was able to differentiate dry eye suffers and changes with punctal plugging in a small group of patients.[65] Dimensionality was not tested.

CONCLUSIONS

Symptomology is critical to the diagnosis of dry eye disease and is what separates it from general ocular surface disease.[1] As the screening element of the diagnosis of dry eye, standardization is essential and the two accepted questionnaires are the OSDI (cut-off $\geq$13 out of 100) or the DEQ-5 (cut-off $\geq$6 out of 22).[4] As shown in Table 1.1, none of the existing questionnaires meet current best practice[5] for patient reported outcome design and none stand out for their sensitivity. Hence, the choice of questionnaire for monitoring treatment should be based on the respondent burden (related to the number of questions) and recall frequency (to fit with the follow-up schedule). If other aspects of treatment, such as its impact on quality of life or the burden of treatment, are of interest, additional unidimensional questionnaires designed to assess these traits should be utilized.

REFERENCES

1. Craig JP, Nichols KK, Akpek E, et al. TFOS DEWS II definition and classification report. *Ocul Surf.* 2017;15: 276–283.
2. The definition and classification of dry eye disease: report of the definition and Classification Subcommittee of the International Dry Eye Workshop. *Ocul Surf.* 2007;5: 75–92.
3. Yazdani M, Chen X, Tashbayev B, et al. Evaluation of the ocular surface disease index questionnaire as a discriminative test for clinical findings in dry eye disease patients. *Curr Eye Res.* 2019;44:941–947.
4. Wolffsohn JSAR, Chalmers R, Djalilian A, et al. TFOS DEWS II diagnostic methodology report. *Ocul Surf.* 2017; 15:539–574.
5. Services USDoHaH. Patient-reported outcome measures: use in medical product development to support labelling claims. Guidance for industry. 2009. Available at: http://www.fda.gov/dowlloads/Drugs/GuidanceCompliance RegulatoryInformation/Guidances/UCM193282.pdf. Center for Drug Evaluaiton and Research; Center for biologics Evaluation and Research; Center for Devices and Radiological Health.
6. Hatch R, Young D, Barber V, Harrison DA, Watkinson P. The effect of postal questionnaire burden on response rate and answer patterns following admission to intensive care: a randomised controlled trial. *BMC Med Res Methodol.* 2017;17:49.
7. Eisele G, Vachon H, Lafit G, et al. The effects of sampling frequency and questionnaire length on perceived burden,

compliance, and careless responding in experience sampling data in a student population. *Assessment.* 2020. https://doi.org/10.1177/1073191120957102.
8. Wolffsohn JS, Cochrane AL, Watt NA. Implementation methods for vision related quality of life questionnaires. *Br J Ophthalmol.* 2000;84:1035–1040.
9. Vianya-Estopa M, Nagra M, Cochrane A, et al. Optimising subjective anterior eye grading precision. *Contact Lens Anterior Eye.* 2020;43:489–492.
10. du Toit R, Pritchard N, Heffernan S, Simpson T, Fonn D. A comparison of three different scales for rating contact lens handling. *Optom Vis Sci.* 2002;79:313–320.
11. Viswanathan M, Kayande U, Bagozzi RP, Riethmuller S, Cheung SYY. Impact of questionnaire format on reliability, validity, and hypothesis testing. *Test Psychometr Methodol Appl Psychol.* 2017;24:465–498.
12. Jibb LA, Khan JS, Seth P, et al. Electronic data capture versus conventional data collection methods in clinical pain studies: systematic review and meta-analysis. *J Med Internet Res.* 2020;22:e16480.
13. Davis TC, Mayeaux EJ, Fredrickson D, Bocchini Jr JA, Jackson RH, Murphy PW. Reading ability of parents compared with reading level of pediatric patient education materials. *Pediatrics.* 1994;93:460–468.
14. Tsang S, Royse CF, Terkawi AS. Guidelines for developing, translating, and validating a questionnaire in perioperative and pain medicine. *Saudi J Anaesth.* 2017;11: S80–S89.
15. Okumura Y, Inomata T, Iwata N, et al. A review of dry eye questionnaires: measuring patient-reported outcomes and health-related quality of life. *Diagnostics.* 2020;10.
16. Klein DF, Cleary TA. Platonic true scores and error in psychiatric rating scales. *Psychol Bull.* 1967;68:77–80.
17. Embretson SE. The continued search for nonarbitrary metrics in psychology. *Am Psychol.* 2006;61:50–55. discussion 62-71.
18. Pesudovs K, Burr JM, Harley C, Elliott DB. The development, assessment, and selection of questionnaires. *Optom Vis Sci.* 2007;84:663–674.
19. Schaumberg DA, Buring JE, Sullivan DA, Dana MR. Hormone replacement therapy and dry eye syndrome. *J Am Med Assoc.* 2001;286:2114–2119.
20. Schiffman RM, Christianson MD, Jacobsen G, Hirsch JD, Reis BL. Reliability and validity of the ocular surface disease index. *Arch Ophthalmol.* 2000;118:615–621.
21. Simpson TL, Situ P, Jones LW, Fonn D. Dry eye symptoms assessed by four questionnaires. *Optom Vis Sci.* 2008;85: 692–699.
22. McAlinden C, Gao R, Wang Q, et al. Rasch analysis of three dry eye questionnaires and correlates with objective clinical tests. *Ocul Surf.* 2017;15:202–210.
23. Dougherty BE, Nichols JJ, Nichols KK. Rasch analysis of the ocular surface disease index (OSDI). *Inv Ophthalmol Vis Sci.* 2011;52:8630–8635.
24. Asiedu K. Rasch analysis of the standard patient evaluation of eye dryness questionnaire. *Eye Contact Lens.* 2017;43: 394–398.

25. Wang MTM, Xue AL, Craig JP. Screening utility of a rapid non-invasive dry eye assessment algorithm. *Contact Lens Anterior Eye*. 2019;42:497–501.

26. Miller KL, Walt JG, Mink DR, et al. Minimal clinically important difference for the ocular surface disease index. *Arch Ophthalmol*. 2010;128:94–101.

27. Wolffsohn JS, Calossi A, Cho P, et al. Global trends in myopia management attitudes and strategies in clinical practice - 2019 Update. *Contact Lens Anterior Eye*. 2020; 43:9–17.

28. Pult H, Wolffsohn JS. The development and evaluation of the new ocular surface disease index-6. *Ocul Surf*. 2019;17: 817–821.

29. Midorikawa-Inomata A, Inomata T, Nojiri S, et al. Reliability and validity of the Japanese version of the Ocular Surface Disease Index for dry eye disease. *BMJ Open*. 2019;9:e033940.

30. Korb DR, Herman JP, Greiner JV, et al. Lid wiper epitheliopathy and dry eye symptoms. *Eye Contact Lens*. 2005;31: 2–8.

31. Ngo W, Situ P, Keir N, Korb D, Blackie C, Simpson T. Psychometric properties and validation of the standard patient evaluation of eye dryness questionnaire. *Cornea*. 2013;32:1204–1210.

32. Greiner JV. A single LipiFlow(R) Thermal Pulsation System treatment improves meibomian gland function and reduces dry eye symptoms for 9 months. *Curr Eye Res*. 2012;37:272–278.

33. Pucker AD, Dougherty BE, Jones-Jordan LA, Kwan JT, Kunnen CME, Srinivasan S. Psychometric analysis of the SPEED questionnaire and CLDEQ-8. *Inv Ophthalmol Vis Sci*. 2018;59:3307–3313.

34. Blackie CA, Solomon JD, Scaffidi RC, Greiner JV, Lemp MA, Korb DR. The relationship between dry eye symptoms and lipid layer thickness. *Cornea*. 2009;28: 789–794.

35. Amparo F, Dana R. Web-based longitudinal remote assessment of dry eye symptoms. *Ocul Surf*. 2018;16:249–253.

36. Amparo F, Schaumberg DA, Dana R. Comparison of two questionnaires for dry eye symptom assessment: the ocular surface disease index and the symptom assessment in dry eye. *Ophthalmology*. 2015;122:1498–1503.

37. Chen SP, Massaro-Giordano G, Pistilli M, Schreiber CA, Bunya VY. Tear osmolarity and dry eye symptoms in women using oral contraception and contact lenses. *Cornea*. 2013;32:423–428.

38. Kheirkhah A, Kobashi H, Girgis J, Jamali A, Ciolino JB, Hamrah P. A randomized, sham-controlled trial of intraductal meibomian gland probing with or without topical antibiotic/steroid for obstructive meibomian gland dysfunction. *Ocul Surf*. 2020;18:852–856.

39. Xue AL, Wang MTM, Ormonde SE, Craig JP. Randomised double-masked placebo-controlled trial of the cumulative treatment efficacy profile of intense pulsed light therapy for meibomian gland dysfunction. *Ocul Surf*. 2020;18: 286–297.

40. Sheppard J, Kannarr S, Luchs J, et al. Efficacy and safety of OTX-101, a novel nanomicellar formulation of cyclosporine A, for the treatment of keratoconjunctivitis sicca: pooled analysis of a phase 2b/3 and phase 3 study. *Eye Contact Lens*. 2020;46(Suppl 1):S14–S19.

41. Craig JP, Cruzat A, Cheung IMY, Watters GA, Wang MTM. Randomized masked trial of the clinical efficacy of MGO Manuka Honey microemulsion eye cream for the treatment of blepharitis. *Ocul Surf*. 2020;18:170–177.

42. Sacchetti M, Lambiase A, Schmidl D, et al. Effect of recombinant human nerve growth factor eye drops in patients with dry eye: a phase IIa, open label, multiple-dose study. *Br J Ophthalmol*. 2020;104:127–135.

43. Kreimei M, Sorkin N, Boutin T, Slomovic AR, Rootman DS, Chan CC. Patient-reported outcomes of autologous serum tears for the treatment of dry eye disease in a large cohort. *Ocul Surf*. 2019;17:743–746.

44. Amparo F, Shikari H, Saboo U, Dana R. Corneal fluorescein staining and ocular symptoms but not Schirmer test are useful as indicators of response to treatment in chronic ocular GVHD. *Ocul Surf*. 2018;16:377–381.

45. Sung J, Wang MTM, Lee SH, et al. Randomized double-masked trial of eyelid cleansing treatments for blepharitis. *Ocul Surf*. 2018;16:77–83.

46. Lambiase A, Sullivan BD, Schmidt TA, et al. A two-week, randomized, double-masked study to evaluate safety and efficacy of lubricin (150 mug/mL) eye drops versus sodium hyaluronate (HA) 0.18% eye drops (vismed(R)) in patients with moderate dry eye disease. *Ocul Surf*. 2017;15:77–87.

47. McMonnies CW. Key questions in a dry eye history. *J Am Optom Assoc*. 1986;57:512–517.

48. Gothwal VK, Pesudovs K, Wright TA, McMonnies CW. McMonnies questionnaire: enhancing screening for dry eye syndromes with Rasch analysis. *Inv Ophthalmol Vis Sci*. 2010;51:1401–1407.

49. Nichols KK, Begley CG, Caffery B, Jones LA. Symptoms of ocular irritation in patients diagnosed with dry eye. *Optom Vis Sci*. 1999;76:838–844.

50. Chalmers RL, Begley CG, Caffery B. Validation of the 5-Item Dry Eye Questionnaire (DEQ-5): discrimination across self-assessed severity and aqueous tear deficient dry eye diagnoses. *Contact Lens Anterior Eye*. 2010;33: 55–60.

51. Begley CG, Caffery B, Nichols KK, Chalmers R. Responses of contact lens wearers to a dry eye survey. *Optom Vis Sci*. 2000;77:40–46.

52. Begley C, Chalmers RL, Abetz L, et al. The relationship between habitual patient-reported symptoms and clinical signs among patients with dry eye of varying severity. *Inv Ophthalmol Vis Sci*. 2003;44:4753–4761.

53. Nichols JJ, Mitchell GL, Nichols KK, Chalmers R, Begley C. The performance of the contact lens dry eye questionnaire as a screening survey for contact lens-related dry eye. *Cornea*. 2002;21:469–475.

54. Chalmers RL, Begley CG, Moody K, Hickson-Curran S. Contact lens dry eye questionnaire-8 and overall opinion of contact lenses. *Optom Vis Sci*. 2012;89:1435–1442.

55. Simmons PA, Carlisle-Wilcox C, Chen R, Liu H, Vehige JG. Efficacy, safety, and acceptability of a lipid-based artificial

tear formulation: a randomized, controlled, multicenter clinical trial. *Clin Therapeut.* 2015;37:858–868.

56. Johnson ME, Murphy PJ. Measurement of ocular surface irritation on a linear interval scale with the ocular comfort index. *Inv Ophthalmol Vis Sci.* 2007;48:4451–4458.

57. Michel M, Sickenberger W, Pult H. The effectiveness of questionnaires in the determination of contact lens induced dry eye. *Ophthalmic Physiol Opt.* 2009;29:479–486.

58. Johnson ME, Ruiz WM, Li JZ. Development of the modified ocular comfort index (MOCI). *Value Health.* 2011: A58.

59. Narayanan S, Miller WL, Prager TC, et al. The diagnosis and characteristics of moderate dry eye in non-contact lens wearers. *Eye Contact Lens.* 2005;31:96–104.

60. Grubbs Jr J, Huynh K, Tolleson-Rinehart S, et al. Instrument development of the UNC dry eye management scale. *Cornea.* 2014;33:1186–1192.

61. Hwang CJ, Ellis R, Davis RM, Tolleson-Rinehart S. Determination of the minimal clinically important difference of the university of North Carolina dry eye management scale. *Cornea.* 2017;36:1054–1060.

62. Abetz L, Rajagopalan K, Mertzanis P, et al. Development and validation of the impact of dry eye on everyday life (IDEEL) questionnaire, a patient-reported outcomes (PRO) measure for the assessment of the burden of dry eye on patients. *Health Qual Life Outcome.* 2011;9:111.

63. Fairchild CJ, Chalmers RL, Begley CG. Clinically important difference in dry eye: change in IDEEL-symptom bother. *Optom Vis Sci.* 2008;85:699–707.

64. Zheng B, Liu XJ, Sun YF, et al. Development and validation of the Chinese version of dry eye related quality of life scale. *Health Qual Life Outcome.* 2017;15:145.

65. Sakane Y, Yamaguchi M, Yokoi N, et al. Development and validation of the dry eye-related quality-of-life score questionnaire. *JAMA Ophthalmol.* 2013;131:1331–1338.

66. Schaumberg DA, Gulati A, Mathers WD, et al. Development and validation of a short global dry eye symptom index. *Ocul Surf.* 2007;5:50–57.

CHAPTER 2

Clinical Assessments of Dry Eye Disease: Tear Film and Ocular Surface Health

KELLY K. NICHOLS, OD, MPH, PHD • MARYAM MOUSAVI, MOPTOM, PHD

INTRODUCTION

Over the last 25 years, our collective knowledge of dry eye disease (DED) has grown exponentially, yet many of the most commonly used clinical diagnostic tests have remained largely the same. What has changed is how we, as clinicians, approach the clinical diagnostic process differently than what was done at the inception of the initial dry eye definition in 1995, published in the Report of the National Eye Institute/Industry workshop on Clinical Trials in Dry Eyes by Lemp et al. At the time, dry eye was largely considered a sign-only–based condition, primarily fluorescein corneal staining. Today, over 25 years later, dry eye screening algorithms begin with an assessment of a patient's dry eye symptoms, including visual disturbances, with the understanding that dry eye symptoms do not always correlate with dry eye signs. In addition, unless a patient is specifically asked about current or episodic dry eye symptoms and associated factors, a diagnostic opportunity may be missed.

The Tear Film and Ocular Surface Society (TFOS) Dry Eye WorkShop (DEWS) II report (2017) defined DED as a multifactorial condition of the ocular surface characterized by a loss of homeostasis of the tear film, accompanied by dry eye symptoms, including visual disturbances. In addition to symptomatology, clinical diagnostic testing should mirror the definition, and assess parameters of tear film homeostasis and known etiologies: tear film instability, hyperosmolarity, ocular surface inflammation and damage, and neurosensory anomalies. This chapter will review available testing across these parameters with the caveat that there will be tests not covered here, but the general concepts and underlying principles will be reviewed. In addition, diagnostic instrumentation and concepts on the horizon with be presented, with a nod to the diagnostic and management future of ocular surface disease.

In the TFOS DEWS report (2007), dry eye testing was often described as two-tiered, whereby a shortened battery of tests could be performed in a general clinical setting, and more advanced procedures and instrumentation were recommended for use in specialty clinics or in research settings. Advances in technology have brought a number of diagnostic instruments and therapeutics to clinical practice in the last 10 to 15 years. In part because of this, specialty clinics solely dedicated to dry eye and ocular surface disease management are becoming more commonplace. However, this can contribute to the perception that DED is becoming more confusing, with more expensive instrumentation required to diagnose and manage the disease. A simplistic approach to screening for dry eye in routine eyecare, followed by an in-depth dry eye assessment when available, is a modern approach, the early detection, prevention, and management of DED. The dry eye screening diagnostic algorithm in the TFOS DEWS II Diagnostic Methodology report utilizes this approach, simplifying dry eye screening so that everyone in an eyecare setting can make an initial diagnosis, followed by additional testing to further classify dry eye subtype. Asking questions, examination with the slit lamp, and making follow-up diagnostic and management symptoms simplifies the process. Critical diagnostic tests are discussed below.

SYMPTOMS

While inquiring about symptoms of dryness and discomfort is the first step in screening for dry eye, the absence of symptoms does not preclude dry eye. The dry eye classification scheme reported in the TFOS DEWS II Diagnosis and Classification report includes pathways to a dry eye diagnosis for asymptomatic or symptomatic patients. Asymptomatic patients can present with no signs of DED and, therefore, no a nondry eye (normal) diagnosis is made and no treatment is required. However, an asymptomatic patient can also present signs with DED, due to a neurotrophic ocular surface or lack of patient report (consider a patient in for a cataract evaluation, for example) and whereby a diagnosis is subsequently made and management is necessary, especially presurgical procedures and in neurotrophic conditions. Patients presenting with symptoms of DED can show signs on the ocular surface as well as showing no signs. Patients with no signs are usually in the preclinical state or have neuropathic pain (nonocular surface disease). Therefore, these patients would need to be carefully observed, offer education/preventative therapy as well as possible referral for pain management. Dry eye is multifactorial, thus every case is different and a practitioner should use both signs and symptoms to diagnose dry eye and be able to design a tailored management approach to fit the patient's level of DED.

Ocular surface symptoms are important to recognize and are often underestimated by clinicians. Symptom screening can help practitioners identify DED. Currently, the presence of ocular symptoms and signs of DED are required to approve therapeutic products for dry eye, and are often evaluated simultaneously in the dry eye exam. There is not a linear relationship between the signs and symptoms of DED as it varies between individuals and types of DED and across disease severity. It is crucial to monitor the progression of DED and its response to treatments and, therefore, a validated symptom questionnaire at the beginning of every clinical assessment with the patient is recommended.

Symptomatic patients usually present with dry and gritty sensation on the ocular surface, often described as discomfort, and in more severe cases, as a burning/ stinging feeling, foreign body sensation, excess tearing, achy/sore eyes and pain, redness, photophobia, and intermittent episodes of blurred vision. These symptoms can be aggravated in environmental conditions such as low humidity and air conditioning, and forced heat in the winter months.

Questionnaires

In clinical research symptoms are gathered by questionnaires which are most often completed by the patient without any input from clinicians. These questionnaires often measure ocular surface discomfort, DED-related visual symptoms, the impact of DED on health-related quality of life, and are also used in clinical care.

Ocular Surface Disease Index

Diagnosis of DED can be initiated by symptom questionnaires such as the Ocular Surface Disease Index (OSDI) which explores different aspects of dry eye symptoms including frequency, identification of precipitation factors, and impact on quality of life. The OSDI questionnaire contains three sections: the frequency of occurrence of several symptoms (e.g., gritty feeling in eye, light sensitivity, and blurred vision), questions indicating limitations on certain activities (reading, driving at night, watching television), and the effect of environmental conditions on ocular surface (wind, low humidity, and air conditioning). The questionnaire has established and validated cutpoints and clinically meaningful changes that have been reported in the literature, and the TFOS DEWS II Diagnostic Methodologies report recommends an OSDI score ≥ 13 as a positive screening for dry eye and a change of ≥ 7 indicative of a meaningful change. This is the most commonly utilized dry eye questionnaire (DEQ-5) in dry eye clinical trials.

Dry Eye Questionnaire

The DEQ-5 consists of five questions which are related to frequency and intensity of ocular symptoms. These include frequency of watery eyes, discomfort and dryness, and the noticeability of late day symptoms. The DEQ-5 (short form) has been validated and is also recommended for dry eye screening by the TFOS DEWS II Diagnostic methodology report with a positive dry eye screening score of ≥ 6.

Impact of Dry Eye on Everyday Living

The Impact of Dry Eye on Everyday Living questionnaire includes two types of visual disturbance queries which are by how much the patient is bothered by "blurry vision" or "sensitivity to light, glare, and/or wind." It shows promise in that it assesses quality of life, but does not have widespread adoption.

National Eye Institute Visual Function Questionnaire

The National Eye Institute's Visual Function Questionnaire is a generic visual function questionnaire which has seven visual sections including general vision, distance vision, peripheral vision, driving, near vision, color vision, and ocular pain. The pain subscale has been correlated positively to dry eye.

Speed Survey

The Standard Patient Evaluation of Eye Dryness Questionnaire (SPEED) questionnaire was designed to quickly track the progression of dry eye symptoms over time in DED and with contact lens wear. Drs. Korb and Blackie reported that this questionnaire gives a score from 0 to 28 that is the result of eight items that assess frequency and severity of symptoms. The survey is validated, and commonly used in optometric practice.

VISUAL DISTURBANCE

The importance of visual disturbance in dry eye is underrated. There are few methodologies to assess visual disturbance and visual function in dry eye beyond the black-on-white visual acuity and contrast sensitivity, but the concept deserves discussion here. In the future, methodology capable of quantifying visual disturbance and tear film quality in real time will aid in both diagnosis and management. Until then, a brief description of existing technology follows.

Computer-Vision Symptom Scale

The Computer-Vision Symptom Scale (CVSS17) is a Rasch-based linear scale that explores 15 different symptoms of computer-related visual and ocular symptoms. With the 17 questions, the CVSS17 includes a broad range of symptoms such as photophobia and "blinking a lot." This has been reported to be valuable in evaluating the computer-related visual and ocular symptoms. Assessing difficulty with prolonged digital screen use, informally or via survey, is increasingly important as the world expands with digital technology. Currently no validated computer use survey for DED exists, although clinicians often collect this information through office surveys or during case history.

Functional Tests of Vision

Functional visual acuity (FVA) is a standardized test for daily activities. It corresponds to the visual acuity measured with the patient's habitual prescription. The visual maintenance ratio is the average FVA divided by the baseline visual acuity. In patients with DED, Sjögren's syndrome, and Stevens Johnson syndrome, the FVA is reduced due to irregularity of the ocular surface and induced higher-order aberrations (HOAs). This technology is not widely available yet the concept is conducive to future development in dry eye diagnosis.

TEAR FILM STABILITY

Tear film stability is a fundamental in the maintenance of tear film homeostasis, and is a critical diagnostic criterion in DED. Some DED diagnostic algorithms are focused around the assessment of tear film stability and other tear film parameters. Tear film stability can be affected by temperature, humidity, and air circulation, even the use of fluorescein in the assessment of tear film stability can impact the tear film. Tear film stability has been included in the definition of DED by TFOS DEWS II, is considered a core mechanism in dry eye, and is critical in maintaining a smooth refractive surface, thus consistent clear vision. There are many techniques to evaluate the stability of the tear film, including invasive and noninvasive methods, which are described below.

Tear Film Break-Up Time

Tear break-up time (TBUT) is one of the most common methods of assessing tear film stability. The time required for the tear film to break up following a blink is called TBUT. It is a quantitative test for measurement of tear film stability. The normal time for tear film break-up is 15–20 s, and abnormal values are generally accepted to be < 10 s using both invasive (with the instillation of fluorescein) and noninvasive techniques. TBUT measured with the addition of fluorescein to the tear film is often described as fluorescein tear break-up time (FTBUT), while when measured noninvasively using a keratography or similar equipment, it is called noninvasive break-up time (NIBUT). It uses a grid or other patterns directed on the precorneal tear film for observation of image distortion and the time from opening the eyes to the first sign of image distortion is measured in seconds.

Fluorescein Break-Up Time

To perform the test, a fluorescein strip is moistened with saline and applied to the inferior cul-de-sac. After several blinks, the tear film is examined using a broad-beam of slit lamp with a cobalt blue filter for the appearance of the first dry (black) spots on the cornea. TBUT values of less than 5–10 s indicate tear instability and are observed in patients with mild to moderate DED. The FTBUT is a very common and simple diagnostic test used in clinical practice to assess DED. Sodium fluorescein enhances tear film visibility. However, it is said fluorescein reduces the stability of the tear film, therefore care should be taken to follow the same protocol for fluorescein instillation, directions, and filters.

Methods of instilling fluorescein include micropipette or impregnated strips. To avoid ocular surface damage, it should be instilled at the inferior or outer canthus with the excess saline on the strip shaken off first. It is important to instruct the patient to blink naturally three times and then stop blinking and hold the eye open until instructed. Viewing should take place within about 1 minute after instillation for the best result, although some argue the best viewing occurs several minutes after instillation with a yellow wratten filter. It has been reported that patients with mild and moderate DED have a wide range of FBUT values. Since this method involves subjective observation, there have been numerous attempts to automate the procedure in taking the measurements. Also, the instillation of fluorescein should follow after osmolarity or other tear sampling diagnostic tests due to its invasive nature.

Noninvasive Tear Break-Up Time

The principles of noninvasive tear film assessment is to measure tear dynamics over time, using video recording to capture a series of images with the videokeratoscope. Modern digital videokeratoscopes allow the clinician to use a Placido disc image to assess the tear film surface. Automated noninvasive methods are preferred for the evaluation of break-up time and tear film surface quality (TFSQ), since invasive procedures involving fluorescein may destabilize the tear film. High-Speed Videokeratoscopy (Medmont International Pty Ltd., Victoria, Australia) can be used to assess the dynamics of the TFSQ. The reflected image indicates the quality of the tear film surface over time. A uniform pattern is observed on a healthy, regular tear film, whereas an irregular pattern is seen when there is tear film thinning and/or break up. Additionally, NIBUT is also measured with a Keratograph (Oculus K5M, Wetzlar, Germany), which can identify localized breaks and disturbances in the Placido disk pattern, projected in infrared, related to changes in TFSQ. Corneal topographers utilizing placido ring images can also be used, although the measurements are not automated.

Interferometry

Oily substances spread to form a thin layer on the surface of water. Exposure of such an oily layer to adequate light results in the generation of an interferometric fringe pattern from interference from the front and back surface refractive index change reflections. Interferometry can allow the thickness of the lipid layer of the tear film to be estimated. Using slit lamp photometry to measure reflectivity (Tearscope; Keeler, Windsor, UK) that uses broadband illumination to visualize the kinetics of the lipid layer of the tear film, showing that different patterns of interferometric fringe are generated according to the lipid layer thickness. The DR-1 system (Kowa, Nagoya, Japan) was also developed as an interferometer for evaluation of the kinetics of the lipid layer of the tear film in both normal subjects and patients with DED. This system has revealed that lipid layer kinetics is related to the tear film condition or blink pattern. Interferometry is now an established technique for clinical examination that allows visualization of the kinetics of the oily layer of the tear film. The TearScience LipiView interferometer (J&J Vision, Jacksonville, FL) and the lateral shearing interferometer have recently been introduced as the first clinically available instruments to allow automated measurements of the thickness of the lipid layer of the tear film. These instruments are expected to provide new understandings into the lipid layer of the tear film and the pathophysiology of dry eye.

Tear Evaporation Rate

A healthy lipid layer is necessary to prevent tear film evaporation as the evaporation rate indicates the level of tear film stability. Evaporation of the tear film can be measured using different techniques such as a vapor pressure gradient and the velocity of relative humidity increase (resistance hygrometry) within a goggle cup placed over the eye. These techniques have shown that reduced tear film stability (poor lipid layer) has been associated with high evaporation rate and DED symptoms. The evaporation rate is temperature and humidity dependent as well as the time of day being a factor. The rate can also be affected by evaporation from the skin surrounding the eye, and the amount of time between blinks, which is reduced with attentive visual behavior, including screen time. Infrared thermography has been used noninvasively, yet despite these advances, a validated diagnostic measuring technique is yet to be established but would show promise.

TEAR VOLUME AND TEAR MEASUREMENTS

An adequate tear film volume is an important factor for ocular surface health. The occurrence of aqueous deficiency and the resultant loss of homeostasis can be a sign of pathogenic mechanism that is observed in a DED patient although it is not stated in the definition of DED directly. Clinically tear volume can be measured with the Schirmer or phenol red thread (PRT) test, or measurement of the tear meniscus as a surrogate measure for aqueous production.

Osmolarity

Osmolarity of normal eye is generally accepted to be < 308mOsm/L, with values between 308 and 316 mOsm/L, an indicator of mild dry eye in the presence of symptoms and/or a differential of >8 mOsm/L between the eyes. Values increase with severity of

DED. Osmolarity gives qualitative information of the status of the tear film, using instruments such as the TearLab Osmolarity System (TearLab Corp, San Diego, CA), which was the first commercially available point-of-care diagnostic for dry eye. The TFOS DEWS II diagnostic algorithm recommends osmolarity measurements as a screening test for dry eye. There are a number of diagnostic hand-held or small instruments available or in development/testing to assess osmolarity alone or in combination with other tear film biomarkers. Instruments of this type are attractive for their ease of use, portability, and quantitative assessment.

Meniscometry (Tear Meniscus Assessment)
Meniscometry assesses the tear meniscus height and cross-sectional volume of the tears. It is perhaps the easiest and most common method to assess tear volume quantitatively. In clinical practice practitioners use slit lamp techniques to study tear meniscus height (TMH), and in some cases curvature (TMR), and cross-sectional area (TMA). These measurements have shown comparable results with other DED tests of aqueous production. The TFOS DEWS II diagnostic report suggests that TMH be used as a measure of aqueous deficiency to further subtype dry eye, TMH <0.2 mm considered mild, and <0.1 mm moderate to severe aqueous deficiency. The DED diagnostic suite in the Oculus Keratograph 5M (Wetzlar, Germany) includes automated TMH measurement. While not all practices will have this instrumentation, all eyecare practices have a slit lamp, and can measure TMH as a surrogate measure of aqueous production. Other meniscometry measures, such as optical coherence tomography meniscometry, are available, yet the analysis of the images may be difficult, time consuming, and practitioner-dependent. Hand-held instrumentation is not yet available.

The Phenol Red Thread Test
This test consists of a thin cotton thread soaked in a pH-sensitive dye know as phenol red, placed over the lower lid margin, and is used to measure tear volume when moistened with tears. The PRT and the Schirmer test are highly correlated, yet poorly reproducible, except at lower values. However, assessing tear volume is important in DED and PRT is a rapid test (15 s per eye) and a wetting length of ≤5 mm is considered indicative of moderate dry eye.

The Schirmer Test
The Schirmer test, first described in 1903, quantitatively measures the tear production by the lacrimal gland during fixed time period. The test is performed by placing a thin strip of filter paper in the inferior cul-de-sac over the lid margin. The patient's eyes are closed for 5 min and the amount of tears that wets the paper is measured in terms of length of wet strip and the value of value of less than 5 mm of strip wetting in 5 min is accepted as diagnostic marker for aqueous tear deficiency, and Sjögren's syndrome—related dry eye.

DAMAGE TO OCULAR SURFACE
Assessment of ocular surface health is a mainstay in DED diagnostic testing. The most common testing is the evaluation of ocular surface damage using vital dyes—fluorescein and lissamine green staining, both of which are readily available in clinical practice. The TFOS DEWS II Diagnostic algorithm recommends the following staining patterns as indicative of a positive DED screening: >5 corneal fluorescein spots, >9 conjunctival lissamine green spots, or lid wiper epitheliopathy (LWE) of the lid margin, ≥2 mm length, ≥25% width. Each is described below.

Ocular Surface Staining
Ocular surface staining includes the cornea and conjunctiva and the most common staining is punctate staining, which can be seen in various ocular surface diseases.[1] Dyes are instilled to the eye surface to assess the quality of tear film, and to diagnose the severity of DED and its management. Sodium fluorescein, rose bengal, and lissamine green are the most common used dyes to assess the integrity of the ocular surface. Rose bengal has cytotoxicity properties and therefore the least preferred dye. Lissamine green has replaced the use of rose Bengal in assessing ocular surfaces. Therefore, lissamine green and fluorescein is used widely in clinical practice as they are equally tolerated. Fluorescein stains the cornea more than the conjunctiva and pools in epithelial erosions, degenerating and dead cells, whereas rose Bengal and lissamine green stain the dead cells and weaken the healthy cells with insufficient protection of the cells. Observing staining of the cornea and conjunctiva between 1 and 4 min post instillation in clinical practice is considered to be a routine part for dry eye assessment as it is a simple and easy procedure to determine the severity of dry eye.

Impression Cytology
Impression cytology is used in the diagnosis of the ocular surface disorders, primarily from a clinical research perspective, and it is a relatively easy and simple technique. Conditions such as limbal stem-cell

deficiency, DED, and ocular surface neoplasia can be diagnosed with impression cytology. The most common method using impression cytology is the Nelson classification system, which considers the ratio of conjunctival epithelial and goblet cells in terms of their density, morphology, cytoplasmic staining affinity, and nucleus/cytoplasm. Clinical devices such as the Eyeprim device (OPIA Technologies, Paris, France) can be used to standardize the area and pressure used in collecting the sample for further analysis (see ocular surface inflammation, below).

Lid-Parallel Conjunctival Folds

Lid-parallel conjunctival folds (LIPCOF) are folds in the adjacent, lower quadrant of the bulbar conjunctiva, parallel to the lower lid margin. LIPCOF may be the first sign of mild stages of conjunctivochalasis and, therefore, encounter the same etiology, but clinically they show slightly different characteristics. Patients with increased LIPCOF severity are likely to suffer from DED. The combination of nasal LIPCOF and NIBUT has been shown to be the most predictive DED test combination, and LIPCOF should not be overlooked, especially DED that is nonresponsive to treatment.

In Vivo Confocal Imaging

In vivo confocal microscopy (IVCM) is a noninvasive technique that allows the evaluation of signs of ocular surface damage in DED at a cellular level, including decreased corneal and conjunctival epithelial cell density, conjunctival squamous metaplasia, decreased corneal nerve density, and increased tortuosity. Laser scanning IVCM allows easy identification of conjunctival goblet cells suggesting it may be a valuable tool in assessing and monitoring DED-related ocular surface damage. The IVCM has not been widely adopted in clinical practice but is used in clinical research settings, although it is a less invasive technique and has shown to be more effective than impression cytology.

Ocular Surface Sensitivity

With the increased focus on neurosensory and pain disorder aspects of dry eye, assessment of ocular surface sensitivity has become more commonplace. It has been documented that loss of corneal sensitivity can give rise to significant corneal disorders such as neurotrophic keratopathy. Cochet–Bonnet or noncontact air-jet esthesiometry can be useful tests to evaluate corneal sensation. In addition, the cotton wisp test can be easily performed in the clinic and should be considered if signs and symptoms are disproportionate to one another.

INFLAMMATION OF THE OCULAR SURFACE

Inflammation is a recognized component of the pathophysiological mechanism of DED and has been shown to be a stable indicator of severity. Clinically, ocular surface injection can be an indicator of inflammation, yet this can be a challenge to assess because baseline injection is rarely established via description in the record or with photography. Assessment of tear film inflammatory markers is common in a lab-based clinical research setting, and to a lesser degree in the clinical office based on available point-of-care technology. This direction, though having point-of-care diagnostics for inflammatory or other biomarkers in the tear film, and a paired treatment that results in measurable change in the diagnostic biomarker, is the future direction of quantitative ocular surface diagnostics. Reproducible and noncost limiting lab-on-chip technology will be the future of DED diagnosis and management.

Clinicians need to be mindful that the ocular inflammation tests are not explicit for DED. For those patients where the history-taking for differential diagnosis suggests that this might not be primary DED, a full differential diagnosis should be performed using a slit lamp biomicroscope to examine the eyelashes for signs of swelling, blepharitis, demodex folliculorum, meibomian gland dysfunction (MGD), and assessing cornea for ulceration. It can be helpful to have published diagnostic score criteria to screen patients who may need further testing or patients free of symptoms, but show an anomalous sign indicative of dry eye and similar diagnoses. It is also helpful if the tests can be readily performed without too many difficulties on technical aspects or time, and some of the tests may be problematic when used in a population without normal reference values. Presently most practitioners do not routinely include any tests for inflammation as an initial screening requirement for clinical diagnosis of DED. However, in practices that focus on ocular surface disease as a specialization, it is reasonable to expect evaluation of the inflammatory status of the ocular surface.

Ocular/Conjunctival Redness (Injection)

Conjunctival redness occurs when conjunctival vessels are dilated, both the fine vasculature and/or larger diameter vessels. Conjunctival injection is likely the most common clinical sign of ocular surface inflammation. A penlight (torch) or standard slit lamp biomicroscopic examination can easily detect the condition. Recently more quantitative documentation methods have been developed using digital imaging analysis for diagnosis and treatment purposes. At least one instrument, the Oculus Keratograph 5M (Wetzlar, Germany) provides a "redness score" that can be used to compare eyes or visit-to-visit changes. Injection of the lid margin can also be assessed photographically for changes between visits and is often evaluated in context with LWE and/or MGD when DED is suspected.

Matrix Metalloproteinase-9

Dry eye is often accompanied by increased osmolarity of the tear film and inflammation of the ocular surface. Hyperosmolarity contributes to the inflammatory cascade, leading to epithelial cell distress and upregulation of inflammatory processes. Increased cytokines and matrix metalloproteinase-9 (MMP-9) levels have been demonstrated in DED. The MMP-9 diagnostic test can detect enzyme activity levels using an in-office rapid assay. The current diagnostic device (InflammaDry, Rapid Pathogen Screening, Inc, Sarasota, FL, USA) can examine tear MMP-9 levels in 10 minutes. This semi-quantitative test provides a positive mark (pink line) if the MMP-9 levels are >42 pg/mL. Some practitioners use this test as a screening tool, while most use the test when an inflammatory dry eye is strongly suspected.

Ocular Surface Immune Markers including Cytokines and Chemokines

The levels of tear cytokines and chemokines are important and reflect the level of epithelial disease. Since collection of tear fluid is relatively noninvasive compared to biopsies or venipuncture for serum assays, it is an attractive idea to include these as diagnostic tools, and several are in development.

In each of these pending diagnostics, tear fluid is collected using a pen-like instrument or glass microcapillary tubes. Glass microcapillary tubes of small volume, typically 0.5–5 μL, are placed in the inferior and temporal tear prism, and capillary action draws the tears into the tube. The tears can be frozen for analysis or expelled onto an appropriate substrate (or into a diagnostic instrument) for analysis. Pen-like devices, similar to the TearLab osmolarity instrument (TearLab Corp, San Diego, CA), can also be platforms for tear collection and analysis. In general, the tip of the device is disposable, and the reaction and/or measurement occurs in or on the surface of the tip.

Impression cytology, described above, is a method for collection of surface cells and is used to collect samples for immune markers. A Class-II MHC antigen, HLA-DR, is the most commonly used ocular surface immune marker and indicates a loss of the normally immune suppressed environment of the ocular surface. The commercially available Eyeprim membrane (Opia

Technology, Paris, France) has shown to be a suitable impression membrane to harvest conjunctival epithelial cells for the quantification of HLA-DR. It has been shown that not all DED cases are equally inflammatory, and other non-DED causes of ocular surface inflammation can be reflected by this nonspecific inflammatory marker.

EYELID EVALUATION

Evaluation of the eyelids and eyelashes is a routine component of the ocular examination. Anterior eyelid conditions, such as anterior blepharitis and demodex blepharitis, are differential diagnoses and comorbidities of DED and should be ruled out in making a diagnosis of DED. Evaluation of posterior eyelid conditions, including MGD, is a critical part of the dry eye examination.

Blink/Lid Closure Analysis

Blinking is essential in maintaining optical performance, the health of the ocular surface, and meibum distribution, which helps reforming a proper tear film lipid layer. Incomplete blinking can result in DED symptoms, exposure keratopathy, and corneal staining. Incomplete blinks can be observed using fluorescein and the pattern is visible as a dark line indicating the movement limit of the upper eyelid due to previous incomplete blink. Complete blink count can be measured in conjunction with tear film/lipid layer interferometry using the TearScience Lipiview (J&J Vision, Jacksonville, FL). The blink can be observed in real time and also via video.

Lid Wiper Epitheliopathy

A small portion of the marginal conjunctiva of the upper and lower lid acts as a wiping surface to spread the tear film over the ocular surface. This contacting surface at the lid margin has been termed the "lid wiper." LWE is a term that describes an insult to the lid wiper epithelia accompanied by subclinical inflammation. This condition is believed to be caused by increased friction between this region and the ocular surface due to poor lubrication and it has been found that dry eye patients suffer from this condition. LWE cannot be identified using white light, therefore, staining techniques using lissamine green and fluorescein need to be applied. LWE can be observed immediately adjacent to the lid margin of the everted eyelid using a slit lamp biomicroscope and is most commonly classified by combining the extent of its staining, in terms of length in mm, and width relative to the lid margin width.

Evaluation and identification of presence or absence of LWE and ocular surface inflammation with tear osmolarity measurements can help to correctly diagnose DED.

Meibometry, Meibography, and Meiboscopy

Meibomian glands are sebaceous glands that can be found in the upper and lower lids. There are approximately 30 meibomian glands in the upper lid and 25 in the lower lid. When meibomian gland ductal epithelium or posterior lid margin tissues undergo keratinization, possibly due to increased osmolarity or low-grade chronic inflammation, alterations in meibomian gland secretions, called meibum, meibomian gland obstruction can occur. MGD is thought to be reflected by quantity, quality, and expressibility of the glands, which can be determined by the application of digital pressure to the glands and evaluation of the meibum expression. Normal meibum is clear and readily expressed with gentle pressure in the normal and healthy eyelid. In contrast, it becomes cloudy and then opaque, losing its viscosity and becoming toothpaste-like, not too easy to express in patients with severe MGD. Gland expression can be done digitally, with cotton tip applicators or with one of a number of small hand-held devices. The most common clinical expression grading scheme is a 0–4 scale, where grade 0 is normal, clear expression, grade 1 is slightly cloudy meibum, grade 2 is cloudy to opaque meibum, grade 3 is opaque "toothpaste sign," and grade 4 is no expression. This is a "summed" gestalt grade across the lid margin. Some clinicians grade expression by the worst grade seen across the lid, and other reports grade each gland within the central eight glands. There is not a validated and widely accepted clinical grading scheme, which is also noted in the TFOS DEWS II diagnostic algorithm, where MGD is graded as "mild, moderate, and severe" without further description. Consistency in technique with good chart notation or photography aids in comparison across visits or with treatment.

It has been suggested that MGD may be the leading cause of DED throughout the world. In recent decades innovations in ocular imaging have advanced significantly to develop techniques, technologies, and methods of image analysis and test for diagnosing MGD. These diagnostic techniques include methods such as meibometry, meibography, and meiboscopy, meibography being the most frequently performed. Meibometry is a simple test for quantifying the amount of lipid at the lid margin. Meibography allows observation of the silhouette of the meibomian gland morphological structure by using photo or video documentation.

Meiboscopy is similar to meibography, and requires a slit lamp and transilluminator without expensive instrumentation.

Recent advances in technology have led to the development of a noncontact, stand-alone, or slit lamp mounted meibography systems. Several different scoring scales, such as the meiboscore, have been proposed for the evaluation of meibography. Meibography has been also used to visualize and evaluate meibomian gland area quantitatively using software that is currently under development, and several studies are underway to validate these quantitative programs. However, other clinical parameters should be considered as meibography alone does not appear to be sufficient when diagnosing MGD. Several instruments can measure more than one tear film parameter, such as lipid layer thickness measured by interferometry (TearScience LipiView, J&J Vision, Jacksonville, FL) and the addition of an instrument that has multiple diagnostic abilities, such as meibography, NIBUT, photography, videography, a meniscus measurement, and lipid layer thickness can be an asset to growing the dry eye practice.

DED DIAGNOSTIC TEST BATTERIES AND TEST ORDER

Unfortunately, there is no single diagnostic test to definitively diagnose DED, and the results of diagnostic tests discussed above do not always correlate with symptoms. Symptoms remain a very important diagnostic test in DED and it is critical to revisit symptomology in the presence of ocular signs, as patients can inadvertently neglect reporting symptoms without a prompt. In addition to symptoms, tear film stability measured by break-up time, corneal integrity assessment via vital dye staining, and osmolality remain the three recommended screening tests. The TFOS DEWS II diagnostic report suggests any one abnormal result, in the presence of symptoms, is adequate for a dry eye diagnosis, and that a diagnosis can be made without expensive instrumentation, as well as in the context of a routine examination. Following a positive dry eye screening, further assessment of aqueous production and MGD help further classify the dry eye subtype and provide direction for treatment. Unfortunately there isn't a single qualitative/quantitative test that is capable of assessing severity of the disease, or response to treatment, but the future is bright with a number of point-of-care in-office diagnostic platforms to measure biomarkers—inflammatory and other. Until that time though, dry eye diagnosis does not have to be difficult. Keep it simple, ask symptom questions, screen for dry eye, exclude conditions that can mimic DED, further classify dry eye as MGD or aqueous deficient (or some amount of both), initiate management, and follow-up. Keeping up with new ocular surface diagnostic technologies can aid in building and growing the dry eye practice of the future.

REFERENCE

1. Wolffsohn J, Arita R, Chalmers R, et al. TFOS DEWS II diagnostic methodology report. *Ocul. Surf.* 2017;15(3): 539–574. https://doi.org/10.1016/j.jtos.2017.05.001.

CHAPTER 3

Clinical Assessment of Dry Eye Disease: Nerve Health

STEPHANIE M. COX, OD • WILLIAM W. BINOTTI, MD • PEDRAM HAMRAH, MD

INTRODUCTION

Dry eye disease (DED) is a multifactorial disease for which the exact pathophysiological mechanism remains unknown.[1] Nevertheless, a combination of a compromised tear film, ocular surface inflammation, and neurosensory abnormalities in the presence of signs and/or symptoms is considered the main pillars of DED.[1,2] This chapter aims to address evaluation of neurosensory abnormalities through assessment of nerve health, as well as the impact the other pillars, the tear film and ocular surface inflammation, have on the nerves and vice versa.

Nerves of the ocular surface have both a sensory function and a physiological function. The first function involves the nociceptive, or sensory, neural pathway system of the body. Our body is in direct contact with the surrounding environment, and the nociceptive neural pathway system provides awareness of the surrounding environment, as well as internal stimuli to the central nervous system, so that if needed, action can be initiated to prevent harm by and/or protect against noxious stimuli that could cause tissue damage.[3,4] However, ocular surface nerves do more than provide sensation. They have a large impact on the tear film, and nerve health can impact both the progression of DED and DED treatment. This chapter will discuss the role that the nerves play in DED and how we can assess these nerves clinically.

ANATOMY OF THE NERVES

To fully understand any aspect that nerves play in DED (sensations, pain, corneal reflex actions, or neuroimmune crosstalk), an understanding of the anatomy of the corneal nerves, their pathways to the brain, and efferent nerves to target organs is necessary. The afferent nerves that innervate the cornea and ocular surface are pseudounipolar neurons, which have their cell bodies within the trigeminal ganglion. The axons innervating the ocular surface travel via the nasociliary branch of the ophthalmic division of the trigeminal nerve (cranial nerve V_1). While conjunctival innervation does contribute to corneal innervation at the limbus and far periphery, the cornea has its own very dense innervation network.[5] Nerve trunks enter the corneal stroma in a radial fashion before branching to form a midstromal plexus, which is most dense in the corneal periphery.[5-7] In addition to the midstromal plexus, branches from the limbal stromal plexus and collaterals of the stromal nerve trunks contribute to a subbasal plexus.[5,6] After penetrating Bowman's membrane, nerve bundle branches and the nerve fibers ultimately converge to form the subbasal plexus.[5-7] As the branches innervate the corneal epithelium, they form terminals throughout all corneal epithelial cell layers (Fig. 3.1).[6]

The nociceptors of the ocular surface are most often characterized by the stimulus or stimuli to which they respond. The three major types of receptors have been identified as mechanical, thermal, and polymodal. Mechanical receptors are stimulated by mechanical stimuli only, especially stimuli with motion.[8] However, it has been shown that the most prominent nociceptors are polymodal receptors, which respond to a variety of stimuli. They respond strongly to changes/initiation of mechanical stimuli and to noxious, but not necessarily painful, mechanical stimuli.[8-10] These receptors also respond to heat stimuli above approximately 39°C, noxious cold stimuli, and changes to pH levels.[8-10] Unlike mechanical and polymodal receptors, studies have shown that cold receptors are constantly active even without stimulation.[11,12] These receptors also show increased activity to cold stimuli, decreased activity to warm stimuli, and increased activity to acidic stimuli, hypertonic stimuli, and certain chemical stimuli.[8,10] Due to the ongoing activity of cold receptors and their increased activity with small reductions in ocular

Dry Eye Disease. https://doi.org/10.1016/B978-0-323-82753-9.00011-4

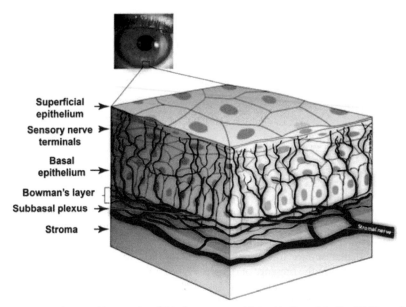

Superficial
epithelium

Sensory nerve
terminals

Basal
epithelium

Bowman's layer

Subbasal plexus

Stroma

FIG. 3.1 Illustration of corneal innervation. (This figure was published in Cruzat A, Qazi Y, Hamrah P, In vivo confocal microscopy of corneal nerves in health and disease. *Ocular Surf.* 2016;15(1):15–47, Copyright Elsevier.)

surface temperature, which could be experienced between blinks, it is theorized that these receptors are important in basal tearing.[12] Evidence in mice supports that the transient receptor potential cation channel subfamily M member 8 (TRPM8) channel, which is associated with cold receptors, specifically is important for this basal tearing.[12]

The first-order neurons of the ocular surface have a second axon branch reaching toward the brainstem. This branch of the axon enters the brainstem at the level of the pons and terminates to form a synapse with the second-order neuron cell bodies within the trigeminal nucleus.[13] The trigeminal nucleus is divided, from rostral to caudal, into the oralis (V_o), the interpolaris (V_i), and the caudalis (V_c). The corneal afferent terminations exist within (1) the caudal region of V_i and the rostral region of V_c (the V_i/V_c complex) and (2) the caudal region of V_c and rostral region of the dorsal horn of the first cervical vertebrae (the $V_c/C1$ complex).[13–20] Here we will focus on the responses within these complexes that are most closely related to DED. When comparing these two regions, one can broadly state that tearing can be altered by V_i/V_c complex stimulation and inhibition, which is not the case for the $V_c/C1$ complex.[21] Further, the $V_c/C1$ complex does not respond to drying or wetting of the cornea, while some neurons within the V_i/V_c complex do respond to corneal dryness.[21] These neurons, which

are sometimes called type II V_i/V_c complex neurons, also show reduced activity when the cornea is moistened with artificial tears.[21,22] These type II neurons also respond to hyperosmolarity and cold temperatures.[23] Preclinical studies suggest that nerves in the V_i/V_c complex and $V_c/C1$ complex become sensitized when the cornea is exposed to hyperosmotic conditions in DED.[24] Responses in the $V_c/C1$ complex are consistently inhibited by analgesics, which suggests that this area is involved in pain sensation; however, this response to analgesics is not present within the V_i/V_c complex.[14,22,25]

Processing of the information transmitted to these complexes contributes to several reflex responses: (1) blinking; (2) corneal-lacrimal reflex tearing; and (3) goblet cell secretion. Studies investigating the contribution of the trigeminal nucleus processing to blinking have shown that the V_i/V_c complex neurons initiate reflex blinking and control their amplitude.[26] Dry eye conditions enhance the typical reflex blinks caused by hypertonic solution. In addition, chemical suppression of the V_i/V_c complex neurons or the $V_c/C1$ complex neurons reduced the blink reflex.[24] Contribution to the second and third reflex responses, corneal-lacrimal reflex tearing and goblet cell secretion, are supported by the neuron projections from the trigeminal nucleus. Projections from both complexes of the trigeminal nucleus travel to the superior salivatory and lacrimal nucleus, which is known to project to the pterygopalatine ganglion and then the tear producing glands. Compared to the V_c/C1 complex, there does appear to be a stronger association between the superior salivatory and lacrimal nucleus and the V_i/V_c complex, which responds to drying/wetting of the cornea, hyperosmolarity, and cold temperatures.[21,25] Both complexes also project to the thalamus, which is often a relay station for further processing within the brain, such as the processing of sensory information within the primary somatosensory cortex. However, the thalamus appears to have a stronger association with the V_c/C1 complex, which responds to analgesics in a way expected for neurons involved in pain processing.[22,25] While the presence of projections to and from the superior salivatory and lacrimal nucleus explains the contribution of the trigeminal nucleus to the reflex responses of corneal-lacrimal reflex tearing and goblet cell secretion, the apparent organization of the information carried specifically from the V_i/V_c complex to the superior salivatory and lacrimal nucleus suggests that the V_i/V_C complex's contribution is of grave importance to these reflexes.

Nerves from the superior salivatory and lacrimal nucleus follow the greater petrosal branch of the facial nerve to synapse in the pterygopalatine ganglion. The postganglionic nerves then join with the zygomatic branch of the trigeminal nerve, and terminate at the tear producing glands, including the lacrimal gland. In addition to parasympathetic innervation from the pterygopalatine ganglion, the lacrimal gland also has sympathetic and sensory innervation from the superior cervical and trigeminal ganglions, respectively.[27-35] However, the parasympathetic system appears to be most closely associated with secretion and tearing.[35,36]

Like the lacrimal gland, the goblet cells also have a diverse innervation, although it should be noted that not all goblet cell clusters are associated with nerves.[33,34,37-41] Like the lacrimal gland, current evidence suggests that the parasympathetic innervation affects secretion.[42] While the response of the lacrimal gland to ocular surface stimuli is well known, evidence suggests that goblet cells also secrete their mucins in response to ocular surface stimulation.[34] The proximal association of nerves with the Meibomian glands[32,41,43-62] and accessory lacrimal glands[41,63] is also well established; however, there is limited evidence to support the hypothesis that these nerves influence the production or secretion of tear contributing substances, although recent evidence demonstrates that neurostimulation does result in release of meibum.[64-66]

The presence of a variety of receptors at the ocular surface and the organization of information at the level of the trigeminal nucleus suggest that this pathway may

also be linked to tear production even at times of homeostasis. While the importance of nerves and their pathways in the pathogenesis of DED is still fully being discovered, it is clear that understanding and assessing nerve health in DED evaluations is critical.

MANIFESTATIONS OF COMPROMISED NERVE HEALTH

The nociceptive neurons are composed of thinly myelinated Aα-fibers (proprioception), Aβ-fibers (mechanoreception), AΩ-fibers (nociception), and unmyelinated C-fibers (polymodal, including nociception).[4,67-69] The nerve terminals of the peripheral tissues, such as the eye, contain high-threshold receptors, ergo nociceptors, responsible for depolarizing cellular ion channels, and initiating communication of the presence of a noxious stimulus from the peripheral to the central nervous system through the nociceptive pathways. In other words, a stimulus, whether thermal, mechanical, or chemical, that exceeds the threshold of nociceptors, is required to generate a noxious stimulus message and reach the brain.[4,67-69]

When pain is experienced from a noxious stimulus, it is considered nociceptive. There are several classifications for pain, such as acute (when the pain lasts 3 months or less) or chronic (when the pain lasts greater than 3 months).[70] There are also different types of pain:[3,68,71]

(a) **Nociceptive pain**: physiologic response to direct noxious stimuli, albeit external (i.e., mechanical, thermal and chemical) or internal (i.e., tissue ischemia or cellular hypoxia), that activates high-threshold nociceptor neurons.[3,67,68]

(b) **Inflammatory pain**: pain hypersensitivity due to detection of active inflammation in peripheral tissue by nociceptors or cytokine receptors of the peripheral nervous system.[72] Local inflammation often triggers both neuronal depolarization and other immune cell depolarization, generating a self-reinforced stimulus called neurogenic inflammation.[4,69]

(c) **Neuropathic pain**: maladaptive response, caused by a neuronal lesion or disease that initially affects either the peripheral or central nervous system, of the somatosensory system that generates a painful response in the absence of a stimulus or an amplified response to innocuous and noxious stimuli.[68,71,73-75]

(d) **Dysfunctional pain/noninflammatory/non-neuropathic pain**: amplification of the nociceptive signaling in the absence of inflammation or neural lesions.[76,77]

It is important to note that these classifications can sometimes overlap, meaning a chronic pain can have an inflammatory component or a neuropathic component, or both.

Both environmental stimuli and tear film hyperosmolarity can trigger the corneal nociceptors resulting in DED symptoms, such as burning sensation, foreign body sensation, light sensitivity, dryness, and ocular pain.[78-80] The activated nociceptors also generate reflex responses, such as corneal-lacrimal reflex tearing, goblet cell secretion, and blink reflex.[79-81] These sensations and reflexes can be augmented in the presence of inflammation often associated with DED. Corneal inflammation can cause a nociceptive hypersensitivity enhancing the nociceptive pathways and exacerbating the noxious stimuli and even innocuous stimuli, such as wind, light (photoallodynia), and palpebral mechanical contact.[2,79,81] Thus, inflammation can cause changes to the ocular surface nerves, which in turn can change the sensations and reflexes experienced by a patient; however, changes to peripheral nerves can also initiate or perpetuate inflammation. Corneal nerve damage, which has been shown in DED,[82] activates inflammation to aid healing and repair.[83] The inflamed tissue area promotes a heightened sensitivity that can be activated by low-threshold innocuous stimuli and noxious stimuli that are both prolonged and exaggerated.[84] It is hypothesized that these continuous stimuli, either from untreated or persistent inflammation, can cause neural sensitization and neuroplasticity. If the stimuli continue within the peripheral nerves and are not addressed, this can result in central sensitization. This can then result in the development of neuropathic pain, where DED symptoms persist despite appropriate treatment and resolution of ocular surface inflammation and tear film stability.[79,81,85] Importantly, both neuropathic and chronic pain are complex and poorly understood neurological phenomena, specifically when involving corneal nerves.[71,86] However, there is a growing consensus within the research and clinical community that neuropathic pain is likely the explanation for patients who present with DED symptoms, but lack signs of DED or those with symptoms that are out of proportion to signs. Nevertheless, neuropathic pain can also occur with severe surface disease such as in early stages of neurotrophic keratopathy. Both neurogenic inflammation and neuropathic pain are examples of the neuroimmune crosstalk that can occur in the cornea, which is discussed next.

NEUROIMMUNE CROSSTALK

An additional key aspect of nerve health involves the impact of inflammation associated with DED on these nerves and vice versa. Corneal inflammation and nerve dysfunction are two important pillars in the pathophysiology of DED.[2,78] Evidence for inflammation in patients has been demonstrated in various types of DED, i.e., evaporative, MGD or aqueous-deficient, and in different stages of severity.[87-89] It has been well-established that desiccation leads to a proinflammatory microenvironment, thus stimulating dendritic cells (DCs), which mature and migrate to draining lymph nodes, subsequently activating T cells that further amplify the inflammatory cascade.[90,91] This process is commonly referred to as the "inflammatory vicious cycle" in DED, affecting the tear film stability, tear osmolarity, ocular surface cytokine activation, cell cycle function (apoptosis), and corneal nerves.[2,92]

Imaging studies have shown that increased density of corneal DCs are correlated with clinical parameters of DED, lacrimal gland lymphocytic infiltration, and increased tear film cytokines levels.[83,93-96] Thus, corneal DCs have been proposed as an imaging biomarker surrogate for treatment response in DED.[97] In addition, greater corneal DC density has shown a correlation with decreased corneal nerve density.[98,99] Corneal nerve alterations have been reported previously in patients with DED, such as decreased density and increased tortuosity, branching and beading,[83,93,96] and the close association of corneal DCs and nerves suggest a neuroimmune crosstalk that may occur in various ocular surface diseases, including DED.[100]

The exact mechanism of how corneal nerves can affect local immune responses in different diseases is not fully understood. Nevertheless, there is growing evidence of the critical role the peripheral nervous system plays in maintaining corneal immune privilege and immune homeostasis.[101-104] Antigen-presenting cells, including DCs and macrophages, as well as T-lymphocytes can directly activate neurons, Schwann cells, and glial cells via cytokines and chemokines, such as interleukin (IL)-1β, tumor necrosis factor (TNF)-α, bradykinin, and nerve growth factor.[69,72,84] Conversely, neuropeptides can modulate or suppress proinflammatory cytokine secretion of leukocytes.[101-104] Thus, dysfunction of corneal nerves can trigger a maladaptive proinflammatory innate immune response, called neurogenic inflammation.[79,81,85]

Preclinical studies have demonstrated that sensory nerve denervation results in a significant increase in activation and migration of DCs into the cornea, increased expression of vascular adhesion molecules followed by an increase of proinflammatory cytokine levels (IL-1β, IL-6, and IL-17), corneal angiogenesis, and lymphangiogenesis.[105-107] In clinical studies, there was an inverse correlation of corneal nerve density and DC density on in vivo confocal microscopy (IVCM) in patients with infectious keratitis, neurotrophic keratitis, and DED.[87,89,98,108,109] Moreover, it has been shown that corneal nerves regenerate 6 months after infection and resolution of inflammation, although they do not fully recover to normal levels.[110] Furthermore, the literature suggests that chronic peripheral nerve injury and inflammation that occur in DED can drive peripheral sensitization of the nociceptive pathways.[74,75] This phenomenon may contribute to many of the DED symptoms, such as photophobia (photoallodynia), burning, foreign body sensation, and pain.[79,81,99] When peripheral sensitization remains present for long periods of time, central sensitization can occur.

Taken together, recent studies suggest that dysfunction or damage to corneal nerves result in an immediate disruption of immune homeostasis and may be an underlying intrinsic part of the pathogenesis of many ocular surface diseases.[100]

CLINICAL ASSESSMENT OF CORNEAL NERVE HEALTH

An assessment of nerve health in DED should involve two major aspects: anatomy and function.

Anatomy

While nerves beyond the ocular surface are out of reach for anatomical assessment, anatomical assessment of corneal nerves can be conducted via IVCM imaging of the subbasal nerve plexus.[111,112] IVCM is a noninvasive tool that allows for real-time, layer-by-layer, and near-histological resolution cellular imaging of the cornea.[87] The main principles consist of utilizing a white or laser light through a pinhole aperture, the light is focused point-by-point and the scattered light is deflected through a second confocal aperture.[113,114] The most common IVCM devices use either a slit-scanning or a laser scanning design. The latter has the advantage of scanning multiple points at a faster rate and higher axial resolution with *en face* visualization and subsequent volumetric imaging of corneal structures.[113,115]

The specifications vary among the different devices commercially available: lateral resolution 1−2 μm, axial resolution 4−27 μm, and field of view 300 × 300 μm or 400 × 400 μm.[113,116] The laser scanning device uses a 670 nm diode laser that generates a 1 μm lateral resolution; however, it requires contact and minor corneal applanation during image acquisition.[116] Thus, utilization of anesthetic eye drops, a disposable contact cap, and gel are recommended.

The different indices of refraction of the various corneal structures allow for visualization of subbasal nerve plexus, epithelial cells, keratocytes, endothelial cells, and immune cells, i.e., DCs.[87,113,114] Quantification of corneal subbasal nerves through IVCM images have been well-established in the literature in DED.[117] Their characteristics and clinical application will be discussed in the following sections (Fig. 3.2).

One common quantitative nerve assessment performed on these IVCM images is total nerve density, which is calculated by summing the length of all the nerves within one image and dividing the sum by the area of the image. Studies have reported group mean total nerve densities of 15,956 $\mu m/mm^2$ to 24,461 $\mu m/mm^2$ for control groups[96,98,118−121] and 9,426 $\mu m/mm^2$ to 18,300 $\mu m/mm^2$ in DED.[96,118,120−124] While there is some overlap in these ranges, most studies report reduced total nerve fiber density in DED subjects compared to controls.[93,96,118,119,121,125] Historically, nerve counts were used, in which the number of nerves were counted within an image and divided by the image area. However, this measure is not commonly used today.

Another anatomical measure assessed via IVCM imaging is nerve tortuosity. This measure is typically graded on a scale of 0−4 where 0 is no tortuosity and 4 is extensive tortuosity. The average normal value for tortuosity is reported as 1.1 grade (grade range 0−4).[111,126,127] In DED, increased tortuosity is reported consistently in numerous studies.[128−130] Previous studies reported grade 2.63−3.18 nerve tortuosity in Sjögren's-related dry eye and grade 2.30−3.01 in non-Sjögren's dry eye, which was significantly different when compared to controls.[128−130]

A third measure that can be made via IVCM is beading of nerves. Subbasal nerve beading frequency varied from 90 to 198 beads/mm in healthy individuals.[128,130,131] Many studies report this is increased in DED.[128−130] Reported values for DED include 332−387/mm in Sjögren's-related DED and 186−323/mm and in non-Sjögren's-related DED.[125,128,129]

A new interest for IVCM assessment is the presence of microneuromas. Microneuromas are known to be the source of ectopic spontaneous excitations in sensory fibers in patients with postsurgical pain.[132] In 2015, Aggarwal et al. first described microneuromas as stumps of severed nerves and abrupt endings of nerve fibers on IVCM and reported their presence in patients with photoallodynia.[133] Recently, the presence of microneuromas has been suggested as a biomarker for neuropathic pain.[134] These microneuromas were found to be more numerous in patients with peripheral pain

Neuropathic Corneal Pain   Dry Eye Disease

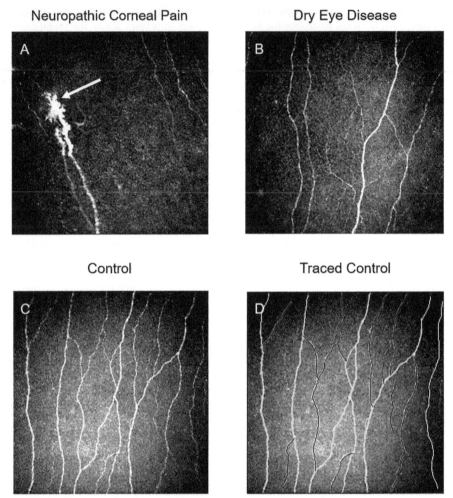

Control   Traced Control

FIG. 3.2 Representative in vivo confocal microscopy (IVCM) images of patients and controls to demonstrate corneal nerve changes. **(A)** Subbasal corneal nerve plexus in a neuropathic corneal pain (NCP) patient. *White arrow* demonstrates a microneuroma. **(B)** Subbasal corneal nerve plexus in a patient with painless conventional dry eye disease (DED). **(C)** Subbasal corneal nerve plexus in a healthy control subject. **(D)** Sample nerve tracing in a healthy subbasal corneal nerve plexus **(C)**. *Yellow lines* represent main nerve trunks and *red lines* represent nerve branches. (This figure was published in Moein H, Akhlaq A, Dieckmann G, Abbouda A, Pondelis N, Salem Z, Muller RT, Cruzat A, Cavalcanti BM, Jamali A, Hamrah P, Visualization of microneuromas by using in vivo confocal microscopy: an objective biomarker for the diagnosis of neuropathic corneal pain? *Ocular Surf.* 18(4): 651–656, Copyright Elsevier.)

compared to those with centralized pain, which suggests that the anatomical appearance of nerves supports the symptomology of patients and the importance of these microneuromas in the pathophysiology of the neuropathic corneal pain.[135,136] As we continue to investigate microneuromas, it is important to ensure thorough corneal mapping, given that microneuromas are not equality distributed throughout the cornea,[135] and that investigations utilize appropriately trained and experienced observes, since research has noted that other corneal structures, such as entry points of stromal nerve fiber bundles through the Bowman's membrane or immune cells associated with nerves can be mistaken as microneuromas (Table 3.1).[137,138]

TABLE 3.1
Table of Select Studies Involving IVCM.

Study	Device Used	Sample	Nerve Density	Beading	Tortuosity	Correlations
Labbe et al.[96]	Heidelberg Retinal Tomograph/ Rostock Cornea Module	10 control eyes 12 DED eyes	• Decreased in DED versus controls	• No difference	• No difference	
Levy et al.[118]	Heidelberg Retinal Tomograph/ Rostock Cornea Module	15 controls 30 SS DED treated with cyclosporine	• Decreased in DED versus controls • Increased in DED with treatment		• Increased in DED versus controls • Decreased in DED with treatment	• Negative correlation of nerve density and DC density
Tepelus et al.[119]	Heidelberg Retinal Tomograph/ Rostock Cornea Module	24 eyes with NSS DED 44 eyes with SS DED 10 control eyes	• Decreased in NSS DED versus controls • Decreased in SS DED versus controls • Decreased in SS DED versus NS DED		• Increased in NS DED versus controls • Increased in SS DED versus controls	• Negative correlation between DC density and nerve density
Tepelus et al.[120]	Heidelberg Retinal Tomograph/ Rostock Cornea Module	30 eyes of GVHD 20 eyes of DED 16 control eyes	• Decreased in GVHD versus control • No difference in DED versus controls • No difference in DED versus GVHD		• No difference in tortuosity	
Kheirkhah et al.[121]	Heidelberg Retinal Tomograph/ Rostock Cornea Module	40 eyes with DED 13 control eyes	• Decreased in DED versus controls • No change in DED with treatment			

Continued

TABLE 3.1
Table of Select Studies Involving IVCM.—cont'd

Study	Device Used	Sample	Nerve Density	Beading	Tortuosity	Correlations
John et al.[123]	Heidelberg Retinal Tomograph/ Rostock Cornea Module	8 DED placebo treated 9 DED treated with amniotic membrane				• Increase in corneal sensitivity correlated to increase in corneal nerve density within treated group
Kheirkhah et al.[124]	Heidelberg Retinal Tomograph/ Rostock Cornea Module	33 DED with GVHD 21 DED without GVHD	• No difference in nerve density			• No significant correlation between Schirmer's and nerve density
Labbe et al.[125]	Heidelberg Retinal Tomograph/ Rostock Cornea Module	14 control pts 43 NSS DED	• Lower density in DED	• More beading in DED versus controls	• More tortuosity in DED versus controls	
Benitez del Castillo et al.[128]	Confoscan	11 controls <60yoa 10 controls ≥60yoa 11 SS DED 10 NSS DED	• Decreased in ≥60 yoa controls versus <60 yoa controls • Decreased in NSS DED versus <60 yoa controls • Decreased in SS DED controls versus <60 yoa controls • No difference between NSS DED, SS DED, and ≥60 yoa controls		• Greater tortuosity in DED groups compared to non-DED groups	• Correlation was present between number of nerves and Schirmer's • Correlation between corneal sensitivity and Schirmer's • Correlation between corneal sensitivity and nerve number

GVHD, Graft-versus-Host Disease; *NSS DED*, Non-Sjögren's Syndrome DED; *SS DED*, Sjögren's Syndrome DED.

Function

Because the presence of nerves does not necessarily indicate appropriate function, evaluation for DED involves functional health assessment. Esthesiometry, measuring corneal sensitivity, attempts to determine the absolute threshold, which is the stimulus intensity at which a patient can first detect a stimulus (i.e., when the patient can feel the stimulus on the cornea or the patient reacts by blinking when the stimulus touches the cornea). There are several methods that can be used to determine thresholds; however, the most relevant for corneal threshold detection is (1) the ascending method of limits and (2) the descending method of limits. In the ascending method of limits, the stimulus is presented in increasing intensity until the patient reports detection (in this case, feels it on the cornea) or has a reaction to the stimulus (in this case, blinks). When using the descending method of limits, the stimulus is presented at its highest intensity to the patient first. Then the stimulus intensity is reduced until the patient reports not detecting the stimulus or stops having a reaction to the stimulus. When testing corneal sensitivity, the most common method of threshold detection is the method of ascending methods of limits.

The most basic stimulus is a cotton-tipped applicator with the fibers pulled and separated to create cotton-wisps. These exposed fibers are touched to the ocular surface to see if a response is elicited. A response is expected from normal subjects, and thus a lack of response suggests reduced sensitivity. The disadvantages of this method are numerous. First, the utilization of a single stimulus provides very limited subjective information to the clinician, especially with regard to DED. For example, the lack of response would suggest that the patient suffers from neurotrophic keratopathy (keratitis). While typically neurotrophic keratopathy patients to lack symptomology, recent evidence suggests that these patients can have concurrent chronic pain, including neuropathic pain.[139] Therefore, cotton-wisp testing, in the absence of the availability of other more sophisticated tests, may provide the only information on corneal nerve sensitivity and could be valuable in assessing corneal nerve function.

The second stimulus often used for corneal sensitivity measurement is a filament of varying lengths provided by Cochet–Bonnet esthesiometer. The corneal sensitivity threshold is determined by exerting a range of pressures on the cornea following the methods of ascending limits.[140] First the filament is fully extended to its longest extent, which is 6.0 cm in length, and touched to the cornea at a 90 degree angle to the corneal apex. Then, pressure is placed on the filament until it bends (Fig. 3.3).

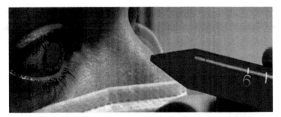

FIG. 3.3 Image showing the Cochet–Bonnet esthesiometer being used to test corneal sensitivity. Notice that the stimulus is applied by causing a bend in the filament while it is at a 90 degree angle to the cornea.

One can look to see if the patient blinks or reports feeling the stimulus. If the patient reports feeling the stimulus or blinks, this is the reading recorded. A lack of response should cause the clinician to bring the slider back to the 5.5 cm mark and repeat the procedure. If a response is still not elicited, the filament should be shortened by moving the slider back in 0.5 cm increments and repeating the testing procedure until the patient blinks or reports a sensation. This first response is the measure to be recorded. In normal patients, 6 cm is normal. Anything less than 6 cm is considered abnormal. The advantage of this method is that patients with reduced but not absent corneal sensitivity can be identified. In addition, it has shown good repeatability for same-day and 3-month measurements of the central cornea.[141] In DED patients the sensitivity response varies.[125,142,143] There is no clear differentiation of whether the sensitivity is increased or decreased compared to normal. One significant disadvantage of this method is that hypersensitivity cannot be assessed. In addition, the method is subjective instead of objective (Table 3.2).

The most sophisticated sensitivity measure comes from the modified Belmonte esthesiometer. This device highlights the various receptors of the ocular surface described previously by having modes for thermal, mechanical, and chemical sensitivity. To use this device the subject sits in front of the device and an air puff delivers the various sensations. The intensity of the air puff tests mechanical sensitivity. Thermal sensitivity is tested by having the air puff temperature changed and maintaining the air puff intensity. Chemical sensitivity is tested by adding CO_2 to the air puff. This device is not commercially available, which makes it valuable as a research tool, but is not valuable for clinical assessment.

Several factors can explain the variable esthesiometry findings within the literature, such as variable repeatability of the measured outcome, lack of consistency of the technique, and subjectivity of patient referred

TABLE 3.2
Table of Select Studies Involving Corneal Sensitivity.

Study	Device Used	Sample	Finding
Labbe et al.[96]	Cochet–Bonnet	10 control eyes 12 DED eyes	• Decreased corneal sensitivity in DED versus controls
Labbe et al.[125]	Cochet–Bonnet	14 control pts 43 NSS DED	• Mean corneal sensitivity (avg of 5 points) lower in DED • No difference in central corneal sensitivity
Boucier et al.[142]	Belmonte esthesiometer	44 DED 42 control	• Decreased mechanical, chemical, and thermal sensitivity in DED versus controls
Adatia et al.[157]	Cochet–Bonnet	18 SS patients	• Negative correlation of sensation with staining
Nepp et al.[158]	Cochet–Bonnet	46 DED subjects	• DED severity was negatively correlated with sensitivity • Sensitivity in DED patients showed high variability over 3 months
Kaido et al.[146]	Cochet–Bonnet	21 symptomatic DED 20 nonsymptomatic patients with reduced TBUT	• Symptomatic group had increased sensitivity when blink response was assessed as endpoint • Symptomatic group had increased sensitivity when pain response was assessed as endpoint • No difference was noted with perception of touch was assessed as the endpoint
Toker et al.[143]	Cochet–Bonnet	37 aqueous deficient DED 35 control subjects	• Corneal sensitivity was reduced in aqueous-deficient DED patients. • Corneal sensitivity was not significantly different from controls after cyclosporine treatment

NSS DED, Non-Sjögren's Syndrome DED; *SS DED*, Sjögren's Syndrome DED.

sensation.[140] Another explanation would be cumulative effect from nerve loss and nerve hypersensitivity that can occur in longstanding damage from DED. In the former, a decreased functional response is expected, whereas in the latter there would be an increased response.[125,144–147]

Another method for assessing corneal nerve function is the Schirmer's wetting test. Schirmer's test can be performed with or without anesthetic drop instillation. The instillation of anesthesia to the ocular surface before Schirmer's testing eliminates ocular surface stimulation caused by the presence of the Schirmer's strip and reflex tearing allowing for measurement of baseline tear production. When performed without anesthetic, reflex tearing is measured. The repeatability and reliability of the Schirmer's test is, however, variable. Nichols et al.[148] found the repeatability of the Schirmer's test is much better at lower values than higher values. Regarding specificity of diagnosis, one study of Sjögren's syndrome patients reported a specificity of approximately 95% when the cut-off for diagnosis was set at 5 mm in 5 min.[149] Another study showed a specificity

of 72.4% at this cut-off value.[150] It has also been shown that a lower Schirmer's test value is associated with severe DED, suggesting better reliability at those low values.[151,152] Anesthesia appears to increase the reliability of dry eye diagnosis.[153] In a study of men over the age of 50, the Schirmer's test was found to be second to tear break-up time at best discriminating healthy and dry eye subjects reporting an area under the receiver operating characteristic curve of 0.891 (95% confidence interval: 0.750, 0.982).[154] Recent evidence suggests that patients with nerve compromise have reduced Schirmer's strip results. Therefore, a patient with reduced Schirmer strip results should be assumed to have nerve compromise.

One final metric for corneal nerve function includes assessment of central versus peripheral pain using anesthetic drops on the cornea. This assessment involves the instillation of a topical anesthetic to the eye. If the anesthetic completely eliminates the patient symptoms, it is known that the corneal nerves are responsible for the symptoms and the patient has peripheral pain. However, if the patient symptoms persist after instillation, the patient likely has nonocular pain, due to ganglionopathy or centralized pain, which cannot be eliminated by topical anesthetic drops. If the patient has an incomplete reduction of pain, they have both ocular and nonocular pain.[155,156]

CONCLUSION

The nerves of the ocular surface have a large impact on sensations experienced by patients and on the tear film integrity. For this reason, the nerves of the ocular surface should be assessed by clinicians to guide their treatment. In addition, researchers should consider how nerves could influence their experiments. For example, including patients in a clinical trial of a DED treatment based on symptoms alone could cause a heterogeneous group of both neuropathic corneal pain patients and DED patients. The results of the study could then lack significance because the treatment only worked on those with true DED. For many years the impact of corneal nerves was not considered; however, more recent work using IVCM and the recognition of neuropathic corneal pain has helped to expand our knowledge in the area of corneal nerve assessment.

REFERENCES

1. Bron AJ, de Paiva CS, Chauhan SK, et al. TFOS DEWS II pathophysiology report. *Ocul Surf*. 2017;15:438–510.
2. Pflugfelder SC, de Paiva CS. The pathophysiology of dry eye disease: what we know and future directions for research. *Ophthalmology*. 2017;124:S4–S13.
3. Woolf CJ, Ma Q. Nociceptors–noxious stimulus detectors. *Neuron*. 2007;55:353–364.
4. Frias B, Merighi A. Capsaicin, nociception and pain. *Molecules*. 2016;21.
5. He J, Bazan NG, Bazan HE. Mapping the entire human corneal nerve architecture. *Exp Eye Res*. 2010;91: 513–523.
6. Marfurt CF, Cox J, Deek S, Dvorscak L. Anatomy of the human corneal innervation. *Exp Eye Res*. 2010;90: 478–492.
7. Al-Aqaba MA, Fares U, Suleman H, Lowe J, Dua HS. Architecture and distribution of human corneal nerves. *Br J Ophthalmol*. 2010;94:784–789.
8. Tanelian DL, Beuerman RW. Responses of rabbit corneal nociceptors to mechanical and thermal stimulation. *Exp Neurol*. 1984;84:165–178.
9. Belmonte C, Giraldez F. Responses of cat corneal sensory receptors to mechanical and thermal stimulation. *J Physiol*. 1981;321:355–368.
10. Gallar J, Pozo MA, Tuckett RP, Belmonte C. Response of sensory units with unmyelinated fibres to mechanical, thermal and chemical stimulation of the cat's cornea. *J Physiol*. 1993;468:609–622.
11. Belmonte C, Aracil A, Acosta MC, Luna C, Gallar J. Nerves and sensations from the eye surface. *Ocul Surf*. 2004;2: 248–253.
12. Parra A, Madrid R, Echevarria D, et al. Ocular surface wetness is regulated by TRPM8-dependent cold thermoreceptors of the cornea. *Nat Med*. 2010;16:1396–1399.
13. Bereiter DA, Hathaway CB, Benetti AP. Caudal portions of the spinal trigeminal complex are necessary for autonomic responses and display Fos-like immunoreactivity after corneal stimulation in the cat. *Brain Res*. 1994;657: 73–82.
14. Meng ID, Hu JW, Benetti AP, Bereiter DA. Encoding of corneal input in two distinct regions of the spinal trigeminal nucleus in the rat: cutaneous receptive field properties, responses to thermal and chemical stimulation, modulation by diffuse noxious inhibitory controls, and projections to the parabrachial area. *J Neurophysiol*. 1997;77:43–56.
15. Meng ID, Bereiter DA. Differential distribution of Fos-like immunoreactivity in the spinal trigeminal nucleus after noxious and innocuous thermal and chemical stimulation of rat cornea. *Neuroscience*. 1996;72:243–254.
16. Lu J, Hathaway CB, Bereiter DA. Adrenalectomy enhances Fos-like immunoreactivity within the spinal trigeminal nucleus induced by noxious thermal stimulation of the cornea. *Neuroscience*. 1993;54:809–818.
17. Marfurt CF. The central projections of trigeminal primary afferent neurons in the cat as determined by the transganglionic transport of horseradish peroxidase. *J Comp Neurol*. 1981;203:785–798.
18. Marfurt CF, Del Toro DR. Corneal sensory pathway in the rat: a horseradish peroxidase tracing study. *J Comp Neurol*. 1987;261:450–459.
19. Marfurt CF, Echtenkamp SF. Central projections and trigeminal ganglion location of corneal afferent neurons in the monkey, *Macaca fascicularis*. *J Comp Neurol*. 1988; 272:370–382.
20. Panneton WM, Burton H. Corneal and periocular representation within the trigeminal sensory complex in the cat studied with transganglionic transport of horseradish peroxidase. *J Comp Neurol*. 1981;199:327–344.
21. Hirata H, Okamoto K, Tashiro A, Bereiter DA. A novel class of neurons at the trigeminal subnucleus interpolaris/caudalis transition region monitors ocular surface fluid status and modulates tear production. *J Neurosci*. 2004;24:4224–4232.
22. Hirata H, Hu JW, Bereiter DA. Responses of medullary dorsal horn neurons to corneal stimulation by CO_2 pulses in the rat. *J Neurophysiol*. 1999;82:2092–2107.
23. Kurose M, Meng ID. Corneal dry-responsive neurons in the spinal trigeminal nucleus respond to innocuous cooling in the rat. *J Neurophysiol*. 2013;109:2517–2522.
24. Rahman M, Okamoto K, Thompson R, Katagiri A, Bereiter DA. Sensitization of trigeminal brainstem pathways in a model for tear deficient dry eye. *Pain*. 2015; 156:942–950.
25. Hirata H, Takeshita S, Hu JW, Bereiter DA. Cornea-responsive medullary dorsal horn neurons: modulation

by local opioids and projections to thalamus and brain stem. *J Neurophysiol.* 2000;84:1050–1061.

26. Henriquez VM, Evinger C. The three-neuron corneal reflex circuit and modulation of second-order corneal responsive neurons. *Exp Brain Res.* 2007;179:691–702.

27. Toth IE, Boldogkoi Z, Medveczky I, Palkovits M. Lacrimal preganglionic neurons form a subdivision of the superior salivatory nucleus of rat: transneuronal labelling by pseudorabies virus. *J Auton Nerv Syst.* 1999;77:45–54.

28. Ruskell GL. Distribution of pterygopalatine ganglion efferents to the lacrimal gland in man. *Exp Eye Res.* 2004; 78:329–335.

29. Ten Tusscher MP, Klooster J, Baljet B, Van der Werf F, Vrensen GF. Pre- and post-ganglionic nerve fibres of the pterygopalatine ganglion and their allocation to the eyeball of rats. *Brain Res.* 1990;517:315–323.

30. van der Werf F, Baljet B, Prins M, Otto JA. Innervation of the lacrimal gland in the cynomolgous monkey: a retrograde tracing study. *J Anat.* 1996;188(Pt 3):591–601.

31. Meneray MA, Bennett DJ, Nguyen DH, Beuerman RW. Effect of sensory denervation on the structure and physiologic responsiveness of rabbit lacrimal gland. *Cornea.* 1998;17:99–107.

32. Uddman R, Alumets J, Ehinger B, Hakanson R, Loren I, Sundler F. Vasoactive intestinal peptide nerves in ocular and orbital structures of the cat. *Invest Ophthalmol Vis Sci.* 1980;19:878–885.

33. Toshida H, Nguyen DH, Beuerman RW, Murakami A. Evaluation of novel dry eye model: preganglionic parasympathetic denervation in rabbit. *Invest Ophthalmol Vis Sci.* 2007;48:4468–4475.

34. Kovacs I, Ludany A, Koszegi T, et al. Substance P released from sensory nerve endings influences tear secretion and goblet cell function in the rat. *Neuropeptides.* 2005;39: 395–402.

35. Ruskell G. Changes in nerve terminals and acini of the lacrimal gland and changes in secretion induced by autonomic denervation. *Cell Tissue Res.* 1969;94:261–281.

36. De Haas E. The response of the lacrimal gland to parasympathicomimetics in keratoconjunctivitis sicca. *Ophthalmologica.* 1964;147:461–466.

37. Kessler TL, Dartt DA. Neural stimulation of conjunctival goblet cell mucous secretion in rats. *Adv Exp Med Biol.* 1994;350:393–398.

38. Kessler TL, Mercer HJ, Zieske JD, McCarthy DM, Dartt DA. Stimulation of goblet cell mucous secretion by activation of nerves in rat conjunctiva. *Curr Eye Res.* 1995;14: 985–992.

39. Diebold Y, Rios JD, Hodges RR, Rawe I, Dartt DA. Presence of nerves and their receptors in mouse and human conjunctival goblet cells. *Invest Ophthalmol Vis Sci.* 2001; 42:2270–2282.

40. Dartt DA, McCarthy DM, Mercer HJ, Kessler TL, Chung EH, Zieske JD. Localization of nerves adjacent to goblet cells in rat conjunctiva. *Curr Eye Res.* 1995;14: 993–1000.

41. Seifert P, Spitznas M. Vasoactive intestinal polypeptide (VIP) innervation of the human eyelid glands. *Exp Eye Res.* 1999;68:685–692.

42. Rios JD, Zoukhri D, Rawe IM, Hodges RR, Zieske JD, Dartt DA. Immunolocalization of muscarinic and VIP receptor subtypes and their role in stimulating goblet cell secretion. *Invest Ophthalmol Vis Sci.* 1999;40:1102–1111.

43. Seifert P, Spitznas M. Immunocytochemical and ultrastructural evaluation of the distribution of nervous tissue and neuropeptides in the meibomian gland. *Graefe's Arch Clin Exp Ophthalmol.* 1996;234:648–656.

44. Kirch W, Horneber M, Tamm ER. Characterization of Meibomian gland innervation in the cynomolgus monkey (*Macaca fascicularis*). *Anat Embryol.* 1996;193:365–375.

45. Montagna W, Ellis RA. Cholinergic innervation of the Meibomian glands. *Anat Rec.* 1959;135:121–127.

46. Leeson T. Tarsal (Meibomian) glands of the rat. *Br J Ophthalmol.* 1963;47:222.

47. Aisa J, Lahoz M, Serrano P, et al. Acetylcholinesterase-positive and paraformaldehyde-induced-fluorescence-positive innervation in the upper eyelid of the sheep (*Ovis aries*). *Histol Histopathol.* 2001;16:487–496.

48. Miraglia T, Gomes NF. The meibomian glands of the marmoset (*Callithrix jacchus*). *Acta Anat.* 1969;74: 104–113.

49. Chung CW, Tigges M, Stone RA. Peptidergic innervation of the primate meibomian gland. *Invest Ophthalmol Vis Sci.* 1996;37:238–245.

50. Perra MT, Serra A, Sirigu P, Turno F. Histochemical demonstration of acetylcholinesterase activity in human Meibomian glands. *Eur J Histochem.* 1996;40:39–44.

51. Simons E, Smith PG. Sensory and autonomic innervation of the rat eyelid: neuronal origins and peptide phenotypes. *J Chem Neuroanat.* 1994;7:35–47.

52. Elsas T, Edvinsson L, Sundler F, Uddman R. Neuronal pathways to the rat conjunctiva revealed by retrograde tracing and immunocytochemistry. *Exp Eye Res.* 1994; 58:117–126.

53. Chanthaphavong RS, Murphy SM, Anderson CR. Chemical coding of sympathetic neurons controlling the tarsal muscle of the rat. *Auton Neurosci.* 2003;105:77–89.

54. Zhu HY, Riau AK, Barathi VA, Chew J, Beuerman RW. Expression of neural receptors in mouse meibomian gland. *Cornea.* 2010;29:794–801.

55. Fan Q, Smith PG. Decreased vasoactive intestinal polypeptide-immunoreactivity of parasympathetic neurons and target innervation following long-term sympathectomy. *Regul Pept.* 1993;48:337–343.

56. LeDoux MS, Zhou Q, Murphy RB, Greene ML, Ryan P. Parasympathetic innervation of the meibomian glands in rats. *Invest Ophthalmol Vis Sci.* 2001;42:2434–2441.

57. Hartschuh W, Reinecke M, Weihe E, Yanaihara N. VIP-immunoreactivity in the skin of various mammals: immunohistochemical, radioimmunological and experimental evidence for a dual localization in cutaneous nerves and merkel cells. *Peptides.* 1984;5:239–245.

58. Hartschuh W, Weihe E, Reinecke M. Peptidergic (neurotensin, VIP, substance P) nerve fibres in the skin. Immunohistochemical evidence of an involvement of neuropeptides in nociception, pruritus and inflammation. *Br J Dermatol.* 1983;109:14−17.

59. Kam WR, Sullivan DA. Neurotransmitter influence on human meibomian gland epithelial cells. *Invest Ophthalmol Vis Sci.* 2011;52:8543−8548.

60. Liu S, Li J, Tan DT, Beuerman RW. The eyelid margin: a transitional zone for 2 epithelial phenotypes. *Arch Ophthalmol.* 2007;125:523−532.

61. Luhtala J, Palkama A, Uusitalo H. Calcitonin gene-related peptide immunoreactive nerve fibers in the rat conjunctiva. *Invest Ophthalmol Vis Sci.* 1991;32:640−645.

62. Luhtala J, Uusitalo H. The distribution and origin of substance P immunoreactive nerve fibres in the rat conjunctiva. *Exp Eye Res.* 1991;53:641−646.

63. Seifert P, Spitznas M. Demonstration of nerve fibers in human accessory lacrimal glands. *Graefe's Arch Clin Exp Ophthalmol.* 1994;232:107−114.

64. Jester JV, Nicolaides N, Kiss-Palvolgyi I, Smith RE. Meibomian gland dysfunction. II. The role of keratinization in a rabbit model of MGD. *Invest Ophthalmol Vis Sci.* 1989;30:936−945.

65. Jester JV, Rife L, Nii D, Luttrull JK, Wilson L, Smith RE. In vivo biomicroscopy and photography of meibomian glands in a rabbit model of meibomian gland dysfunction. *Invest Ophthalmol Vis Sci.* 1982;22:660−667.

66. Pondelis N, Dieckmann GM, Jamali A, Kataguiri P, Senchyna M, Hamrah P. Infrared meibography allows detection of dimensional changes in meibomian glands following intranasal neurostimulation. *Ocul Surf.* 2020;18:511−516.

67. Sneddon LU. Comparative physiology of nociception and pain. *Physiology.* 2018;33:63−73.

68. Tracey Jr WD. Nociception. *Curr Biol.* 2017;27:R129−R133.

69. Woller SA, Eddinger KA, Corr M, Yaksh TL. An overview of pathways encoding nociception. *Clin Exp Rheumatol.* 2017;35(Suppl 107):40−46.

70. Treede RD, Rief W, Barke A, et al. A classification of chronic pain for ICD-11. *Pain.* 2015;156:1003−1007.

71. Costigan M, Scholz J, Woolf CJ. Neuropathic pain: a maladaptive response of the nervous system to damage. *Annu Rev Neurosci.* 2009;32:1−32.

72. Juhl GI, Jensen TS, Norholt SE, Svensson P. Central sensitization phenomena after third molar surgery: a quantitative sensory testing study. *Eur J Pain.* 2008;12:116−127.

73. St John Smith E. Advances in understanding nociception and neuropathic pain. *J Neurol.* 2018;265:231−238.

74. Chiu IM, von Hehn CA, Woolf CJ. Neurogenic inflammation and the peripheral nervous system in host defense and immunopathology. *Nat Neurosci.* 2012;15:1063−1067.

75. Scholz J, Woolf CJ. The neuropathic pain triad: neurons, immune cells and glia. *Nat Neurosci.* 2007;10:1361−1368.

76. Nielsen CS, Stubhaug A, Price DD, Vassend O, Czajkowski N, Harris JR. Individual differences in pain sensitivity: genetic and environmental contributions. *Pain.* 2008;136:21−29.

77. Staud R, Craggs JG, Perlstein WM, Robinson ME, Price DD. Brain activity associated with slow temporal summation of C-fiber evoked pain in fibromyalgia patients and healthy controls. *Eur J Pain.* 2008;12:1078−1089.

78. Belmonte C, Nichols JJ, Cox SM, et al. TFOS DEWS II pain and sensation report. *Ocul Surf.* 2017;15:404−437.

79. Aggarwal S, Colon C, Kheirkhah A, Hamrah P. Efficacy of autologous serum tears for treatment of neuropathic corneal pain. *Ocul Surf.* 2019;17:532−539.

80. Kim J, Yoon HJ, You IC, Ko BY, Yoon KC. Clinical characteristics of dry eye with ocular neuropathic pain features: comparison according to the types of sensitization based on the Ocular Pain Assessment Survey. *BMC Ophthalmol.* 2020;20:455.

81. Galor A, Zlotcavitch L, Walter SD, et al. Dry eye symptom severity and persistence are associated with symptoms of neuropathic pain. *Br J Ophthalmol.* 2015;99:665−668.

82. Cox SM, Kheirkhah A, Aggarwal S, et al. Alterations in corneal nerves in different subtypes of dry eye disease: an in vivo confocal microscopy study. *Ocul Surf.* 2021;22:135−142.

83. Cruzat A, Pavan-Langston D, Hamrah P. In vivo confocal microscopy of corneal nerves: analysis and clinical correlation. *Semin Ophthalmol.* 2010;25:171−177.

84. Hucho T, Levine JD. Signaling pathways in sensitization: toward a nociceptor cell biology. *Neuron.* 2007;55:365−376.

85. Hamrah P, Qazi Y, Shahatit B, et al. Corneal nerve and epithelial cell alterations in corneal allodynia: an in vivo confocal microscopy case series. *Ocul Surf.* 2017;15:139−151.

86. Finnerup NB, Kuner R, Jensen TS. Neuropathic pain: from mechanisms to treatment. *Physiol Rev.* 2021;101:259−301.

87. Cruzat A, Qazi Y, Hamrah P. In vivo confocal microscopy of corneal nerves in health and disease. *Ocul Surf.* 2017;15:15−47.

88. Qazi Y, Aggarwal S, Hamrah P. Image-guided evaluation and monitoring of treatment response in patients with dry eye disease. *Graefes Arch Clin Exp Ophthalmol.* 2014;252:857−872.

89. Qazi Y, Kheirkhah A, Blackie C, et al. Clinically relevant immune-cellular metrics of inflammation in meibomian gland dysfunction. *Invest Ophthalmol Vis Sci.* 2018;59:6111−6123.

90. Hikichi T, Yoshida A, Tsubota K. Lymphocytic infiltration of the conjunctiva and the salivary gland in Sjogren's syndrome. *Arch Ophthalmol.* 1993;111:21−22.

91. Wakamatsu TH, Sato EA, Matsumoto Y, et al. Conjunctival in vivo confocal scanning laser microscopy in patients with Sjogren syndrome. *Invest Ophthalmol Vis Sci.* 2010;51:144−150.

92. Yamaguchi T. Inflammatory response in dry eye. *Invest Ophthalmol Vis Sci.* 2018;59:DES192−DES199.

93. Alhatem A, Cavalcanti B, Hamrah P. In vivo confocal microscopy in dry eye disease and related conditions. *Semin Ophthalmol.* 2012;27:138−148.

94. Yamaguchi T, Hamrah P, Shimazaki J. Bilateral alterations in corneal nerves, dendritic cells, and tear cytokine levels in ocular surface disease. *Cornea.* 2016;35(Suppl 1):S65−S70.

95. Kheirkhah A, Dohlman TH, Amparo F, et al. Effects of corneal nerve density on the response to treatment in dry eye disease. *Ophthalmology.* 2015;122:662−668.

96. Labbe A, Alalwani H, Van Went C, Brasnu E, Georgescu D, Baudouin C. The relationship between subbasal nerve morphology and corneal sensation in ocular surface disease. *Invest Ophthalmol Vis Sci.* 2012;53:4926−4931.

97. Qazi YK A, Dohlman TH, Cruzat A, et al. *Corneal Dendritic Cells as a Surrogate Biomarker of Therapeutic Efficacy in Dry Eye-Associated Corneal Inflammation.* Denver, CO: ARVO Annual Meeting Abstract; 2015.

98. Cruzat A, Witkin D, Baniasadi N, et al. Inflammation and the nervous system: the connection in the cornea in patients with infectious keratitis. *Invest Ophthalmol Vis Sci.* 2011;52:5136−5143.

99. Hamrah P, Cruzat A, Dastjerdi MH, et al. Corneal sensation and subbasal nerve alterations in patients with herpes simplex keratitis: an in vivo confocal microscopy study. *Ophthalmology.* 2010;117:1930−1936.

100. Hamrah P, Seyed-Razavi Y, Yamaguchi T. Translational immunoimaging and neuroimaging demonstrate corneal neuroimmune crosstalk. *Cornea.* 2016;35(Suppl 1):S20−s24.

101. Kawashima H, Prasad SA, Gregerson DS. Corneal endothelial cells inhibit T cell proliferation by blocking IL-2 production. *J Immunol.* 1994;153:1982−1989.

102. Hori J, Joyce NC, Streilein JW. Immune privilege and immunogenicity reside among different layers of the mouse cornea. *Invest Ophthalmol Vis Sci.* 2000;41:3032−3042.

103. Streilein JW, Okamoto S, Sano Y, Taylor AW. Neural control of ocular immune privilege. *Ann N Y Acad Sci.* 2000;917:297−306.

104. Hamrah P, Haskova Z, Taylor AW, Zhang Q, Ksander BR, Dana MR. Local treatment with alpha-melanocyte stimulating hormone reduces corneal allorejection. *Transplantation.* 2009;88:180−187.

105. Paunicka KJ, Mellon J, Robertson D, Petroll M, Brown JR, Niederkorn JY. Severing corneal nerves in one eye induces sympathetic loss of immune privilege and promotes rejection of future corneal allografts placed in either eye. *Am J Transplant.* 2015;15:1490−1501.

106. Yamaguchi T, Turhan A, Harris DL, et al. Bilateral nerve alterations in a unilateral experimental neurotrophic keratopathy model: a lateral conjunctival approach for trigeminal axotomy. *PLoS One.* 2013;8:e70908.

107. Yamaguchi T, Harris DL, Higa H, Shimazaki J, Andrian UV, Hamrah P. Neurogenic immune homeostasis: peripheral innervation maintains avascularity and immune privilege of the cornea. *Investig Ophthalmol Vis Sci.* 2015;56:4034.

108. Aggarwal S, Cavalcanti BM, Regali L, et al. In vivo confocal microscopy shows alterations in nerve density and dendritiform cell density in fuchs' endothelial corneal dystrophy. *Am J Ophthalmol.* 2018;196:136−144.

109. Cavalcanti BM, Cruzat A, Sahin A, Pavan-Langston D, Samayoa E, Hamrah P. In vivo confocal microscopy detects bilateral changes of corneal immune cells and nerves in unilateral herpes zoster ophthalmicus. *Ocul Surf.* 2018;16:101−111.

110. Muller RT, Abedi F, Cruzat A, et al. Degeneration and regeneration of subbasal corneal nerves after infectious keratitis: a longitudinal in vivo confocal microscopy study. *Ophthalmology.* 2015;122:2200−2209.

111. Oliveira-Soto L, Efron N. Morphology of corneal nerves using confocal microscopy. *Cornea.* 2001;20:374−384.

112. Patel DV, Tavakoli M, Craig JP, Efron N, McGhee CN. Corneal sensitivity and slit scanning in vivo confocal microscopy of the subbasal nerve plexus of the normal central and peripheral human cornea. *Cornea.* 2009;28:735−740.

113. Guthoff R, Baudouin C, Stave J. *Atlas of Confocal Laser Scanning In-Vivo Microscopy in Opthalmology − Principles and Applications in Diagnostic and Therapeutic Ophtalmology.* Springer Science & Business Media; 2006.

114. Lemp MA, Dilly PN, Boyde A. Tandem-scanning (confocal) microscopy of the full-thickness cornea. *Cornea.* 1985;4:205−209.

115. McLaren JW, Nau CB, Patel SV, Bourne WM. Measuring corneal thickness with the ConfoScan 4 and z-ring adapter. *Eye Contact Lens.* 2007;33:185−190.

116. Niederer RL, McGhee CN. Clinical in vivo confocal microscopy of the human cornea in health and disease. *Prog Retin Eye Res.* 2010;29:30−58.

117. Binotti WW, Bayraktutar B, Ozmen MC, Cox SM, Hamrah P. A review of imaging biomarkers of the ocular surface. *Eye Contact Lens.* 2020;46(Suppl 2):S84−s105.

118. Levy O, Labbe A, Borderie V, et al. Increased corneal subbasal nerve density in patients with Sjogren syndrome treated with topical cyclosporine A. *Clin Exp Ophthalmol.* 2017;45:455−463.

119. Tepelus TC, Chiu GB, Huang J, et al. Correlation between corneal innervation and inflammation evaluated with confocal microscopy and symptomatology in patients with dry eye syndromes: a preliminary study. *Graefe's Arch Clin Exp Ophthalmol.* 2017;255:1771−1778.

120. Tepelus TC, Chiu GB, Maram J, et al. Corneal features in ocular graft-versus-host disease by in vivo confocal microscopy. *Graefe's Arch Clin Exp Ophthalmol.* 2017;255:2389−2397.

121. Kheirkhah A, Satitpitakul V, Hamrah P, Dana R. Patients with dry eye disease and low subbasal nerve density are at high risk for accelerated corneal endothelial cell loss. *Cornea.* 2017;36:196−201.

122. Chinnery HR, Naranjo Golborne C, Downie LE. Omega-3 supplementation is neuroprotective to corneal nerves

in dry eye disease: a pilot study. *Ophthalmic Physiol Opt.* 2017;37:473–481.

123. John T, Tighe S, Sheha H, et al. Corneal nerve regeneration after self-retained cryopreserved amniotic membrane in dry eye disease. *J Ophthalmol.* 2017;2017:6404918.

124. Kheirkhah A, Qazi Y, Arnoldner MA, Suri K, Dana R. In vivo confocal microscopy in dry eye disease associated with chronic graft-versus-host disease. *Invest Ophthalmol Vis Sci.* 2016;57:4686–4691.

125. Labbe A, Liang Q, Wang Z, et al. Corneal nerve structure and function in patients with non-sjogren dry eye: clinical correlations. *Invest Ophthalmol Vis Sci.* 2013;54:5144–5150.

126. Wu T, Ahmed A, Bril V, et al. Variables associated with corneal confocal microscopy parameters in healthy volunteers: implications for diabetic neuropathy screening. *Diabet Med.* 2012;29:e297–303.

127. Kim G, Singleton JR, Mifflin MD, Digre KB, Porzio MT, Smith AG. Assessing the reproducibility of quantitative in vivo confocal microscopy of corneal nerves in different corneal locations. *Cornea.* 2013;32:1331–1338.

128. Benitez del Castillo JM, Wasfy MA, Fernandez C, Garcia-Sanchez J. An in vivo confocal masked study on corneal epithelium and subbasal nerves in patients with dry eye. *Invest Ophthalmol Vis Sci.* 2004;45:3030–3035.

129. Villani E, Galimberti D, Viola F, Mapelli C, Ratiglia R. The cornea in Sjogren's syndrome: an in vivo confocal study. *Invest Ophthalmol Vis Sci.* 2007;48:2017–2022.

130. Zhang M, Chen J, Luo L, Xiao Q, Sun M, Liu Z. Altered corneal nerves in aqueous tear deficiency viewed by in vivo confocal microscopy. *Cornea.* 2005;24:818–824.

131. Patel DV, McGhee CN. In vivo confocal microscopy of human corneal nerves in health, in ocular and systemic disease, and following corneal surgery: a review. *Br J Ophthalmol.* 2009;93:853–860.

132. Kehlet H, Jensen TS, Woolf CJ. Persistent postsurgical pain: risk factors and prevention. *Lancet.* 2006;367:1618–1625.

133. Aggarwal S, Kheirkhah A, Cavalcanti BM, et al. Autologous serum tears for treatment of photoallodynia in patients with corneal neuropathy: efficacy and evaluation with in vivo confocal microscopy. *Ocul Surf.* 2015;13:250–262.

134. Moein HRD G, Abbouda A, Pondelis N, Jamali A, Salem Z, Hamrah P. *In Vivo Confocal Microscopy Demonstrates the Presence of Microneuromas and May Allow Differentiation of Patients with Corneal Neuropathic Pain from Dry Eye Disease.* Baltimore, MA: The Association for Research in Vision and Ophthalmology; 2017.

135. Ross AR, Al-Aqaba MA, Almaazmi A, et al. Clinical and in vivo confocal microscopic features of neuropathic corneal pain. *Br J Ophthalmol.* 2019;104(6):768–775.

136. Dermer H, Hwang J, Mittal R, Cohen AK, Galor A. Corneal sub-basal nerve plexus microneuromas in individuals with and without dry eye. *Br J Ophthalmol.* 2021.

137. Chinnery HR, Rajan R, Jiao H, et al. Identification of presumed corneal neuromas and microneuromas using

138. Stepp MA, Pal-Ghosh S, Downie LE, et al. Corneal epithelial "neuromas": a case of mistaken identity? *Cornea.* 2020;39:930–934.

139. Yavuz Saricay L, Bayraktutar BN, Kenyon BM, Hamrah P. Concurrent ocular pain in patients with neurotrophic keratopathy. *Ocul Surf.* 2021;22:143–151.

140. Martin XY, Safran AB. Corneal hypoesthesia. *Surv Ophthalmol.* 1988;33:28–40.

141. Chao C, Stapleton F, Badarudin E, Golebiowski B. Ocular surface sensitivity repeatability with Cochet-Bonnet esthesiometer. *Optom Vis Sci.* 2015;92:183–189.

142. Bourcier T, Acosta MC, Borderie V, et al. Decreased corneal sensitivity in patients with dry eye. *Invest Ophthalmol Vis Sci.* 2005;46:2341–2345.

143. Toker E, Asfuroglu E. Corneal and conjunctival sensitivity in patients with dry eye: the effect of topical cyclosporine therapy. *Cornea.* 2010;29:133–140.

144. Benitez-Del-Castillo JM, Acosta MC, Wassfi MA, et al. Relation between corneal innervation with confocal microscopy and corneal sensitivity with noncontact esthesiometry in patients with dry eye. *Invest Ophthalmol Vis Sci.* 2007;48:173–181.

145. De Paiva CS, Pflugfelder SC. Corneal epitheliopathy of dry eye induces hyperesthesia to mechanical air jet stimulation. *Am J Ophthalmol.* 2004;137:109–115.

146. Kaido M, Kawashima M, Ishida R, Tsubota K. Relationship of corneal pain sensitivity with dry eye symptoms in dry eye with short tear break-up time. *Invest Ophthalmol Vis Sci.* 2016;57:914–919.

147. Tagawa Y, Noda K, Ohguchi T, Tagawa Y, Ishida S, Kitaichi N. Corneal hyperalgesia in patients with short tear film break-up time dry eye. *Ocul Surf.* 2019;17:55–59.

148. Nichols KK, Mitchell GL, Zadnik K. The repeatability of clinical measurements of dry eye. *Cornea.* 2004;23:272–285.

149. de Monchy I, Gendron G, Miceli C, Pogorzalek N, Mariette X, Labetoulle M. Combination of the schirmer I and phenol red thread tests as a rescue strategy for diagnosis of ocular dryness associated with sjögren's syndrome. *Invest Ophthalmol Vis Sci.* 2011;52:5167–5173.

150. Vitali C, Moutsopoulos HM, Bombardieri S. The European Community Study Group on diagnostic criteria for Sjögren's syndrome. Sensitivity and specificity of tests for ocular and oral involvement in Sjögren's syndrome. *Ann Rheum Dis.* 1994;53:637–647.

151. Sullivan BD, Crews LA, Messmer EM, et al. Correlations between commonly used objective signs and symptoms for the diagnosis of dry eye disease: clinical implications. *Acta Ophthalmol.* 2014;92:161–166.

152. Sullivan BD, Whitmer D, Nichols KK, et al. An objective approach to dry eye disease severity. *Invest Ophthalmol Vis Sci.* 2010;51:6125–6130.

153. Li N, Deng X-G, He M-F. Comparison of the Schirmer I test with and without topical anesthesia for diagnosing dry eye. *Int J Ophthalmol.* 2012;5:478.

154. See C, Bilonick RA, Feuer W, Galor A. Comparison of two methods for composite score generation in dry eye syndrome. *Invest Ophthalmol Vis Sci.* 2013;54:6280–6286.

155. Dieckmann G, Goyal S, Hamrah P. Neuropathic corneal pain: approaches for management. *Ophthalmology.* 2017;124:S34–s47.

156. Crane AM, Feuer W, Felix ER, et al. Evidence of central sensitisation in those with dry eye symptoms and neuropathic-like ocular pain complaints: incomplete response to topical anaesthesia and generalised heightened sensitivity to evoked pain. *Br J Ophthalmol.* 2017;101:1238–1243.

157. Adatia FA, Michaeli-Cohen A, Naor J, Caffery B, Bookman A, Slomovic A. Correlation between corneal sensitivity, subjective dry eye symptoms and corneal staining in Sjogren's syndrome. *Can J Ophthalmol.* 2004;39:767–771.

158. Nepp J, Wirth M. Fluctuations of corneal sensitivity in dry eye syndromes—a longitudinal pilot study. *Cornea.* 2015;34:1221–1226.

CHAPTER 4

Pathophysiology of Dry Eye Disease Using Animal Models

YIHE CHEN, MD • REZA DANA, MD, MSC, MPH

INTRODUCTION

Dry eye disease (DED) is a multifactorial condition of the ocular surface, characterized by chronic inflammatory damages of the cornea and conjunctiva, along with the involvement of Meibomian and lacrimal glands, and neurosensory system innervating the ocular surface. The key underlying pathophysiological process driving the disease is due to the loss of immune homeostasis at the ocular surface, with subsequent disruptions of the tear film stability, corneal epithelial barrier, and corneal sensation.[1] DED can be broadly classified into two categories based on the lack of aqueous tears or not—aqueous-deficient form (with reduced tear quantity) and evaporative form (with reduced tear quality),[2,3] and accordingly various animal models have been created to mimic DED through decreasing the tear production or increasing the tear evaporation. It is worth to be noted that the two types of DED are not mutually exclusive, and one model that primarily falls into one category may still possess some features of the other. In fact, coexistence of deficiencies of tear quality and quantity is not uncommon in human patients with DED,[4] and recent report from the Dry Eye Work Shop (DEWS II) has advocated a continuum classification scheme to highlight such overlap between the two primary types of DED.[1] Therefore, it is suggested that no matter how the disease is initially induced, characteristic features of both types of DED may occur as the disease progresses, and common pathophysiological processes are shared among various etiologies of DED in both human and animal models.

It is well known that continued inflammation plays a key role in DED,[5] and significant advancement has been achieved in the past 2 decades in our understanding of the precise pathogenesis, particularly the immune mechanisms underlying the disease, primarily through the valuable animal models including the transgenic mouse models of Sjögren's syndrome and the popular desiccation stress-induced non-Sjögren's DED mouse models that were established independently by both Pflugfelder (Baylor College of Medicine)[6] and Dana (Harvard Medical School)[7] groups in early 2000s. Mouse models are the most popular in corneal research, including DED, although rat, rabbit, and dog DED models have also been reported.[8-13] Mice are particularly useful to study the disease pathogenesis given their similar ocular surface structures with humans, well-defined immunogenetics in inbred strains, abundant availability of reagents and various transgenic and knockout strains, as well as small size and ease of husbandry. Anatomically, mouse cornea has similar layers to human cornea, including epithelium, stroma, posterior limiting lamina (Descemet's membrane), and endothelium, despite the presence of anterior limiting lamina (Bowman's membrane) in mice is questionable (Fig. 4.1).[14] However, major discrepancies also exist—the diameter and thickness of mouse cornea are much smaller than human cornea. Unlike the oval shape in human, mouse cornea is round in shape and its diameter measured from limbus to limbus is about 2.6 mm in adult (6–8 weeks) C57BL/6 strain,[14] the most commonly used strain for murine DED model. The central corneal full thickness in adult C57BL/6 is about 140 μm, higher than peripheral thickness of about 90 μm; the individual epithelium and stroma layer shows similarly thicker center than periphery.[14] In contrast, human cornea is thinner in the center (535 ± 20 μm) than periphery (657 ± 71 μm).[15] Clinically, corneal epitheliopathy is the most evaluated sign of DED, and is examined by corneal fluorescein staining (CFS), which stains areas of epithelial defect or where the epithelial barrier is lacking.[2,16,17] Corneal epithelial barrier in both mouse and human is similarly formed by desmosomal junctions, hemidesmosomes, and basement membrane, except there are more layers of epithelial cells in mouse than in human,[14,18] and thus CFS is similarly used for evaluating disease severity in mouse

Dry Eye Disease. https://doi.org/10.1016/B978-0-323-82753-9.00001-1

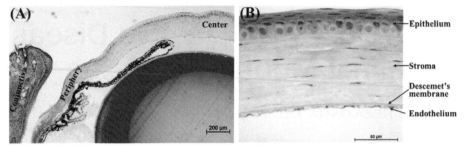

FIG. 4.1 **Histology of Adult C57BL/6 Mouse Cornea Aged 6–8 Weeks.** H & E staining shows **(A)** thicker central cornea than peripheral with individual epithelial and stromal layer thickness tapering from center toward periphery; and **(B)** four layers of corneal structures including epithelium, stroma, posterior limiting lamina (Descemet's membrane), and endothelium.

DED models. In addition to epithelial layer, corneal stroma is also critically involved in the pathogenesis of DED, as it is the principal site where bone marrow—derived immune cells reside in healthy cornea (with a few residing in epithelial layer) which are in resting status in normal but become activated in DED.[19,20] The mouse stroma is similarly arranged into lamellae with scattered keratocytes as observed in human, with some different fiber organization patterns in the anterior part of the stroma.[14] The corneal resident immune cells are characterized as primarily $CD11b^+CD3^-CD19^-$ myeloid but not lymphoid lineage cells, including dendritic cells (Langerhans cells within epithelium), macrophages, and monocytes.[19,21–24] Furthermore, the distribution pattern and functional status of corneal immune cells are consistent between human and mouse: significantly more myeloid cells are localized in the corneal periphery (throughout the entire stroma) than in the center (primarily in anterior stroma), and these cells represent phenotypically "immature" status that contributes to the immune homeostasis in normal cornea.[19,21,23,25] Lastly, corneal nerve is substantially involved in DED pathogenesis, due to its critical roles in corneal pain sensation, epithelial integrity, and release of neuroinflammatory substances. Nerves enter the corneal stroma at the limbal circumference from the ophthalmic branch of the trigeminal ganglion, and extends anteriorly toward corneal epithelium, forming the subbasal nerve plexus that supplies the overlying corneal epithelium.[26,27] A major difference in corneal nerves between mouse and human is that the nerve fibers distribute deeper in mouse (closer to endothelium) than in human.[14] In summary, it is important to be aware of both similarities and differences in histological structures and cellular components between mouse and human cornea for us to correctly extend research findings from mouse models of DED to human patients.

CLINICAL FINDINGS IN ANIMAL MODELS OF DRY EYE DISEASE

The common ocular symptoms in DED patients include ocular discomfort, visual disturbance, burning sensation, or pain.[17,28] However, subjective symptoms are hardly assessed in animal models due to the issue of feasibility. On the other hand, the recommended diagnostic tests in patients by the most recent DEWS II reports include tear film break-up time, tear osmolarity, tear volume, and ocular surface fluorescein staining.[17] All of these objective criteria, through various combinations, have been used in evaluating DED-related signs in animal models.

Desiccating Stress-Induced Dry Eye Disease

Desiccating stress, including environmental and pharmacologic ways, has been a popular method to induce DED in animals since it was initially validated in mice 2 decades ago.[6,7] The advantages of this model over others include relatively localized eye disease with minimally systemic effects, use of wild-type animals without genetic modifications, reliable and reversible (i.e., treatable) disease induction. Initial efforts to test the effect of desiccating stress on cornea were made by preventing eye blinking through placement of lid specula in rabbits for 2 h, which led to methylene blue staining on cornea, a sign of corneal epithelial defect, and corneal epithelial thinning demonstrated by scanning electron microscopy.[10] However, this model presents a very acute process lasting only hours, and animals have to receive anesthetics which themselves can affect tear secretion. Other researchers used a pharmacologic way by topical application of 1% atropine sulfate, an anticholinergic agent which inhibits aqueous tear secretion by lacrimal glands, in rabbits three times daily for 5 days, and they observed significantly decreased tear production and increased CFS as early as day 2.[11] Pflugfelder group (Baylor College of

Medicine) later combined continuous airflow with transdermal scopolamine patch, an inhibitor of muscarinic acetylcholine receptors, to induce DED in female CBA mice.[6] After 4-day's stress, mice showed significant reduction of tear secretion using cotton thread test (CTT) and increased punctate CFS; however, environmental desiccating stress alone (continuous airflow alone without scopolamine) generated in this model through an air fan placed at 6 inches in front of the mice's cage did not effectively induce significant ocular surface changes, suggesting that the environmental desiccating stress created in this model may not be adequate. Subsequently, Dana group (Harvard Medical School) optimized several key environmental factors by creating a more stable and efficient Controlled-Environment Chamber (CEC) which provided continuous dry airflow with low humidity (via filtering through desiccant columns) directly into the chamber where mice were housed (via airlines connected to an air pump outside the chamber and regulated by a flow meter) as well as a constant temperature of 21°C to 23°C inside the chamber.[7] All these environmental parameters were monitored by a probe. Combined with subcutaneous scopolamine injection, the CEC led to significantly decreased tear secretion and increased CFS in female BALB/c mice as early as day 3 post desiccating stress and throughout to the end of observation at day 28.[7] Further studies from Dana group demonstrated that C57BL/6 mouse strain showed more severe tear reduction than BALB/c strain under the stress, while the CFS severity remained comparable between the two strains[29]; this is probably related to the differential biased immune response in C57BL/6 (prone to Th1 response) and BALB/c (prone to Th2 response)[30] that are relevant to the pathogenesis of DED (to be discussed later in the following sections). This study has made C57BL/6 the most frequently used mouse strain in basic and translational DED research.[20,31–37] Since the beginning of the development of DED models, female animals were exclusively selected given the fact that the significant majority of human patients suffering from DED are women,[38–40] and a recent study using the combined environmental and pharmacologic desiccating stress model confirmed that female C57BL/6 mice presented with significantly higher CFS scores and lower tear production than male counterparts.[37] Since the creation of CEC, continuous efforts have been made to improve the stability of the low humanity inside the chamber including the use of an intelligent dehumidifying device.[41,42] By replacing the air-drying desiccant columns with a digitally controlled dry cabinet inside which the circulating air

was supplied from atmosphere air that was first dried via membrane dryers before entering the chamber (Fig. 4.2), the daily variation of the humidity observed in the original CEC system was significantly reduced, and thus a constant low humidity below 15% was achieved throughout different seasons in a year. Additionally, the dry air is continuously pumped into the mouse cage through four air lines connected to two opposite walls of each cage. With such improvement, mice developed a severe corneal epitheliopathy evidenced by all quadrants thick punctate CFS with 14-day's desiccating stress; and importantly, after mice were transferred to nondesiccated vivarium without any further pharmacologic desiccating stress, the epitheliopathy gradually regressed to lower levels, but never normalized, for more than 4 months observation period, despite the resolution of aqueous tear deficiency.[42] Thus, for the first time, a *chronic* DED model was established, which is critical because DED is generally encountered as a chronic disorder (months to years) in the clinical setting, and experimental data derived from a chronic model are more related to humans than that from an acute model.

Scopolamine or other anticholinergics are able to effectively suppress tear production by lacrimal glands via blocking acetylcholine receptors and thus induce DED without concomitant environmental desiccating stress.[6,43] However, there have been concerns regarding the use of the anticholinergics due to the existence of an independent, nonneuronal cholinergic system in lymphocytes.[44] Animal study has shown that in vivo treatment with systemic scopolamine in C57BL/6 mice leads to general enhancement of Th2 (type 2 T helper cell) and Treg (regulator T cell) responses but inhibition of Th17 (type 17 T helper cell) response, which are consequences of direct pharmacologic effects of scopolamine on T cells but not DED pathogenesis relevant.[43] Therefore, pharmacologic desiccating stress may not be a suitable model for DED pathophysiology investigations, and care should be taken in interpreting research findings in those models created through systemic acetylcholine receptor blockade. In fact, the improved, digitally controlled CEC system has been shown to effectively induce both acute[43,45,46] and chronic DED[47–49] in mice without the use of scopolamine. These DED mice exhibit consistently high CFS scores and ocular pain, a common symptom seen in human patients, as demonstrated by increased eye wipe response to topical hypertonic saline stimulation (R. Dana, unpublished data). Ocular surface sensory nerves express polymodal nociceptors, mechanonociceptors, and cold thermoreceptors, and all of them contribute

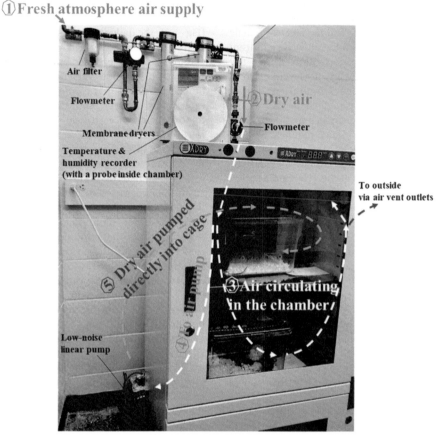

FIG. 4.2 **The Up-to-Date Controlled-Environment Chamber (CEC) with Stable Relative Humidity Below 20% and Temperature Between 21°C and 23°C, 24 h a Day.**   Fresh atmosphere air **(1)** is regulated by a flowmeter and filtered through two membrane dryers to generate dry air **(2)** that enters the digitally controlled dry cabinet, inside which mouse cages are housed. The pressure dry air inside the CEC circulates **(3)** and exchanges via dozens of air vents on the back wall of the cabinet at a rate of at least 10 times per hour that is required for healthy mouse housing. Meanwhile, the pressure dry air is also supplied to a low-noise linear pump outside the cabinet **(4)**, and pumped back directly into the mouse cages **(5)** via four air lines connected to two opposite walls of each cage, allowing a continuous dry air blow to the mouse eye at about 10 L/min monitored by a flowmeter placed inside the cabinet. The temperature and humidity inside the CEC are constantly monitored by a probe (placed inside CEC) and recorded on circular charts by a recorder (placed outside the CEC).

to pain sensation with the cold thermoreceptors also functioning to regulate basal tear production and blinking.[50] The hyperosmolarity formed by hypertonic saline at the mouse ocular surface activates both transient receptor potential cation channel subfamily V member 1 (TRPV1) channel (expressed by substantial proportions of corneal nerve endings and mediating polymodal nociceptor sensory transduction) and transient receptor potential cation channel subfamily M member 8 (TRPM8) channel (expressed by relatively smaller proportions of corneal nerve endings and mediating cold thermoreceptor sensory transduction).[51-53]

Surgical or Medical Destruction of Lacrimal Gland

The lacrimal gland is the main contributor to the aqueous layer of the tear film by secreting water, electrolytes, and proteins.[54] Mechanically obstructing or removing the lacrimal glands has thus been used to induce aqueous-deficient DED. After lacrimal gland duct was closed via cauterization in rabbits, tear film osmolarity was progressively increased, but there was no changes in Schirmer's test probably due to the compensatory secretion from the accessory lacrimal glands.[55,56] Similarly, gland obstruction achieved by excretory duct ligation in mice led to increased CFS.[57] Surgical removal of bilateral extraorbital lacrimal glands is a more aggressive way to induce severe DED. Both rats[8,9] and mice[58–61] were used to establish this type of model, and animals showed decreased aqueous tear production and increased CFS scores, more severe than that observed in desiccating stress-induced DED.[58] Consistent with the sexual predisposition in desiccating stress-induced models, extraorbital lacrimal gland excision led to more severe corneal epitheliopathy and ocular pain (measured by eye wipe response to capsaicin, an activator of TRPV1 channel) in females than in males.[9,60,61] Cold allodynia demonstrated by eye closing response to innocuous cold air flow was also reported in the mouse model of extraorbital lacrimal gland excision.[62] In addition, combined extraorbital and intraorbital lacrimal glands excision resulted in a comparable or more severe clinical DED.[9,60]

Systemic delivery of scopolamine or topical application of atropine eye drops have been described above as pharmacologic desiccating stress via inhibiting lacrimal gland function. Additional methods of medical inhibition of lacrimal glands have also been reported to induce DED, including direct intralacrimal gland injection of toxins or cytokines. Female mice receiving one single intralacrimal gland injection of botulinum toxin-B, a well-known antiacetylcholine toxin, presented with significantly decreased tear production as early as day 3 postinjection and lasting for 4 weeks; after 4 weeks, despite normalized tear production, the animals showed persisting, significantly increased CFS,[63–66] suggesting that this model represents another form of chronic DED with similar clinical findings from CEC-induced chronic DED.[47–49] On the other hand, injection of a neurotrophin receptor antibody-conjugated saporin toxin into lacrimal glands of rats led to the damage of nerves within the glands and decreased eye wipe response to corneal menthol stimulus (assessment of polymodal nociceptor-mediated pain); however, basal tear production and eye wipe response to corneal application of capsaicin (assessment of cold nociceptor-mediated pain) remained normal in animals.[67] Such corneal hypoalgesia observed in this saporin toxin model was also a commonly seen symptom in DED patients.[68,69] In addition to toxins, injection of proinflammatory cytokine IL-1α into lacrimal glands was used to induce DED. A single injection led to rapid reduction of basal tear secretion in both C57BL/6 and BALB/c strains; however, this effect disappeared spontaneously by day 13 in C57BL/6 and by day 7 in BALB/c, respectively.[70] Lastly, an autoimmune rabbit model was reported by intralacrimal injection of in vitro–stimulated autologous peripheral blood lymphocytes with lacrimal epithelial cells. Animal developed decreased tear production (by Schirmer's test) and tear stability (by tear break-up time) and increased corneal rose Bengal staining.[71,72]

Genetic Manipulation–Induced Dry Eye Disease

Various types of selectively inbred or genetically modified mice demonstrate DED phenotypes in addition to other co-existing systemic immunoinflammatory disorders, and most of them are generated on the C57BL/6 background.

Mouse models of Sjögren's syndrome

Mouse models of Sjögren's syndrome are among the earliest animal models established for DED study, and these models show common lymphatic infiltration in both lacrimal and salivary (submandibular) glands, termed dacryoadenitis and sialadenitis, respectively. Nonobese diabetic (NOD) mouse, the most commonly used Sjögren's syndrome model, was developed through a highly selective inbred process. They develop spontaneous insulitis leading to type 1 diabetes, which occurs before the development of exocrinopathy, and thus the Sjögren's syndrome in this model is considered to be secondary.[73,74] In contrast to human patients and wild-type animal DED models, autoimmune dacryoadenitis in NOD mice is more prone to develop in male than female, evidenced by much earlier onset and higher incidence of dacryoadenitis in male animals.[75] Clinical DED develops subsequent to the lymphatic infiltration of lacrimal glands, and the relevant findings in NOD male mice include decreased tear production and tear film break-up time, as well as increased CFS.[76] With aging, NOD mice showed not only increased corneal permeability measured with the fluorescent Oregon green dextran dye but also increased tear volume measured with cotton thread technique.[77] Further studies have developed new strains of NOD mice that develop glandular infiltrates but not overt diabetes, including C57BL/6.NOD-Aec1Aec2 and NOD.H2[b]; however, no significant change in corneal permeability was detected in either strain.[78,79]

MRL/lpr mouse is another important model of Sjögren's syndrome, which carries the *lpr* (lymphoproliferation) mutation leading to defective expression of Fas, a critical molecule mediating cell apoptosis. Distinct to NOD mouse, MRL/lpr mouse has a female predisposition to develop dacryoadenitis, accompanied with systemic lupus erythematosus and arthritis. Despite similar focal lymphocytic infiltrates in lacrimal and salivary glands as that in human Sjögren's syndrome, the clinical tear production as measured by Schirmer's test in MRL/lpr mice was nearly normal.[80–82] However, CTT, a more accurate and sensitive measurement of tears in small animals like mice,[83] showed reduced aqueous tear production in MRL/lpr mice.[84]

CD25 is the cytokine IL-2 binding receptor alpha chain and serves as the limiting factor of IL-2 signaling,[85] which is critical for the survival and function of immunoregulatory T cells that essentially suppress abnormal immune activation. It is thus expected that absence of CD25 signaling will lead to inappropriate immune response, including autoimmunity to self-tissue. In fact, CD25 knockout (KO) mice spontaneously develop Sjögren's syndrome-like lymphocytic infiltration in exocrine glands, including the salivary and lacrimal glands[86]; in addition, they develop autoimmune inflammatory bowel disease and hemolytic anemia that leads to early mortality.[87] The development of dacryoadenitis in CD25 KO mice was observed as early as 8 week of age without sex predilection, and it got worse when the mice became aged.[88] The ocular surface findings in CD25 KO mice include increased corneal staining with Oregon green dextran dye and decreased corneal surface smoothness.[89,90]

Thrombospondin-1 (TSP-1) is a matricellular protein that activates latent TGF-β1, an important antiinflammatory cytokine. Thus, mice deficient in TSP-1 develop inflammatory infiltrates in multiple organs, including in lacrimal glands that leads to a Sjögren's syndrome-like pathology, but in a milder degree than TGF-β1 KO mouse.[91] In addition, unlike TGF-β1 KO mouse which has a shortened life span, TSP-1 KO mouse exhibits a normal life span, making them more suitable for scientific study. TSP-1 KO mice of both sexes develop progressively increased CFS and even dry crusty eyes in severe cases. There is no significant changes in tear production.[92]

Autoimmune regulator *(Aire)*-deficient mice develop spontaneous multiorgan autoimmune disorders, involving retina (uveitis), the salivary and lacrimal glands (Sjögren's syndrome), and others. Accompanied by inflammatory destruction of lacrimal glands in *Aire*-deficient mice, stimulated tear production was significantly reduced and corneal lissamine green staining was profound.[93,94] Other Sjögren's syndrome—related models associated with lymphocytic infiltration in

lacrimal glands have been described such as NZB/W F1 mouse, TGF-β1 knockout mouse, and *aly/aly* mouse[80,95–97]; however, impact on ocular surface tissues in these mouse strains is unclear due to the lack of relevant reports.

SPDEF knockout and mucin knockout mice
Conjunctival goblet cells are the major source of ocular surface mucins which are critical to maintain the homeostasis of the tear film, such as MUC5AC the most abundant mucin in the tear film. Decreased number of conjunctival goblet cells has been identified in multiple animal models of DED and is used as one of the histological features for DED.[48,98–102] SAM-pointed domain epithelial-specific transcription factor (SPDEF) is the transcription factor essential for goblet cell differentiation in mucosal epithelium, and *Spdef* KO mice which lack conjunctival goblet cells show significantly increased CFS and tear volume (measured by CTT) that progress with aging,[103] suggesting an evaporative type of DED. Relatedly, *Muc5ac* KO mice showed decreased tear break-up time and increased CFS without aqueous tear production change,[104] although another study did not find increased CFS in either *Muc5ac* KO or *Muc5b* KO mice.[105]

Neurokinin-1 receptor (NK1R) knockout mouse
NK1R is the preferred receptor for substance P (SP), a neuropeptide mediating corneal pain and promoting corneal inflammation when upregulated in diseased status.[46,62,106] However, basal levels of SP in tears may play a critical physiological role in maintaining ocular surface homeostasis,[107–109] and mice genetically deficient for functional NK1R showed reduced level of aqueous tear secretion, without significant increase of CFS.[110]

Animal Models of Meibomian Gland Dysfunction
The Meibomian gland is a specialized sebaceous gland located in the eyelids. The gland produces a lipid secretion called meibum that constitutes the lipid layer of the tear film and prevents the underlying aqueous layer from evaporation, thus maintaining the homeostasis of the tear film.[50] Meibomian gland dysfunction (MGD) is one of the major causes of DED, and various animal models of MGD have been developed, including rabbit models and a variety of transgenic mouse strains.

Obstruction of Meibomian gland
Mechanical obstruction of Meibomian gland duct resulting from epithelial hyperkeratinization and/or

increased viscosity of the secretion (meibum) is considered the most common cause leading to MGD.[111] Using larger animals such as rabbit, electrocauterization was used to cause mechanical damage to Meibomian gland orifices and subsequent keratinization and fibrosis of orifices, leading to the blockade of the gland. Animals showed significantly increased tear osmolality without significant changes of CFS or aqueous tear production except a short temporary reduction by CTT at day 1 postcautery.[112,113] In a similar rat model of Meibomian gland orifice obstruction, animals showed significantly reduced tear break-up time, increased CFS, but stable tear production by Schirmer's test.[114] In addition, earlier studies using chronic topical application of 2% epinephrine over a period of months to 1 year led to orifice plugging in rabbits, but there is no tear film or CFS data available.[115,116]

Mutant and transgenic mouse models
HR-1 hairless mice were used to develop MGD model by feeding them with HR-AD diet (a special diet with limited lipid content). In addition to atopic dermatitis-like symptoms, these mice presented markedly plugged orifices and a toothpaste-like meibum.[117] Apolipoprotein E knockout ($ApoE^{-/-}$) mice are characterized by increased blood cholesterol levels, and they were found to present with the typical clinical MGD manifestations of Meibomian gland dropout (progressive loss) and increased CFS.[118] X-linked anhidrotic-hypohidrotic ectodermal dysplasia (EDA) mice resulting from *Eda* gene mutation completely lacks Meibomian gland, and they develop corneal neovascularization, keratitis, ulceration, and keratinization, as well as blepharitis and conjunctivitis.[119] Relevant DED signs in this extreme MGD model include increased CFS and decreased tear break-up time, while aqueous tear secretion is normal.[120] Other transgenic mouse models leading to defective Meibomian gland development ranging from gland absence to atrophy or dystrophy include ectoderm-targeted overexpression of the glucocorticoid receptor (GR),[121] epithelial cell–conditional fibroblast growth factor receptor 2 (FGFR2) knockout,[122] acyl-CoA:cholesterol acyltransferase-1 (ACAT-1) knockout,[123] conditional deletion of Krüppel-like factor (KLF),[124] homeobox transcription factor Barx2 knockout,[125] and among others, and the DED-relevant ocular surface signs have not been evaluated in any of them.

Age-related Meibomian gland dysfunction
Studies of human and mouse Meibomian glands have shown decreased acinar cell proliferation and increased glandular atrophy during aging, which leads to Meibomian gland dropout and abnormal lipid excretion without epithelial hyperkeratinization, referred to as age-related Meibomian gland dysfunction (ARMGD).[126–128] Meibomian gland dropout is seen in wild-type C57BL/6 mice over 1 year of age,[129] and ARMGD has been documented in 2 years old C57BL/6 mice showing increased Meibomian gland dropout and CFS, and decreased tear secretion.[129,130] However, the clinical DED signs in aged mice are not entirely due to the changes of Meibomian glands, other changes in lacrimal glands, immune homeostasis, and hormone levels also critically contribute to the DED phenotypes in the aged.[130,131]

Other Models
Spontaneous canine DED
Spontaneous DED is commonly seen in dogs, and the incidence is estimated about 35% with more prevalent in the aged and equally involving male and female. The disease is considered mainly autoimmune-driven and tends to be more severe than that observed in humans. It is diagnosed with aqueous tear deficiency by Schirmer's test.[12] This model has been used to test the therapeutic effect of topical cyclosporin A eye drops,[13] the first and one of only two US FDA-approved drugs currently for treating DED patients.

Benzalkonium chloride–induced DED
Benzalkonium chloride (BAC), in its low concentration (<0.02%), is a commonly used preservative in ophthalmic medications.[132] In patients using BAC-preserved eye drops, DED-associated symptoms and signs are more prevalent.[133] Rabbits treated with topical 0.1% BAC twice daily for 14 days exhibited significant reduction of tear production (Schirmer's test) and increase of CFS and rose Bengal staining.[134,135] Female C57BL/6 mice treated with topical 0.075% BAC twice daily for 7 days showed significantly increased corneal staining with Oregon green dextran dye and decreased tear production measured by CTT.[136]

Androgen deficiency–related DED models
As seen in most autoimmune disorders, DED predominantly affects women than men,[38–40] and the female sex is a significant risk factor for the development of DED with sex hormones believed to be critically involved.[50] Androgen deficiency in castrated rabbits was associated with lipid content alterations in the Meibomian gland.[137] Male rats and rabbits with bilateral orchiectomy showed significantly reduced tear production measured by Schirmer's test and shortened tear

break-up time.[138,139] In addition, ovariectomy in female mice led to decreased estradiol and testosterone levels, as well as DED signs of reduced tear production and increased CFS.[140]

High fat diet–induced DED

A recent study reported that C57BL/6 mice subjected to high fat diet for up to 4 months developed overweight, hyperlipidemia, and DED-like clinical changes, including deceased tear production and increased Oregon green dextran staining, which were correlated with oxidative stress at both ocular surface and lacrimal glands.[141,142]

Ocular surface hyperosmolarity–induced DED

Tear hyperosmolarity ($\geq$308 mOsm/L) is frequently detected and used as one of the diagnostic tests in DED patients.[50] Tear hyperosmolarity can result from decreased aqueous tear production or increased tear evaporation. Topical application of hypertonic saline (900 or 3000 mOsm/L, four times daily for 5 days) to the ocular surface of BALB/c and C57BL/6 mice did not lead to significant changes in CFS or tear production, but caused decrease in corneal nerve density and led to immune cell activation.[53,143] Another report using much longer stressing time (500 mOsm/L, six times daily for 28 days) found that mice developed significantly increased CFS.[144]

PATHOPHYSIOLOGY OF DRY EYE DISEASE LEARNED FROM ANIMAL MODELS

Characteristic pathologies in ocular surface of DED animals include (i) changes in corneal epithelial thickness/cell shape, (ii) decreased numbers and atrophy of conjunctival goblet cells,[48,98,136] (iii) apoptosis of corneal and conjunctival epithelia,[145] and (iv) basal acinar cell proliferation and altered lipid production in Meibomian gland.[146] The central mechanisms leading to these pathological consequences are believed to be driven by a vicious cycle of ocular surface inflammation that is initiated by various intrinsic or extrinsic triggers, such as desiccating stress,[147] and thus the underlying immunopathogenesis is discussed in this section.

Immune Homeostasis of Normal Ocular Surface

The ocular surface comprises of a continuous mucosal lining of cornea and conjunctiva, extending to the mucocutaneous junctions of the lid margins.[147] Despite being constantly exposed to outside environment, the ocular surface remains integrated and uninflamed while keeping its visual function. This ability to maintain immune homeostasis is mediated through both physical barrier function and active mechanisms, encompassing epithelium, stroma, nerve, and resident immune cells. The avascular nature of normal cornea is essential for its transparency and the "immune privileged" status by creating an access barrier for circulating immune cells to enter the site.[148] To maintain the avascularity, corneal epithelium constitutively expresses soluble vascular endothelial growth factor receptor-1 (sVEGFR-1) to inhibit VEGF-A-mediated new blood vessel formation (hemangiogenesis),[149] and VEGFR-3, serving as a trap, to prevent VEGF-C- and VEGF-D-mediated new blood and lymphatic vessels formation (lymphangiogenesis).[150]

Normal cornea has no T or B lymphocytes, but is endowed with a significant population of $CD11b^+CD11c^-$ macrophages/monocytes in the deep stroma, along with some $CD11b^+CD11c^+$ dendritic cells in the anterior stroma and $CD11b^{lo/-}CD11c^+$ Langerhans cells in the epithelium.[19,24,151] These cells are collectively believed to be capable of functioning as antigen-presenting cells (APCs) in immune response, and they are phenotypically "immature" characterized as low expression levels of MHC class II (MHC-II) along with absence of costimulatory molecules B7 (CD80 and CD86) and CD40. These immature APC predominantly reside at corneal periphery and decrease in number gradually toward the corneal center.[23] The immature status of corneal-resident APC along with absence of lymphocytes in normal cornea contributes to the immune quiescence by not only avoiding effector cell activation but inducing immune tolerance.[151,152]

Corneal epithelium also constitutively expresses a variety of critical immunoregulatory factors, including programmed death-ligand 1 (PD-L1), Fas ligand (FasL), pigment epithelial-derived factor (PEDF), and thrombospondin-1 (TSP-1).[45,153–155] PD-L1 is a newer member of B7 family, and its ligation with the receptor programmed death (PD)-1 on activated T cells leads to suppression of T cells.[156] PD-L1 KO mice show spontaneously significant T-cell infiltration in cornea.[157] In addition, PD-L1 actively inhibits corneal hemangiogenesis and thus contributes to corneal avascularity.[158] Similarly, FasL, a member of tumor necrosis factor (TNF) family, can lead to apoptotic cell death by binding to its receptor Fas that is expressed by a variety of cells and tissues, including T cells, and prevent neovascularization.[159,160] Two forms of FasL have been identified including the antiinflammatory, soluble form (sFasL) that can antagonize the function of the other proinflammatory, membrane-bound form (mFasL).[161] Although sFasL is the predominant form of FasL expressed in the retina of mice,[162] it remains unclear what form(s) of FasL that is constitutively expressed in the cornea. Both PD-L1 and FasL constitutively expressed in corneal epithelium may trigger apoptosis of invading effector T cells that infiltrate in the cornea in response to inflammation. PEDF is a ubiquitously expressed glycoprotein belonging to the serine protease inhibitor family.[163] TSP-1 is a major activator of latent TGF-β, and only activated TGF-β can serve as an antiinflammatory cytokine.[91,164] Normal corneal epithelium–derived PEDF and TSP-1 have both been shown to potently suppress APC activation.[45,155] Both factors exert antiangiogenic function[163,165] with PEDF showing additional neurotropic roles.[166]

The cornea is among the most densely innervated tissues, and corneal nerves play a crucial role for ocular surface homeostasis by protecting the cornea from irritants (by regulating tear secretion and the blink reflex) and by secreting a variety of neuropeptides that are essential for epithelial and stromal cells.[167] Healthy innervation in cornea has been shown to regulate corneal epithelial cell and stem cell survival,[168,169] and suppress corneal neovascularization.[170] Corneal neuropathy has been observed in DED patients and animal models.[53,100,171,172] Specifically, among various nerve-derived factors, neuropeptides SP and vasoactive intestinal peptide (VIP) are constitutively secreted by nerve endings in normal cornea, with SP contributing to corneal epithelial homeostasis and VIP playing antiinflammatory functions.[109,173]

Innate Immunity Activation

The immune homeostasis of ocular surface is disrupted in DED, mediated by both innate and adaptive immunity. Innate response serves as the immediate, nonspecific reaction to various insults, and the involving components include mucosal barriers, cytokines, chemokines, and innate immune cells.

Innate inflammatory cytokines release by ocular surface tissues

Desiccating or hyperosmolar stress on ocular surface, either direct or consequent to lacrimal or Meibomian glands damage that results from extrinsic insults or intrinsic changes, can be the initiating factors driving the development of DED by triggering immunoinflammatory cascades at the ocular surface. Stressed ocular surface epithelial cells quickly upregulate the levels of activated mitogen-activated protein kinases (MAPK), including c-jun N-terminal kinases (JNK)-1/2,

extracellular-regulated kinases (ERK)-1/2, and p38 in hours,[35,143,174] which may subsequently activate downstream kinases and transcription factors such as NFκB, leading to the early expression of proinflammatory cytokines TNF-α, IL-1β, and IL-6 at the ocular surface.[20,143,174,175] In addition, desiccating stress can elicit the cellular signal of damage-associated molecular patterns, which activate toll-like receptor 4 (TLR4)—a critical innate immune mechanism—in cornea, demonstrated by translocation of TLR4 in epithelial cells (from cell inside to cell surface) and upregulation in stroma cells.[176] TLR4 activation further leads to downstream caspase-8 activation facilitating the assembly and activation of inflammasomes NLRP12 and NLRC4, thereby promoting the activation and secretion of proinflammatory cytokines such as IL-1β.[177] In addition to TLR4-mediated pathway, increased reactive oxygen species upon desiccating stress exposure induced activation of caspase-8 and NLRP3 inflammasome, further promoting the production of bioactive IL-1β.[178] Both IL-1β and TNF-α have been shown to promote corneal expression of matrix metalloproteinase-9 (MMP-9),[174,179] a critical proteolytic enzyme cleaving epithelial basement membrane components and tight junction proteins (such as ZO-1 and occludin) and thus leading to corneal barrier disruption.[174,180]

Innate immune cell infiltration and activation at the ocular surface

Early infiltration of CD11b$^+$ monocytes and macrophages in DED corneas is a hallmark consistently found in various animal models.[20,176,181] Influx of these innate inflammatory cells relies on the chemotactic gradient between the periphery and corneal tissues created by higher expression of various chemokines on the ocular surface in DED, including macrophage inflammatory protein 1α (MIP-1α, or CCL3) and MIP-1β (CCL4).[182] Chemokines are small molecular weight cytokines with chemoattractant properties that serve an essential function in immunity by coordinating the trafficking of immune cells between different anatomic sites.[183] In some cases, multiple chemokines may interact with the same chemokine receptor. Increased levels of these chemokines at ocular surface in DED can lead to tissue-specific recruitment of peripheral circulating monocytes that express corresponding specific receptors, including those expressing CCR1 for chemokine MIP-1α, and CCR5 for both chemokines MIP-1α and MIP-1β.[184] In addition, chemokine monocyte chemotactic protein 1 (MCP-1, or CCL2) and its receptor CCR2 are also involved in the recruitment of CD11b$^+$ cells in DED.[185] In fact, the corneal infiltrating

CD11b$^+$ cells in DED have shown significant upregulation of CCR1, CCR2, and CCR5.[186] These infiltrated monocytes and macrophages become activated under the stimulation of environmental TNF-α and IL-1β, and can subsequently produce the same inflammatory cytokines by themselves, thus amplifying the ocular surface inflammation.[176,185]

Another important innate cells called natural killer (NK) cells are also significantly increased in the conjunctiva of mice shortly after desiccating stress, and these NK cells are in activated status by expressing the critical cytokine—interferon-γ (IFN-γ), which not only directly disrupts ocular surface barrier but also promotes corneal APC maturation by upregulating their expressions of MHC-II and costimulators B7—a function bridging adaptive T-cell response in DED.[32] In fact, depletion of NK cells has been shown to lead to decreased levels of cytokines and chemokines responsible for T-cell differentiation and trafficking, thereby resulting in defects in generation and infiltration of activated T cells in DED.[187,188]

Adaptive Immunity Activation

Innate immunity activation causes direct tissue damages as well as facilitates the following antigen-specific, long-lasting adaptive immune response. Essential components bridging the innate and adaptive immunity in DED include NK cells (as described above) and more importantly APC that encompass monocytes and macrophages, dendritic cells, and Langerhans cells. The effectors exerting adaptive immunity comprise of T and B lymphocytes, and a substantial of experimental data demonstrate that CD4$^+$ T-cell immunity plays a central pathogenic role in both Sjögren's syndrome and non-Sjögren's DED.[34,136,189,190]

Ocular surface APC activation and migration

Antigen capture and subsequent presentation by APC to naive T cells is an essential initial step to activate T-cell response.[191] Accordingly, depletion of ocular surface APC has been shown to prevent T-cell activation in DED.[192] In normal healthy cornea, the preponderance of APC is in an "immature" status that is critical to maintain ocular surface immune quiescence and contributes to immune privilege of cornea.[193] However, in DED, significantly increased inflammatory cytokines, such as IL-1β and TNF-α in the ocular surface overcome the existing antiinflammatory factors such as TSP-1 and PEDF[45,155] and promote resident APC to acquire "mature" phenotypes by upregulating their MHC-II expression,[20] which is required for APC presentation of antigenic epitopes to T cells. This maturing process

is accompanied by the presumed "autoantigen" uptake and processing. To date, the nature of autoantigen(s) in DED remains unclear although kallikrein-13 has been proposed as a putative autoantigen based on its reactivity with sera from Sjögren's syndrome mice (IQI/Jic mice).[194] The study showed kallikrein-13 expression in multiple tissues where there was coincident lymphocyte infiltration in this transgenic mouse model, including the lacrimal glands, however, the ocular surface tissue was not examined.[194] Further, immunization of rats with a kallikrein family protein led to marked lymphocytic infiltration of the lacrimal glands.[195] In desiccating stress-induced DED mice, increased serum antibodies against kallikrein-13 were detected, and ocular surface tissue expression of kallikrein-13 was reported.[196] Further studies are required to elucidate the endogenous ocular surface antigen(s) that is hypothesized to be exposed upon desiccating stress and provides "danger signals" to resident APC.

To present antigen to and activate naive T cells which primarily reside in secondary draining lymphoid tissues, mature, antigen-bearing APC in ocular surface have to acquire the ability to travel from ocular surface to draining lymph nodes of the eye. This trafficking process once again is tightly regulated by the specific chemokine-receptor axis. Corneal mature MHC-II$^+$ APC in DED show significantly enhanced expression of CCR7, a chemokine receptor guiding APC egress toward the draining lymph nodes through enriched environmental CCR7 ligands—CCL19 and CCL21.[186,197] Topical blockade of CCR7 has been shown to sufficiently prevent the migration of corneal APC to draining lymph nodes and subsequent T-cell activation in DED.[186] In addition to chemokines, ocular surface APC gain access to lymphoid compartment via newly-formed afferent lymphatic vessels which are lack in normal uninflamed cornea. Interestingly, there is considerable and exclusive growth of lymphatic, but not blood, vessels in DED cornea, that starts early after DED induction from peripheral cornea and advances into central cornea as disease progresses. The selective corneal lymphangiogenesis in DED is dependent on lymphangiogenic-specific vascular endothelial growth factor-C and D (VEGF-C and VEGF-D) and their receptor VEGFR-3.[198–200] Colocalization of CCR7$^+$ cells with CCL19/21 within corneal lymphatic vessels has been demonstrated in DED cornea.[197]

T-cell activation and expansion in local draining lymph nodes

The central role of adaptive immunity in DED pathogenesis was first demonstrated in the middle of 2000s by an elegant study from the Pflugfelder–Stern–Niederkorn collaboration showing that DED can be induced in healthy mice by adoptive transfer of CD4[+] T lymphocytes derived from dry eye mice.[34] In addition, topical cyclosporine-A (CsA), a selective T cell immunosuppressive agent, is one of the first FDA-approved medications to treat DED, providing a strong support for T cells as principal effectors in DED pathogenesis. Recent animal studies have shed considerable light on the precise mechanisms by which how and what subsets of T cells are activated and cause DED via coordinating with an array of other cellular and molecular immune factors. These preclinical studies have significantly facilitated the development of novel therapeutic strategies that are more targeted with less side effects than topical CsA.

Differentiation and activation of naive T cells and expansion of effector T cells. Local draining lymph nodes are the primary site of T-cell activation in DED. Mature migratory CCR7[+] APC in local draining lymph nodes express high levels of MHC-II which provides antigenic peptide to cognate naive T cells, as well as B7 (CD80 and CD86) and CD40 costimulatory molecules, which function together with antigen to stimulate T cells.[32,186,201] Thus, these APC are efficient in priming T cells by upregulating activation markers of CD69 and CD154 (CD40 ligand, CD40L) on T cells (predominantly on CD4[+] T subset).[202] Once the immune synapse between APC and T cells is formed, the environmental cytokines, primarily secreted by APC, are predominant factors determining the differentiation fate of primed CD4[+] T cells. It is known that the ligation of CD154 with CD40 on APC promotes the production of IL-12 by APC,[203] and increased levels of IL-12 in the milieu of draining lymph nodes of DED mice have been shown.[48] Accordingly, CD4[+] T cells show upregulation of IL-12 receptor (IL-12R) expression,[202] and signaling of IL-12/IL-12R promotes naive CD4[+] T to differentiate to IFN-γ-expressing Th1 cells, supported by increased levels of the Th1 signature cytokine IFN-γ in DED lymph nodes and conjunctiva,[43,202,204] despite no confirmation of the cellular source of IFN-γ. Subsequently, the concept of classical Th1 dominance in DED was revised with the characterization of a newly defined CD4[+] T-cell subset—IL-17-expressing Th17 cells in DED.[31,36,205] Initial differentiation of naive T cells toward Th17 lineage is driven by the proinflammatory cytokine IL-6 in the presence of TGF-β,[206,207] and increased expression of IL-6 in DED lymph nodes has been demonstrated.[31,208]

Subsequently, the heightened levels of IL-2 and IL-23 in the lymphoid compartment[48,49] further promotes differentiated Th17 cells to proliferate and become activated to gain full function. Unlike most T-cell differentiating and activating cytokines that are mainly produced by APC, the heightened IL-2 is principally from activated effector T cells themselves and acts in an autocrine fashion. In DED, mature APC have been suggested to be the major microenvironmental source of IL-6, TGF-β, and IL-23.[175] Fully activated Th17 cells are capable of secreting effector cytokines, including the signature IL-17 and others such as granulocyte-macrophage colony-stimulating factor (GM-CSF), rendering them pathogenic in DED.[31,209] Interestingly, unlike Th1 subset that is regarded as a terminally differentiated CD4[+] T-cell lineage and stays relatively stable, the Th17 cells show significant phenotypic and functional plasticity characterized by their ability of acquiring features of other lineages under stimulation of certain signals in the microenvironment.[210] In DED, two subsets of effector Th17 cells have been identified, including IFN-γ[−]IL-17[+] "single-positive" Th17 and IFN-γ[+]IL-17[+] "double-positive" Th17/1.[48] In fact, quantitative analysis of IFN-γ[+]IL-17[−]CD4[+] Th1 cells showed no number changes in DED,[43,48] suggesting that simple link of increased IFN-γ levels in DED to classic Th1 lineage without examining its cellular source may be inaccurate; instead, the major source of IFN-γ in DED could be the double-positive Th17/1 cells in the disease progression stage while NK cells serve as the primary source in early disease induction phase when adaptive immunity has not been activated. In fact, recent findings have demonstrated that the increased IFN-γ in DED is indeed an integral part of Th17 immunity, as evidenced by the ability of single-positive Th17 cells to convert into double-positive Th17/1 cells with stimulation of environmental IL-12 and IL-23 in DED.[48] Furthermore, double-positive Th17/1 cells are more pathogenic than single-positive Th17 cells, and are required to induce severe acute ocular surface inflammation in DED; in contrast, the classic IL-17[−]IFN-γ[+] Th1 cells isolated from DED are unable to transfer the disease phenotype to normal animals.[48] Taken together, effector Th17 response characterized by their dynamic and coordinated production of various cytokines including IL-17, IFN-γ, and GM-CSF plays a major pathogenic role in DED.

Modulation of effector T-cell activation by regulatory T cells. The dominant players on the immunoregulatory arm that restricts and suppresses excessive inflammation are specialized CD4$^+$ regulatory T cells (Treg), characterized by high expression of CD25 (the high affinity receptor subunit for IL-2 to maintain survival and proliferation of Treg) and Foxp3 (the master transcriptional factor for the development and function of Treg), which are in contrast to proinflammatory CD4$^+$ effector T-cell subsets Th1, Th2, or Th17. To date, two types of Treg have been defined, including the larger population that is developed during the normal process of T-cell maturation in the thymus (termed "natural Treg," nTreg or tTreg) and the smaller but more specific population that is induced in the periphery from naive T cells in the presence of IL-2 and TGF-β or after encounters with foreign antigens (termed "induced Treg," iTreg or pTreg).[211,212] Both subsets of Treg work in synchrony to maintain peripheral tolerance and immune homeostasis through dampening naive T cell priming or attenuating effector T-cell function.[213,214] In DED the regulatory function of Treg is compromised demonstrated by the inability of Treg to suppress IL-17 or IFN-γ production by effector CD4$^+$ T cells despite that the number of Treg is minimally affected.[31,43] Furthermore, complete depletion of Treg using an anti-CD25 antibody led to exacerbated DED while reconstitution of normal Treg in mice conferred the recipients resistance to disease induction,[34] suggesting that Treg, probably nTreg, play important regulatory roles in DED pathogenesis. The characteristic phenotype of dysfunctional Treg is downregulation of Foxp3 expression,[215] which has been demonstrated in DED mice.[31] It remained to be elucidated whether other critical Treg function-associated molecules are altered in DED, including surface expression of cell contact-dependent coinhibitory molecules CTLA-4 and GITR as well as secreted antiinflammatory cytokines IL-10 and TGF-β by Treg. It is known that TGF-β is required for the generation of both Treg and Th17, and the presence or absence of the other cytokine IL-6 is a key determinant skewing the immune balance between the two reciprocally interconnected and functionally opposed cell subsets.[216,217] As increased IL-6 levels have been consistently observed in both ocular surface and draining lymphoid tissue in DED,[20,31,143,174,208] it is plausible to attribute IL-6 as one of the critical factors leading to Treg dysfunction while promoting Th17 in DED. In addition, in vivo blockade of IL-17 effectively restores Treg function in DED,[31] suggesting that IL-17 may also directly or indirectly contributes to Treg dysfunction. Nevertheless, the detailed mechanisms underlying Treg dysfunction in DED,

especially their interaction with Th17-associated factors, have yet to be investigated.

CD8$^+$ regulatory T cells have also been implicated in DED pathogenesis by a study demonstrating that depletion of CD8$^+$ T cells in mice promoted the generation of Th17 response and led to a more severe ocular surface disease.[218] The precise subset is assumed to be CD8$^+$CD103$^+$ cells, which are presumably to limit the Th17 immunity in DED via suppressing the process of APC-mediated Th17 generation, but not restricting already activated Th17 cells.[218]

Ocular surface homing of effector T cells

In addition to the acquisition of the ability to producing inflammatory cytokines, activated effector T cells in the draining lymphoid compartment have to upregulate specific chemokine receptors, thus facilitating their interaction with blood vessel endothelium and their migration to peripheral targeting tissues. In DED, increased conjunctival infiltration of CD3$^+$ T cells has been demonstrated.[136,185] These effector CD4$^+$ T cells in DED preferentially upregulate expressions of CCR5, CXCR3, and CCR6,[202,219,220] directing them to migrate toward ocular surface where higher levels of corresponding chemokines are present, including CCR5 ligands MIP-1α (CCL3), MIP-1β (CCL4), and regulated on activation, normal T-cell expressed and secreted (RANTES, or CCL5); CXCR3 ligands monokine induced by interferon-γ (MIG, or CXCL9), interferon-γ inducible protein 10 (IP-10, or CXCL10); and CCR6 ligand CCL20.[36,182,220] Among these various T-cell–associated chemokine/receptor axis, CCR6 is discretely expressed by Th17 and CCR6/CCL20 axis has been shown functionally critical for the homing of effector Th17 cells to the ocular surface from the lymphoid compartment, demonstrated by significant abolishment of T-cell infiltration in conjunctiva in the absence of CCR6 (knockout) or after topical neutralization of CCL20 in DED mice.[219,220] CCR2, a receptor expressed by monocytes, is also expressed by Th17 cells,[221] particularly on the highly pathogenic IFN-γ$^+$GM-CSF$^+$ Th17 subset,[222] and thus CCR2 also contributes to Th17-cell trafficking in DED as demonstrated by decreased T-cell infiltration in conjunctiva after topical blockade of CCR2 in DED mice.[185] In addition to the requirement of guidance by chemokine-receptor axis, peripheralization of T cells needs additional expression of adhesion molecules, such as integrins, which facilitate their binding to extracellular matrix components. In DED, two important pairs including lymphocyte function–associated antigen-1(LFA-1, or integrin α$_L$β$_2$) and its binding ligand intercellular adhesion molecule-1 (ICAM-1), as well as very late antigen-4 (VLA-4, integrin $\alpha_4\beta_1$) and its binding ligands such as vascular cell adhesion molecule-1 (VCAM-1) have been demonstrated to mediate T-cell journey to the ocular surface. Specifically, topical application of LFA-1 or VLA-4 small molecule antagonists to DED mice led to significant inhibition of T-cell response in ocular surface.[201,223] Lifitegrast, a topical LFA-1 antagonist, has been recently approved by FDA for DED therapy.[224]

Effector T-cell—mediated ocular surface damage

It is widely documented that there are significant infiltration of both IFN-γ^-IL-17$^+$ "single-positive" Th17 and IFN-γ^+IL-17$^+$ "double-positive" Th17/1, but not IFN-γ^+IL-17$^-$ Th1, in DED conjunctiva,[48,220] as well as consistently enhanced expressions of IFN-γ and IL-17 in ocular surface of DED.[20,30,31,36] A series of elegant adoptive transfer experiments have further undoubtedly demonstrated that both Th17 and Th17/1 cells are pathogenic effectors in DED with Th17/1 capable of causing more severe tissue destructions due to their ability to additionally secrete IFN-γ.[48] Although lack of new blood vessel formation in DED cornea[198] may limit the direct access of effector T cells to the cornea, cytokines secreted by these cells in the adjacent conjunctiva can diffuse throughout the ocular surface and thus play a major pathogenic role in DED. In fact, IL-17 has been shown to promote corneal production of both MMP-9 and MMP-3 by binding to its receptor IL-17RA that is constitutively expressed by ocular surface epithelia,[31] resulting in corneal epithelial barrier disruption.[36] In addition, IL-17 efficiently induces endothelial and epithelial tissues to secret IL-6, TNF-α, IL-1β, and IL-8,[225,226] thus potentially inducing a cytokine cascade at the ocular surface that can propagate tissue damage, further promoting epitope spreading to a more diverse set of target antigens. Furthermore, IL-17 is critical in promoting corneal lymphangiogenesis via inducing expression of prolymphangiogenic VEGF-D by corneal epithelial cells in DED,[199] thus driving progressive ingrowth of lymphatic vessels that allows continuous trafficking of corneal APC to lymphoid compartment and promotes a vicious cycle of autoimmune response.[42] The other pathogenic T-cell cytokine IFN-γ can cause significant conjunctival epithelial squamous metaplasia characterized by loss of goblet cells and decrease of mucin production, accompanied by epithelial apoptosis.[204,227] Goblet cells are not only the primary source of mucins for tear film that contributes to the physical barrier[104] but also can directly induce

immune tolerance via conditioning APC, and thus loss of conjunctival goblet cells may further exacerbate ocular surface inflammation in DED.[228] Additional fundamental evidence establishing the pathogenic functions of IL-17 and IFN-γ in DED is from preclinical therapeutic tests. In vivo blockade of either IL-17 or IFN-γ leads to significant improvement of corneal epitheliopathy demonstrated by decreased CFS, improved pathological changes, and reduced ocular expression of inflammatory factors.[31,36,48,199,229] Besides IL-17 and IFN-γ, Th17-produced GM-CSF also contributes to ocular surface inflammation in DED primarily through promoting ocular surface APC maturation and migration.[209]

Transition of effector T cells to memory T cells and development of chronic inflammation

Clinical DED often presents as a chronic disease, while a majority of experimental data from wild-type animal models reflect an acute inflammatory process; and thus a major gap between experimental models and clinical setting has been identified. Most recent studies accomplished by Dana group have aimed to address this critical question. Frist, they found that when acute DED mice induced by a period of desiccation was transferred to a normal-humidity environment, corneal epitheliopathy in mice gradually regressed to lower levels, but never normalized, for many months, despite absence of tear deficiency, thus establishing a critical murine model of chronic DED.[42] Significant resolution of acute corneal epitheliopathy was seen in the first week of deprivation of desiccation, during which period the previously expanded effector Th17 pool in acute stage dramatically contracted, accompanied by the emergence of a prominent memory Th17 population (CD4$^+$CD44^{high}CD62L$^-$IL-17$^+$).[49] Memory T-cell—mediated "immunological memory" is a distinct feature of adaptive immunity, and has been shown to play critical pathogenic roles in autoimmunity and chronic inflammation.[230,231] Further, it is revealed that these emerging memory Th17 cells during the contraction phase are generated from a small fraction of surviving effector Th17 cells driven by persisting environmental IL-23 stimulation and diminished IL-2 signaling.[49] These memory Th17 cells are functionally pathogenic demonstrated by their ability of transferring DED phenotypes to healthy naive mice.[42] Subsequent work shows that the major effector precursors of memory Th17 cells are double-positive effector Th17/1 cells with single-positive effector Th17 cells contributing relatively less to the memory pool.[232] Along with the chronic low-grade corneal epitheliopathy, memory

Th17 cells persist for prolonged period in both conjunctiva and draining lymphoid tissues, and they do not produce IFN-γ. Consistently, only heightened levels of IL-17, but not IFN-γ are expressed in the ocular surface in chronic DED.[42,48] In vivo topical blockade of IL-17 in chronic DED can significantly improve the disease severity,[47] demonstrating IL-17 as the principal cytokine sustaining chronicity of DED. The next question is why memory Th17 cells are long-lived in contrast to the short-lived effector Th17 cells. In this regard, two cytokines IL-7 and IL-15 and the distinct expression of their receptors by memory Th17 cells are revealed to be the critical surviving factors for memory Th17 cells via maintaining their robust proliferative and antiapoptotic capabilities.[47] Reactivation of memory Th17 cells by a second desiccating stress on chronic DED mice leads to the development of a more rapid and severe disease exacerbation, suggesting that memory Th17-cell–mediated recall response is responsible for the acute-on-chronic disease exacerbation, akin to intermittent disease "flare" in clinical patients. Blockade of either IL-7 or IL-15 efficiently abolishes memory Th17 cells and the subsequent recall response, preventing the disease flare in chronic DED.[47]

B-cell immunity

B cell is the other major cellular component of adaptive immunity, and B-cell–mediated humoral immunity may participate in disease pathogenicity by primarily differentiating to plasma cells that secret autoantibodies causing self-tissue damages. Autoreactive B cells are known crucial effectors mediating Sjögren's syndrome evidenced by the presence of autoantibodies directed to ribonuclear proteins SS-A/Ro and SS-B/La in both patients and TSP-1 KO Sjögren's syndrome mice.[92,233] In NOD mouse model of Sjögren's syndrome, antinuclear antibody (ANA) and type 3 muscarinic acetylcholine receptor (mAChR) autoantibodies (anti-M_3R) are present in the sera,[78,234] which has also been identified as a marker for Sjögren's syndrome–DED patients.[235] The mAChR is responsible for glandular secretion, and thus the anti-M_3R autoantibodies are suggested to contribute to the glandular dysfunction in Sjögren's syndrome together with the glandular infiltrating effector T cells.[80] In fact, immunization of mice with M_3R peptides led to increased serum levels of anti-M_3R antibodies and low saliva volume, accompanied by $CD4^+$ T-cell and B-cell infiltrates in the salivary glands.[236] The precise functional relevance of anti-M_3R antibodies in lacrimal gland dysfunction in Sjögren's syndrome remains to be determined. In addition, detection of autoantibodies against kallikrein-13 in sera

from IQI/Jic mice also suggests potential roles of B-cell immunity in Sjögren's syndrome–DED.[194] In *Aire*-deficient mouse model of Sjögren's syndrome, autoantibody against odorant binding protein 1a (OBP1a) within lacrimal glands is present in the sera, in association with a large proportion of B cell infiltrates in the glands. However, with individual depletion of $CD4^+$ T cells, $CD8^+$ T cells, or B cells, only $CD4^+$ T-cell–depleted group showed significant improvement of lacrimal gland pathology, and further those $CD4^+$ T cells were capable of recognizing OBP1a, suggesting that B-cell immunity in this model plays a limited pathogenic role.[93] In contrast, in Id3 knockout mouse model of Sjögren's syndrome, depletion of B cells led to disease improvement.[237]

In non-Sjögren's DED, increased serum antibodies against kallikrein-13 was also detected in mice that were subjected to a long period (3 weeks) of desiccating stress, suggesting that humoral immunity may participate in the pathogenesis of DED subsequent to the initiation of cell-mediated immunity (T-cell immunity). Adoptive transfer of serum or purified IgG collected from the desiccating stress-induced DED mice to T-cell–deficient nude mice led to decreased tear production along with increased cytokines IL-1β, TNF-α, IFN-γ, and IL-17 in tears, as well as reduced conjunctival goblet cells,[196] indicating that autoantibodies contribute to T-cell–dominant pathogenesis in non-Sjögren's DED. T-cell–dependent B-cell activation is further demonstrated by a recent study showing that $CD4^+$ T cells isolated from desiccation-induced DED mice promote B-cell proliferation and activation primarily via secreted IL-17, and activated B cells further upregulate expression of IL-17 receptor, through which IL-17 further induces B-cell class switching and differentiation to plasma cells.[238]

In addition to their major function of producing autoantibodies in autoimmunity, B cells may functionally serve as APC and secrete various inflammatory cytokines that facilitate T-cell immunity; these areas have yet to be explored in DED pathogenesis.

Lymphocytic inflammation in lacrimal gland

Lacrimal gland, proposed as an integral part of Lacrimal Functional Unit (LFU) along with the ocular surface,[239] can be another target organ of immune attack in DED, supported by data primarily generated from Sjögren's syndrome–DED models. In both NOD and MRL/lpr mice, significant focal inflammatory infiltrates in lacrimal glands have been shown, and the infiltrating cells consist of dominant $CD3^+CD4^+$ T cells along with small numbers of $CD8^+$ T cells and $B220^+$ B cells, with all of them expressing CD69 activation marker. In addition, there is progressive increase of inflammatory cytokines IL-1β, TNF-α, IL-2, IL-6, IFN-γ, and IL-12, as well as chemokines CCL5, CXCL10, and adhesion molecule ICAM-1 in the lacrimal glands in these genetically modified mice.[75,78,81,240–243] Blockade of either ICAM-1 or LFA-1 with antibodies can significantly reduce glandular inflammation.[243] These findings suggest a pathogenic role of Th1 response in destroying lacrimal glands. In CD25 KO mice, there are more CD8+ than CD4+ T-cell infiltrates in the lacrimal glands with increased expression of both Th1 (IFN-γ and IL-12) and Th17 (IL-17 and CCL20) cytokines, accompanied by ductal epithelial apoptosis.[88] In TSP-1 KO mice, significant infiltration of CD4+ T cells in the lacrimal glands is noted, and they are active IL-17-secreting Th17 cells, which may further promote the release of inflammatory cytokines IL-1β, TNF-α, and IL-6 by glandular cells.[92] Essential role of Th17 in Sjögren's syndrome is further illustrated by the ability of IL-17 to promote autoreactive B-cell response and autoantibodies production in NOD mice.[244] Experimental data focusing on salivary glands pathology in Sjögren's syndrome suggest that T-cell response is critical in inducing disease development, while B-cell response gets involved later in maintaining chronic inflammation,[190,245] however, further studies are required to dissect the temporal T- and B-cell responses, as well as differential contributions of Th17 versus Th1, including whether the increased IFN-γ is part of plastic Th17 response, to lacrimal gland destruction in Sjögren's syndrome–DED. To date, data on lacrimal gland inflammation in non-Sjögren's DED mice are very limited. A recent study showed in desiccation-induced DED mice increased infiltration of CD11c+ dendritic cells in lacrimal glands with activated morphology features observed with a series of intravital multiphoton microscopy in live animals,[246] however, the precise functions of these professional APC in lacrimal gland inflammation remain to be explored.

Disruption of Neuroimmune Homeostasis

Cornea is the most densely innervated tissue in the body, and corneal sensory signals controlled by the trigeminal ganglion neurons are critical in maintaining the ocular surface homeostasis via regulating lacrimation, secretion of epitheliotropic factors, and the blink reflex. Corneal degenerative neuropathy is a frequently encountered pathology in DED, associated with the ocular surface inflammation. In DED induced with either desiccating stress or lacrimal gland excision, acute inflammation of overexpressed inflammatory cytokines

IL-1β, IL-6, and TNF-α, sensitizes various nociceptors expressed by sensory nerve terminals at the ocular surface, increases their activity and excitation, and evokes nociceptive pain[9,60–62] resulting from increased activation and discharges of nerves and subsequent release of substance P (SP)—the principal pain mediator. In addition, central sensitization of trigeminal neurons is demonstrated involved in ocular pain sensation in a lacrimal gland excision model.[247] However, with inflammation progression or in severe inflammatory cases, structural damage of corneal nerves occurs evidenced by reduced intraepithelial nerve terminals in the epithelium as well as the decrease of their originating subbasal nerves in both Sjögren's and non-Sjögren's DED animals,[100,248,249] along with the reduced corneal sensitivity or hypoalgesia.[53,67,100,248] Topical blockade of IL-1β with an interleukin-1 receptor antagonist (IL-1Ra) effectively prevents corneal nerve degeneration in DED (Fig. 4.3). On the other hand, altered gene expression and disturbed regeneration of corneal nerves subsequent to acute nerve damage, along with memory Th17-mediated chronic inflammation, may lead to persistent sensory hypersensitivity, thus potentially contributing to chronic pain or discomfort in DED; however, the exact process including both peripheral and central mechanisms remains to be resolved.

The increased levels of neuropeptide SP produced by corneal innervating neurons can in turn induce neurogenic inflammation thus propagating inflammatory cascade in ocular surface in DED. Although physiological levels of SP at the ocular surface is essential for maintaining ocular surface homeostasis[107–109] and mice genetically deletion of functional SP receptor, neurokinin-1 receptor (NK1R) develop corneal epitheliopathy,[110] abnormally increased expression of SP at both ocular surface and trigeminal ganglion neurons has been noted in DED mice.[46] The heightened levels of sensory nerve–derived SP promotes corneal APC mobilization and maturation, which subsequently induces effector Th17 response in DED.[46] Recent data also suggest a direct role of SP in promoting effector Th17 to convert to memory Th17 in DED.[232] Interestingly, consistently increased expression of SP is also detected in DED draining lymph nodes, along with an increased proportion of NK1R+ Treg which show significantly compromised regulatory function. Furthermore, coculture of normal Treg with SP leads to the loss of function of Treg, demonstrating that SP directly contributes to Treg dysfunction in DED.[106] Additionally, trigeminal neuron-derived SP from DED mice shows pro-hemangiogenesis function,[249] suggesting a

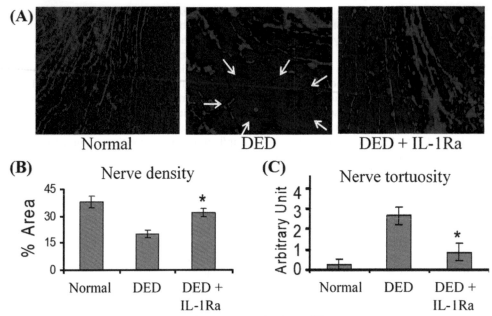

FIG. 4.3 IL-1—Mediated Corneal Nerve Damage in DED Mice. **(A)** Representative confocal micrographs of wild-type C57BL/6 corneal wholemount immunostained with tubulin-III showing decreased density and increased tortuosity of nerve fibers (area surrounded by *white arrows*) in untreated DED corneas compared to DED. Topical treatment with IL-1 receptor antagonist (IL-1Ra) significantly reduced corneal nerve dropout **(B)** and tortuosity **(C)** in DED with computer-assisted quantification. *, $P < .05$ compared to untreated DED (n = 5/group).

potential role of SP in regulating corneal lymphangiogenesis in DED that has yet to be investigated. In addition to SP, calcitonin gene–related peptide (CGRP), a wound healing promoting and antiinflammatory neuropeptide, may also participate in structural and functional changes of corneal nerves in DED, as shown by significantly reduced CGRP-containing corneal sensory nerves in older TSP-1 KO mouse, a model of Sjögren's syndrome, indicating that decreased CGRP may contribute to the dysregulation of ocular surface immune homeostasis and subsequent persisting inflammation.

Effect of Aging on DED

Age-related changes can result in a shift in the balance between protective and pathogenic immune responses, collectively termed "immunosenescence." Advancing age has been shown a risk factor for autoimmunity,[250] including DED supported by evidence of increased prevalence of DED in the elderly[251] and the animal model findings including spontaneous DED in aged canine (decreased tear production) and mouse (ARMGD),[12,129,130] and progressively worsened ocular surface disease with aging in various Sjögren's syndrome mice such as NOD, CD25 KO, *Spdef* KO, and TSP-1 KO mice.[77,88,103,252] In elderly wild-type mice, dry eye phenotypes including increased corneal surface irregularity, conjunctival goblet cell loss, as well as decreased intraepithelial and subbasal corneal nerve density along with reduced corneal sensitivity have been observed[99–101]; however, evaluation of corneal barrier function and relevant corneal epitheliopathy shows only moderately increased permeability to the fluorescent 70-kDa molecule Oregon green dextran, but no significant changes to the smaller ~300 Da carboxyfluorescein dye that is widely used for CFS scoring.[99,253] Interestingly, there is no decreased, but paradoxically increased tear production with aging in wild-type mice,[99,101] and aging-associated higher susceptibility to more severe DED is thus independent on tear deficiency and mainly attributed to an "imbalance" between proinflammatory and antiinflammatory pathways in elderly, with amplified T effector response and failed immunoregulatory mechanisms. Increased matured APC in conjunctiva with enhanced antigen uptaking ability has been shown in aged mice; consistently, APC in eye draining lymph nodes also show higher mature status and a strong capability of priming naive T cells to effector Th1 cells in vitro.[254] Relatedly, increased Th1 and Th17 cells in the local draining lymph nodes, high expression of IL-17, IFN-γ, and CCL20 at the ocular surface, and significant CD4[+], CD8[+], and B cells infiltration in the lacrimal glands have been identified in wild-type aged mice, suggesting involvement of enhanced Th1 and Th17 immunity in age-related DED. Furthermore, adoptive transfer of total CD4[+] T cells or the CD4[+]CXCR3[+] subset (predominantly IFN-γ-expressing cells) isolated from draining lymph nodes and spleen of aged mice effectively leads to T-cell infiltration in conjunctiva and lacrimal glands as well as reduced conjunctival goblet cell density in naive T-cell–deficient recipients, demonstrating the critical pathogenic function of CD4[+] T cells in age-related DED.[99,254] Most recently, it has been shown that wild-type aged mice previously exposed to a dry environment maintain a significantly larger memory Th17 pool as compared to young mice, and develop more severe corneal epitheliopathy (evaluated by CSF scoring) upon secondary exposure to desiccating stress, which is associated with enhanced Th17 recall response; furthermore, depletion of the enlarged memory Th17 pool in the aged prevents the exacerbation of disease, thus demonstrating the additional important role of long-lived memory Th17-cell population in predisposing the aged to DED.[253]

The expanded Th17 immunity in the aged has been linked to functional defects of Treg, the major player of the immunoregulatory arm. Wild-type aged mice show increased frequency of Treg than young mice; however, the Treg from aged exhibit decreased expression of Foxp3 and impaired suppression on effector CD4[+] T cells (Fig. 4.4). In NOD mice, similar findings including increase in the frequency of Treg with age in the eye-draining lymph nodes, spleen, and lacrimal glands, along with the loss of suppressive function were reported.[77] This study further showed that Treg in aged NOD mice were not only incapable of suppressing inflammation but even became pathogenic by coproducing inflammatory cytokines IL-17 and IFN-γ,[77] demonstrating the well-recognized functional plasticity of Treg. The precise molecular mechanisms by which dysfunctional Treg in the aged contribute to expanded memory Th17 compartment remain to be elucidated.

Role of Microbiome in DED
Commensal bacteria colonize all exposed body surfaces among which gut is the most densely populated organ; in contrast, ocular surface is a relatively sterile site with low bacterial load.[147,255] The inhabited bacterial communities are collectively referred to microbiota, and their collective genomes are referred to microbiome.[147] There has been recently increasing interest in studying the effect of microbiome on immune homeostasis in health and disease, and it has been demonstrated that gut microbiota impact not only intestinal diseases but also diseases in other sites, including the eye, a phenomenon referred to as the gut–eye axis.[256,257] Gut microbiota are shown as a trigger of autoreactive T-cell activation and the subsequent autoimmune uveitis (inflammation of eye in the posterior segment), possibly via the antigenic mimic mechanisms[258]; however, they play protective roles in the anterior segment of eye—the ocular surface. Depletion of commensal bacteria by breeding and maintaining wild-type C57BL/6 mice in germ-free environment leads to spontaneous development of DED, evidenced by increased

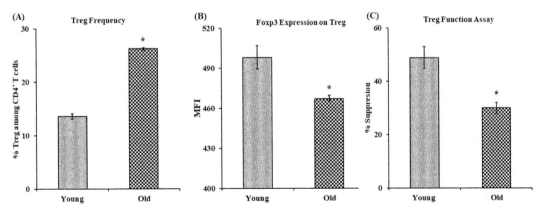

FIG. 4.4 Analysis of Treg in Old Versus Young Wild-Type Mice. Flow cytometry analysis of eye-draining lymph nodes in old mice shows increased frequency of Treg **(A)** but reduced expression levels of Foxp3 by Treg, measured by mean fluorescence intensity (MFI) **(B)**. In addition, Treg suppressive function on effector T-cell proliferation is compromised in old mice compared to young mice **(C)**. *, $P < .05$ (n = 6/group).

CFS, loss of conjunctival goblet cells, and lacrimal infiltration of $CD4^+$ T cells; and fecal microbiota transplant from conventional mice to these germ-free mice ameliorates DED severity and decreases T-cell infiltration.[102] Similar findings have been demonstrated in CD25 KO mice—a Sjögren's syndrome—DED model.[89] In addition, wild-type mice subjected to desiccating stress develop more severe DED when treated with oral antibiotics cocktail that induces intestinal dysbiosis characterized by decrease in *Clostridium* and increase in *Enterobacter*, *Escherichia/Shigella*, and *Pseudomonas*.[259] These findings suggest fecal microbial transplant a potentially novel therapy for DED, and currently a clinical trial using this strategy to treat Sjögren's Syndrome DED is ongoing (ClinicalTrials.gov Identifier: NCT03926286). However, serious adverse effects of fatal infections with multidrug resistant organisms from fecal microbiota transplant have been recently reported in clinical trials. An alternative approach of modulating gut microbiome is oral supplement with probiotics, which are selective live microorganisms that can provide beneficial effects. In antibiotic cocktail-treated germ-free NOD mice (a transgenic model of Sjögren's syndrome), probiotic treatment significantly improves corneal barrier function and tear production, along with increased Treg population,[260] indicating probiotics an appealing approach to treat autoimmune DED, despite its definitive benefits in patients are to be determined by extensive human studies.

CONCLUSIONS AND PERSPECTIVES

Essential data generated from both Sjögren's and non-Sjögren's DED models clearly demonstrate $CD4^+$ T-cell—centered pathogenesis in causing the persisting ocular surface inflammation that leads to a myriad of ocular surface damages involving tear film, epithelium, and nerves. Precise delineation of autoimmune attack to lacrimal glands and Meibomian glands within the concept of ocular surface—local lymphoid compartment cycle is required by further investigations. The understanding on the interplay between immunity and nervous system, sex hormones, angiogenesis, microbiome in DED pathophysiology is rapidly evolving with the use of novel animal tools, such as reporter mice. Specific immunomodulation that targets effector memory T cells or harnesses Treg by virtue of various new approaches is expected to efficiently restore ocular surface homeostasis while avoiding immune suppression, and thus holds a promise in future translational and clinical studies.

REFERENCES

1. Craig JP, Nichols KK, Akpek EK, et al. TFOS DEWS II definition and classification report. *Ocul Surf.* 2017;15(3):276—283. https://doi.org/10.1016/j.jtos.2017.05.008.
2. Lemp MA. Report of the National Eye Institute/Industry Workshop on clinical trials in dry eyes. *Contact Lens Assoc Ophthalmol J.* 1995;21:221—232.
3. Lemp MA, Baudouin C, Baum J, et al. The definition and classification of dry eye disease: report of the definition and classification subcommittee of the International Dry Eye WorkShop (2007). *Ocul Surf.* 2007;5:75—92. https://doi.org/10.1016/s1542-0124(12)70081-2.
4. Lemp MA, Crews LA, Bron AJ, Foulks GN, Sullivan BD. Distribution of aqueous-deficient and evaporative dry eye in a clinic-based patient cohort: a retrospective study. *Cornea.* 2012;31(5):472—478. https://doi.org/10.1097/ICO.0b013e318225415a.
5. Wei Y, Asbell PA. The core mechanism of dry eye disease is inflammation. *Eye Contact Lens.* 2014;40(4):248—256. https://doi.org/10.1097/ICL.0000000000000042.
6. Dursun D, Wang M, Monroy D, et al. A mouse model of keratoconjunctivitis sicca. *Investig Ophthalmol Vis Sci.* 2002;43(3):632—638.
7. Barabino S, Shen LL, Chen L, Rashid S, Rolando M, Dana MR. The controlled-environment chamber: a new mouse model of dry eye. *Investig Ophthalmol Vis Sci.* 2005;46(8):2766—2771. https://doi.org/10.1167/iovs.04-1326.
8. Fujihara T, Murakami T, Fujita H, Nakamura M, Nakata K. Improvement of corneal barrier function by the P2Y2 agonist INS365 in a rat dry eye model. *Investig Ophthalmol Vis Sci.* 2001;42(1):96—100.
9. Skrzypecki J, Tomasz H, Karolina C. Variability of dry eye disease following removal of lacrimal glands in rats. *Adv Exp Med Biol.* 2019;1153:109—115. https://doi.org/10.1007/5584_2019_348.
10. Fujihara T, Nagano T, Nakamura M, Shirasawa E. Establishment of a rabbit short-term dry eye model. *J Ocul Pharmacol Therapeut.* 1995;11(4):503—508. https://doi.org/10.1089/jop.1995.11.503.
11. Burgalassi S, Panichi L, Chetoni P, Saettone MF, Boldrini E. Development of a simple dry eye model in the albino rabbit and evaluation of some tear substitutes. *Ophthalmic Res.* 1999;31(3):229—235. https://doi.org/10.1159/000055537.
12. Kaswan R, Pappas C, Wall K, Hirsh SG. Survey of canine tear deficiency in veterinary practice. *Adv Exp Med Biol.* 1998;438:931—939. https://doi.org/10.1007/978-1-4615-5359-5_132.
13. Gao J, Schwalb TA, Addeo JV, Ghosn CR, Stern ME. The role of apoptosis in the pathogenesis of canine keratoconjunctivitis sicca: the effect of topical cyclosporin A therapy. *Cornea.* 1998;17(6):654—663. https://doi.org/10.1097/00003226-199811000-00014.
14. Henriksson JT, McDermott AM, Bergmanson JPG. Dimensions and morphology of the cornea in three strains

of mice. *Investig Ophthalmol Vis Sci.* 2009;50(8): 3648–3654. https://doi.org/10.1167/iovs.08-2941.

15. Doughty MJ, Zaman ML. Human corneal thickness and its impact on intraocular pressure measures: a review and meta-analysis approach. *Surv Ophthalmol.* 2000;44(5): 367–408. https://doi.org/10.1016/S0039-6257(00)00110-7.

16. Mokhtarzadeh M, Casey R, Glasgow BJ. Fluorescein punctate staining traced to superficial corneal epithelial cells by impression cytology and confocal microscopy. *Investig Ophthalmol Vis Sci.* 2011;52(5):2127–2135. https://doi.org/10.1167/iovs.10-6489.

17. Wolffsohn JS, Arita R, Chalmers R, et al. TFOS DEWS II diagnostic methodology report. *Ocul Surf.* 2017;15(3): 539–574. https://doi.org/10.1016/j.jtos.2017.05.001.

18. Bergmanson JPG, Texas Eye Research and Technology Center. *Clinical Ocular Anatomy and Physiology.* 15th ed. Texas Eye Research and Technology Center; 2009.

19. Hamrah P, Liu Y, Zhang Q, Dana MR. The corneal stroma is endowed with a significant number of resident dendritic cells. *Investig Ophthalmol Vis Sci.* 2003;44(2): 581–589. https://doi.org/10.1167/iovs.02-0838.

20. Rashid S, Jin Y, Ecoiffier T, Barabino S, Schaumberg DA, Dana MR. Topical omega-3 and omega-6 fatty acids for treatment of dry eye. *Arch Ophthalmol.* 2008;126(2): 219–225. https://doi.org/10.1001/archophthalmol.2007.61.

21. Yamagami S, Ebihara N, Usui T, Yokoo S, Amano S. Bone marrow-derived cells in normal human corneal stroma. *Arch Ophthalmol.* 2006;124(1):62–69. https://doi.org/10.1001/archopht.124.1.62.

22. Yamagami S, Yokoo S, Usui T, Yamagami H, Amano S, Ebihara N. Distinct populations of dendritic cells in the normal human donor corneal epithelium. *Investig Ophthalmol Vis Sci.* 2005;46(12):4489–4494. https://doi.org/10.1167/iovs.05-0054.

23. Hamrah P, Zhang Q, Liu Y, Dana MR. Novel characterization of MHC class II-negative population of resident corneal Langerhans cell-type dendritic cells. *Investig Ophthalmol Vis Sci.* 2002;43(3):639–646.

24. Hattori T, Chauhan SK, Lee H, et al. Characterization of langerin-expressing dendritic cell subsets in the normal cornea. *Investig Ophthalmol Vis Sci.* 2011;52(7): 4598–4604. https://doi.org/10.1167/iovs.10-6741.

25. Barabino S, Chen Y, Chauhan S, Dana R. Ocular surface immunity: homeostatic mechanisms and their disruption in dry eye disease. *Prog Retin Eye Res.* 2012;31(3): 271–285. https://doi.org/10.1016/j.preteyeres.2012.02.003.

26. Müller LJ, Marfurt CF, Kruse F, Tervo TMT. Corneal nerves: structure, contents and function. *Exp Eye Res.* 2003;76(5):521–542. https://doi.org/10.1016/S0014-4835(03)00050-2.

27. Cruzat A, Qazi Y, Hamrah P. In vivo confocal microscopy of corneal nerves in health and disease. *Ocul Surf.* 2017; 15(1):15–47. https://doi.org/10.1016/j.jtos.2016.09.004.

28. Amparo F, Schaumberg DA, Dana R. Comparison of two questionnaires for dry eye symptom assessment: the ocular surface disease index and the symptom assessment in dry eye. *Ophthalmology.* 2015;122(7):1498–1503. https://doi.org/10.1016/j.ophtha.2015.02.037.

29. Barabino S, Rolando M, Chen L, Dana MR. Exposure to a dry environment induces strain-specific responses in mice. *Exp Eye Res.* 2007;84(5):973–977. https://doi.org/10.1016/j.exer.2007.02.003.

30. Corrales RM, Villarreal A, Farley W, Stern ME, Li DQ, Pflugfelder SC. Strain-related cytokine profiles on the murine ocular surface in response to desiccating stress. *Cornea.* 2007;26(5):579–584. https://doi.org/10.1097/ICO.0b013e318033a729.

31. Chauhan SK, El Annan J, Ecoiffier T, et al. Autoimmunity in dry eye is due to resistance of Th17 to Treg suppression. *J Immunol.* 2009;182(3):1247–1252. https://doi.org/10.4049/jimmunol.182.3.1247.

32. Chen Y, Chauhan SK, Saban DR, Sadrai Z, Okanobo A, Dana R. Interferon-γ-secreting NK cells promote induction of dry eye disease. *J Leukoc Biol.* 2011;89(6): 965–972. https://doi.org/10.1189/jlb.1110611.

33. Strong B, Farley W, Stern ME, Pflugfelder SC. Topical cyclosporine inhibits conjunctival epithelial apoptosis in experimental murine keratoconjunctivitis sicca. *Cornea.* 2005;24(1):80–85. https://doi.org/10.1097/01.ico.0000133994.22392.47.

34. Niederkorn JY, Stern ME, Pflugfelder SC, et al. Desiccating stress induces T cell-mediated sjögren's syndrome-like lacrimal keratoconjunctivitis. *J Immunol.* 2006;176(7): 3950–3957. https://doi.org/10.4049/jimmunol.176.7.3950.

35. De Paiva CS, Corrales RM, Villarreal AL, et al. Corticosteroid and doxycycline suppress MMP-9 and inflammatory cytokine expression, MAPK activation in the corneal epithelium in experimental dry eye. *Exp Eye Res.* 2006;83(3):526–535. https://doi.org/10.1016/j.exer.2006.02.004.

36. De Paiva CS, Chotikavanich S, Pangelinan SB, et al. IL-17 disrupts corneal barrier following desiccating stress. *Mucosal Immunol.* 2009;2(3):243–253. https://doi.org/10.1038/mi.2009.5.

37. Gao Y, Min K, Zhang Y, Su J, Greenwood M, Gronert K. Female-specific downregulation of tissue polymorphonuclear neutrophils drives impaired regulatory T cell and amplified effector T cell responses in autoimmune dry eye disease. *J Immunol.* 2015;195(7):3086–3099. https://doi.org/10.4049/jimmunol.1500610.

38. Schaumberg DA, Uchino M, Christen WG, Semba RD, Buring JE, Li JZ. Patient reported differences in dry eye disease between men and women: impact, management, and patient satisfaction. *PLoS One.* 2013;8(9). https://doi.org/10.1371/journal.pone.0076121.

39. Schaumberg DA, Sullivan DA, Buring JE, Dana MR. Prevalence of dry eye syndrome among US women. *Am J Ophthalmol.* 2003;136(2):318–326. https://doi.org/10.1016/S0002-9394(03)00218-6.

40. Schaumberg DA, Dana R, Buring JE, Sullivan DA. Prevalence of dry eye disease among US men: estimates from the physicians' health studies. *Arch Ophthalmol.* 2009;

127(6):763−768. https://doi.org/10.1001/archophthalmol.2009.103.

41. Chen W, Zhang X, Zhang J, et al. A murine model of dry eye induced by an intelligently controlled environmental system. *Investig Ophthalmol Vis Sci.* 2008;49(4):1386−1391. https://doi.org/10.1167/iovs.07-0744.

42. Chen Y, Chauhan SK, Soo Lee H, Saban DR, Dana R. Chronic dry eye disease is principally mediated by effector memory Th17 cells. *Mucosal Immunol.* 2014;7(1):38−45. https://doi.org/10.1038/mi.2013.20.

43. Chen Y, Chauhan SK, Lee HS, et al. Effect of desiccating environmental stress versus systemic muscarinic AChR blockade on dry eye immunopathogenesis. *Investig Ophthalmol Vis Sci.* 2013;54(4):2457−2464. https://doi.org/10.1167/iovs.12-11121.

44. Fujii T, Takada-Takatori Y, Kawashima K. Basic and clinical aspects of non-neuronal acetylcholine: expression of an independent, non-neuronal cholinergic system in lymphocytes and its clinical significance in immunotherapy. *J Pharmacol Sci.* 2008;106(2):186−192. https://doi.org/10.1254/jphs.FM0070109.

45. Tan X, Chen Y, Foulsham W, et al. The immunoregulatory role of corneal epithelium-derived thrombospondin-1 in dry eye disease. *Ocul Surf.* 2018;16(4):470−477. https://doi.org/10.1016/j.jtos.2018.07.005.

46. Yu M, Lee SM, Lee H, et al. Neurokinin-1 receptor antagonism ameliorates dry eye disease by inhibiting antigen-presenting cell maturation and T helper 17 cell activation. *Am J Pathol.* 2020;190(1):125−133. https://doi.org/10.1016/j.ajpath.2019.09.020.

47. Chen Y, Chauhan SK, Tan X, Dana R. Interleukin-7 and -15 maintain pathogenic memory Th17 cells in autoimmunity. *J Autoimmun.* 2017;77:96−103. https://doi.org/10.1016/j.jaut.2016.11.003.

48. Chen Y, Chauhan SK, Shao C, Omoto M, Inomata T, Dana R. IFN-γ−Expressing Th17 cells are required for development of severe ocular surface autoimmunity. *J Immunol.* 2017;199(3):1163−1169. https://doi.org/10.4049/jimmunol.1602144.

49. Chen Y, Shao C, Fan NW, et al. The functions of IL-23 and IL-2 on driving autoimmune effector T-helper 17 cells into the memory pool in dry eye disease. *Mucosal Immunol.* 2020. https://doi.org/10.1038/s41385-020-0289-3. Published online.

50. Craig JP, Nelson JD, Azar DT, et al. TFOS DEWS II report executive summary. *Ocul Surf.* 2017;15(4):802−812. https://doi.org/10.1016/j.jtos.2017.08.003.

51. Straub RH. TRPV1, TRPA1, and TRPM8 channels in inflammation, energy redirection, and water retention: role in chronic inflammatory diseases with an evolutionary perspective. *J Mol Med.* 2014;92(9):925−937. https://doi.org/10.1007/s00109-014-1175-9.

52. Alamri AS, Brock JA, Herath CB, Rajapaksha IG, Angus PW, Ivanusic JJ. The effects of diabetes and high-fat diet on polymodal nociceptor and cold thermoreceptor nerve terminal endings in the corneal

epithelium. *Investig Ophthalmol Vis Sci.* 2019;60(1):209−217. https://doi.org/10.1167/iovs.18-25788.

53. Guzmán M, Miglio M, Keitelman I, et al. Transient tear hyperosmolarity disrupts the neuroimmune homeostasis of the ocular surface and facilitates dry eye onset. *Immunology.* 2020;161(2):148−161. https://doi.org/10.1111/imm.13243.

54. Zoukhri D. Effect of inflammation on lacrimal gland function. *Exp Eye Res.* 2006;82(5):885−898. https://doi.org/10.1016/j.exer.2005.10.018.

55. Gilbard JP, Rossi SR, Gray KL. A new rabbit model for keratoconjunctivitis sicca. *Investig Ophthalmol Vis Sci.* 1987;28(2):225−228.

56. Gilbard JP, Rossi SR, Gray KL, Hanninen LA, Kenyon KR. Tear film osmolarity and ocular surface disease in two rabbit models for keratoconjunctivitis sicca. *Investig Ophthalmol Vis Sci.* 1988;29(3):374−378.

57. Dietrich J, Schlegel C, Roth M, et al. Comparative analysis on the dynamic of lacrimal gland damage and regeneration after Interleukin-1α or duct ligation induced dry eye disease in mice. *Exp Eye Res.* 2018;172:66−77. https://doi.org/10.1016/j.exer.2018.03.026.

58. Stevenson W, Chen Y, Lee SM, et al. Extraorbital lacrimal gland excision: a reproducible model of severe aqueous tear-deficient dry eye disease. *Cornea.* 2014;33(12):1336−1341. https://doi.org/10.1097/ICO.0000000000000264.

59. Guzmán M, Keitelman I, Sabbione F, Trevani AS, Giordano MN, Galletti JG. Mucosal tolerance disruption favors disease progression in an extraorbital lacrimal gland excision model of murine dry eye. *Exp Eye Res.* 2016;151:19−22. https://doi.org/10.1016/j.exer.2016.07.004.

60. Mecum NE, Cyr D, Malon J, Demers D, Cao L, Meng ID. Evaluation of corneal damage after lacrimal gland excision in male and female mice. *Investig Ophthalmol Vis Sci.* 2019;60(10):3264−3274. https://doi.org/10.1167/iovs.18-26457.

61. Mecum NE, Demers D, Sullivan CE, Denis TE, Kalliel JR, Meng ID. Lacrimal gland excision in male and female mice causes ocular pain and anxiety-like behaviors. *Sci Rep.* 2020;10(1). https://doi.org/10.1038/s41598-020-73945-w.

62. Li F, Yang W, Jiang H, et al. TRPV1 activity and substance P release are required for corneal cold nociception. *Nat Commun.* 2019;10(1). https://doi.org/10.1038/s41467-019-13536-0.

63. Suwan-Apichon O, Rizen M, Rangsin R, et al. Botulinum toxin B-induced mouse model of keratoconjunctivitis sicca. *Investig Ophthalmol Vis Sci.* 2006;47(1):133−139. https://doi.org/10.1167/iovs.05-0380.

64. Lekhanont K, Park CY, Smith JA, et al. Effects of topical anti-inflammatory agents in a botulinum toxin B-induced mouse model of keratoconjunctivitis sicca. *J Ocul Pharmacol Therapeut.* 2007;23(1):27−34. https://doi.org/10.1089/jop.2006.0071.

65. Lekhanont K, Park CY, Combs JC, Suwan-Apichon O, Rangsin R, Chuck RS. Effect of topical olopatadine and

epinastine in the botulinum toxin B-induced mouse model of dry eye. *J Ocul Pharmacol Therapeut.* 2007; 23(1):83—88. https://doi.org/10.1089/jop.2006.0097.

66. Park CY, Zhuang W, Lekhanont K, et al. Lacrimal gland inflammatory cytokine gene expression in the botulinum toxin B-induced murine dry eye model. *Mol Vis.* 2007;13: 2222—2232.

67. Aicher SA, Hermes SM, Hegarty DM. Denervation of the lacrimal gland leads to corneal hypoalgesia in a novel rat model of aqueous dry eye disease. *Investig Ophthalmol Vis Sci.* 2015;56(11):6981—6989. https://doi.org/10.1167/iovs.15-17497.

68. Labbé A, Alalwani H, Van Went C, Brasnu E, Georgescu D, Baudouin C. The relationship between sub-basal nerve morphology and corneal sensation in ocular surface disease. *Investig Ophthalmol Vis Sci.* 2012;53(8): 4926—4931. https://doi.org/10.1167/iovs.11-8708.

69. Bourcier T, Acosta MC, Borderie V, et al. Decreased corneal sensitivity in patients with dry eye. *Investig Ophthalmol Vis Sci.* 2005;46(7):2341—2345. https://doi.org/10.1167/iovs.04-1426.

70. Zoukhri D, Macari E, Kublin CL. A single injection of interleukin-1 induces reversible aqueous-tear deficiency, lacrimal gland inflammation, and acinar and ductal cell proliferation. *Exp Eye Res.* 2007;84(5):894—904. https://doi.org/10.1016/j.exer.2007.01.015.

71. Zhu Z, Stevenson D, Schechter JE, Mircheff AK, Atkinson R, Trousdale MD. Lacrimal histopathology and ocular surface disease in a rabbit model of autoimmune dacryoadenitis. *Cornea.* 2003;22(1):25—32. https://doi.org/10.1097/00003226-200301000-00007.

72. Guo Z, Song DH, Azzarolo AM, et al. Autologous lacrimal-lymphoid mixed-cell reactions induce dacryoadenitis in rabbits. *Exp Eye Res.* 2000;71(1):23—31. https://doi.org/10.1006/exer.2000.0855.

73. Atkinson MA, Leiter EH. The NOD mouse model of type 1 diabetes: as good as it gets? *Nat Med.* 1999;5(6): 601—604. https://doi.org/10.1038/9442.

74. Humphreys-Beher MG, Hu Y, Nakagawa Y, Wang PL, Purushotham KR. Utilization of the non-obese diabetic (NOD) mouse as an animal model for the study of secondary Sjogren's syndrome. *Adv Exp Med Biol.* 1994; 350:631—636. https://doi.org/10.1007/978-1-4615-2417-5_105.

75. Takahashi M, Ishimaru N, Yanagi K, Haneji N, Saito I, Hayashi Y. High incidence of autoimmune dacryoadenitis in male non-obese diabetic (NOD) mice depending on sex steroid. *Clin Exp Immunol.* 1997;109(3): 555—561. https://doi.org/10.1046/j.1365-2249.1997.4691368.x.

76. Xiao W, Wu Y, Zhang J, Ye W, Xu GT. Selecting highly sensitive non-obese diabetic mice for improving the study of Sjögren's syndrome. *Graefes Arch Clin Exp Ophthalmol.* 2009;247(1):59—66. https://doi.org/10.1007/s00417-008-0941-1.

77. Coursey TG, Bian F, Zaheer M, Pflugfelder SC, Volpe EA, De Paiva CS. Age-related spontaneous lacrimal keratoconjunctivitis is accompanied by dysfunctional T regulatory cells. *Mucosal Immunol.* 2017;10(3):743—756. https://doi.org/10.1038/mi.2016.83.

78. Cha S, Nagashima H, Brown VB, Peck AB, Humphreys-Beher MG. Two NOD Idd-associated intervals contribute synergistically to the development of autoimmune exocrinopathy (Sjögren's syndrome) on a healthy murine background. *Arthritis Rheum.* 2002;46(5):1390—1398. https://doi.org/10.1002/art.10258.

79. Yoon KC, De Paiva CS, Qi H, et al. Desiccating environmental stress exacerbates autoimmune lacrimal keratoconjunctivitis in non-obese diabetic mice. *J Autoimmun.* 2008;30(4):212—221. https://doi.org/10.1016/j.jaut.2007.09.003.

80. Van Blokland SCA, Versnel MA. Pathogenesis of Sjögren's syndrome: characteristics of different mouse models for autoimmune exocrinopathy. *Clin Immunol.* 2002; 103(2):111—124. https://doi.org/10.1006/clim.2002.5189.

81. Fujita H, Fujihara T, Takeuchi T, Saito I, Tsubota K. Lacrimation and salivation are not related to lymphocytic infiltration in lacrimal and salivary glands in MRL lpr/lpr mice. *Adv Exp Med Biol.* 1998;438:941—948. https://doi.org/10.1007/978-1-4615-5359-5_133.

82. Hoffman RW, Alspaugh MA, Waggie KS, Durham JB, Walker SE. Sjögren's syndrome in MRL/l and MRL/n mice. *Arthritis Rheum.* 1984;27(2):157—165. https://doi.org/10.1002/art.1780270206.

83. Barabino S, Chen W, Dana MR. Tear film and ocular surface tests in animal models of dry eye: uses and limitations. *Exp Eye Res.* 2004;79(5):613—621. https://doi.org/10.1016/j.exer.2004.07.002.

84. Verhagen C, Rowshani T, Willekens B, Van Haeringen NJ. Spontaneous development of corneal crystalline deposits in MRL/Mp mice. *Investig Ophthalmol Vis Sci.* 1995;36(2): 454—461.

85. Taniguchi T, Minami Y. The IL-2 IL-2 receptor system: a current overview. *Cell.* 1993;73(1):5—8. https://doi.org/10.1016/0092-8674(93)90152-G.

86. Sharma R, Zheng L, Guo X, Fu SM, Ju ST, Jarjour WN. Novel animal models for Sjögren's syndrome: expression and transfer of salivary gland dysfunction from regulatory T cell-deficient mice. *J Autoimmun.* 2006;27(4): 289—296. https://doi.org/10.1016/j.jaut.2006.11.003.

87. Willerford DM, Chen J, Ferry JA, Davidson L, Ma A, Alt FW. Interleukin-2 receptor α chain regulates the size and content of the peripheral lymphoid compartment. *Immunity.* 1995;3(4):521—530. https://doi.org/10.1016/1074-7613(95)90180-9.

88. Rahimy E, Pitcher JD, Pangelinan SB, et al. Spontaneous autoimmune dacryoadenitis in aged CD25KO mice. *Am J Pathol.* 2010;177(2):744—753. https://doi.org/10.2353/ajpath.2010.091116.

89. Zaheer M, Wang C, Bian F, et al. Protective role of commensal bacteria in Sjögren Syndrome. *J Autoimmun.* 2018;93:45—56. https://doi.org/10.1016/j.jaut.2018.06.004.

90. de Paiva CS, Hwang CS, Pitcher JD, et al. Age-related T-cell cytokine profile parallels corneal disease severity in

Sjögren's syndrome-like keratoconjunctivitis sicca in CD25KO mice. *Rheumatology*. 2010;49(2):246–258. https://doi.org/10.1093/rheumatology/kep357.

91. Crawford SE, Stellmach V, Murphy-Ullrich JE, et al. Thrombospondin-1 is a major activator of TGF-β1 in vivo. *Cell*. 1998;93(7):1159–1170. https://doi.org/10.1016/S0092-8674(00)81460-9.

92. Turpie B, Yoshimura T, Gulati A, Rios JD, Dartt DA, Masli S. Sjögren's syndrome-like ocular surface disease in thrombospondin-1 deficient mice. *Am J Pathol*. 2009; 175(3):1136–1147. https://doi.org/10.2353/ajpath.2009.081058.

93. DeVoss JJ, LeClair NP, Hou Y, et al. An autoimmune response to odorant binding protein 1a is associated with dry eye in the Aire -deficient mouse. *J Immunol*. 2010;184(8):4236–4246. https://doi.org/10.4049/jimmunol.0902434.

94. Vijmasi T, Chen FYT, Chen YT, Gallup M, McNamara N. Topical administration of interleukin-1 receptor antagonist as a therapy for aqueous-deficient dry eye in autoimmune disease. *Mol Vis*. 2013;19:1957–1965.

95. Gilbard JP, Hanninen LA, Rothman RC, Kenyon KR. Lacrimal Gland, cornea, and tear film in the NZB/NZW f1 hybrid mouse. *Curr Eye Res*. 1987;6(10):1237–1248. https://doi.org/10.3109/02713688709025234.

96. Shull MM, Ormsby I, Kier AB, et al. Targeted disruption of the mouse transforming growth factor-β1 gene results in multifocal inflammatory disease [14]. *Nature*. 1992;359(6397):693–699. https://doi.org/10.1038/359693a0.

97. Tsubata R, Tsubata T, Hiai H, et al. Autoimmune disease of exocrine organs in immunodeficient alymphoplasia mice: a spontaneous model for Sjogren's syndrome. *Eur J Immunol*. 1996;26(11):2742–2748. https://doi.org/10.1002/eji.1830261129.

98. Fabiani C, Barabino S, Rashid S, Dana MR. Corneal epithelial proliferation and thickness in a mouse model of dry eye. *Exp Eye Res*. 2009;89(2):166–171. https://doi.org/10.1016/j.exer.2009.03.003.

99. McClellan AJ, Volpe EA, Zhang X, et al. Ocular surface disease and dacryoadenitis in aging C57BL/6 mice. *Am J Pathol*. 2014;184(3):631–643. https://doi.org/10.1016/j.ajpath.2013.11.019.

100. Stepp MA, Pal-Ghosh S, Tadvalkar G, Williams A, Pflugfelder SC, de Paiva CS. Reduced intraepithelial corneal nerve density and sensitivity accompany desiccating stress and aging in C57BL/6 mice. *Exp Eye Res*. 2018;169:91–98. https://doi.org/10.1016/j.exer.2018.01.024.

101. De Silva MEH, Hill LJ, Downie LE, Chinnery HR. The effects of aging on corneal and ocular surface homeostasis in mice. *Investig Ophthalmol Vis Sci*. 2019;60(7): 2705–2715. https://doi.org/10.1167/iovs.19-26631.

102. Wang C, Zaheer M, Bian F, et al. Sjögren-like lacrimal Keratoconjunctivitis in germ-free mice. *Int J Mol Sci*. 2018;19(2). https://doi.org/10.3390/ijms19020565.

103. Marko CK, Menon BB, Chen G, Whitsett JA, Clevers H, Gipson IK. Spdef null mice lack conjunctival goblet cells and provide a model of dry eye. *Am J Pathol*. 2013; 183(1):35–48. https://doi.org/10.1016/j.ajpath.2013.03.017.

104. Floyd AM, Zhou X, Evans C, et al. Mucin deficiency causes functional and structural changes of the ocular surface. *PLoS One*. 2012;7(12). https://doi.org/10.1371/journal.pone.0050704.

105. Marko CK, Tisdale AS, Spurr-Michaud S, Evans C, Gipson IK. The ocular surface phenotype of Muc5ac and Muc5b null mice. *Investig Ophthalmol Vis Sci*. 2014; 55(1):291–300. https://doi.org/10.1167/iovs.13-13194.

106. Taketani Y, Marmalidou A, Dohlman TH, et al. Restoration of regulatory T-cell function in dry eye disease by antagonizing substance P/Neurokinin-1 receptor. *Am J Pathol*. 2020;190(9):1859–1866. https://doi.org/10.1016/j.ajpath.2020.05.011.

107. Yamada M, Ogata M, Kawai M, Mashima Y, Nishida T. Substance P and its metabolites in normal human tears. *Investig Ophthalmol Vis Sci*. 2002;43(8):2622–2625.

108. Yamada M, Ogata M, Kawai M, Mashima Y, Nishida T. Substance P in human tears. *Cornea*. 2003;22. https://doi.org/10.1097/00003226-200310001-00007.

109. Suvas S. Role of substance P neuropeptide in inflammation, wound healing, and tissue homeostasis. *J Immunol*. 2017;199(5):1543–1552. https://doi.org/10.4049/jimmunol.1601751.

110. Gaddipati S, Rao P, Jerome AD, Burugula BB, Gerard NP, Suvas S. Loss of neurokinin-1 receptor alters ocular surface homeostasis and promotes an early development of herpes stromal keratitis. *J Immunol*. 2016;197(10): 4021–4033. https://doi.org/10.4049/jimmunol.1600836.

111. Foulks GN, Bron AJ. Meibomian gland dysfunction: a clinical scheme for description, diagnosis, classification, and grading. *Ocul Surf*. 2003;1(3):107–126. https://doi.org/10.1016/S1542-0124(12)70139-8.

112. Gilbard JP, Rossi SR, Heyda KG. Tear film and ocular surface changes after closure of the meibomian gland orifices in the rabbit. *Ophthalmology*. 1989;96(8): 1180–1186. https://doi.org/10.1016/S0161-6420(89)32753-9.

113. Eom Y, Han JY, Kang B, et al. Meibomian glands and ocular surface changes after closure of meibomian gland orifices in rabbits. *Cornea*. 2018;37(2):218–226. https://doi.org/10.1097/ICO.0000000000001460.

114. Dong ZY, Ying M, Zheng J, Hu LJ, Xie JY, Ma Y. Evaluation of a rat meibomian gland dysfunction model induced by closure of meibomian gland orifices. *Int J Ophthalmol*. 2018;11(7):1077–1083. https://doi.org/10.18240/ijo.2018.07.01.

115. Jester JV, Nicolaides N, Kiss-Palvolgyi I, Smith RE. Meibomian gland dysfunction. II. The role of keratinization in a rabbit model of MGD. *Investig Ophthalmol Vis Sci*. 1989; 30(5):936–945.

116. Jester JV, Rife L, Nii D, Luttrull JK, Wilson L, Smith RE. In vivo biomicroscopy and photography of meibomian glands in a rabbit model of meibomian gland dysfunction. *Investig Ophthalmol Vis Sci*. 1982;22(5): 660–667.

117. Miyake H, Oda T, Katsuta O, Seno M, Nakamura M. Meibomian gland dysfunction model in hairless mice fed a special diet with limited lipid content. *Investig Ophthalmol Vis Sci.* 2016;57(7):3268–3275. https://doi.org/10.1167/iovs.16-19227.

118. Bu J, Wu Y, Cai X, et al. Hyperlipidemia induces meibomian gland dysfunction. *Ocul Surf.* 2019;17(4):777–786. https://doi.org/10.1016/j.jtos.2019.06.002.

119. Cui CY, Smith JA, Schlessinger D, Chan CC. X-linked anhidrotic ectodermal dysplasia disruption yields a mouse model for ocular surface disease and resultant blindness. *Am J Pathol.* 2005;167(1):89–95. https://doi.org/10.1016/S0002-9440(10)62956-2.

120. Wang YC, Li S, Chen X, et al. Meibomian gland absence related dry eye in ectodysplasin A mutant mice. *Am J Pathol.* 2016;186(1):32–42. https://doi.org/10.1016/j.ajpath.2015.09.019.

121. Cascallana JL, Bravo A, Donet E, et al. Ectoderm-targeted overexpression of the glucocorticoid receptor induces hypohidrotic ectodermal dysplasia. *Endocrinology.* 2005;146(6):2629–2638. https://doi.org/10.1210/en.2004-1246.

122. Reneker LW, Wang L, Irlmeier RT, Huang AJW. Fibroblast growth factor receptor 2 (FGFR2) is required for meibomian gland homeostasis in the adult mouse. *Investig Ophthalmol Vis Sci.* 2017;58(5):2638–2646. https://doi.org/10.1167/iovs.16-21204.

123. Yagyu H, Kitamine T, Osuga JI, et al. Absence of ACAT-1 attenuates atherosclerosis but 'causes dry eye and cutaneous xanthomatosis mice with congenital hyperlipidemia. *J Biol Chem.* 2000;275(28):21324–21330. https://doi.org/10.1074/jbc.M002541200.

124. Kenchegowda D, Swamynathan S, Gupta D, Wan H, Whitsett J, Swamynathan SK. Conditional disruption of mouse Klf5 results in defective eyelids with malformed meibomian glands, abnormal cornea and loss of conjunctival goblet cells. *Dev Biol.* 2011;356(1):5–18. https://doi.org/10.1016/j.ydbio.2011.05.005.

125. Tsau C, Ito M, Gromova A, Hoffman MP, Meech R, Makarenkova HP. Barx2 and Fgf10 regulate ocular glands branching morphogenesis by controlling extracellular matrix remodeling. *Development.* 2011;138(15):3307–3317. https://doi.org/10.1242/dev.066241.

126. Jester JV, Parfitt GJ, Brown DJ. Meibomian gland dysfunction: hyperkeratinization or atrophy? *BMC Ophthalmol.* 2015;15(1). https://doi.org/10.1186/s12886-015-0132-x.

127. Nien CJ, Massei S, Lin G, et al. Effects of age and dysfunction on human meibomian glands. *Arch Ophthalmol.* 2011;129(4):462–469. https://doi.org/10.1001/archophthalmol.2011.69.

128. Parfitt GJ, Xie Y, Geyfman M, Brown DJ, Jester JV. Absence of ductal hyper-keratinization in mouse age-related meibomian gland dysfunction (ARMGD). *Aging.* 2013;5(11):825–834. https://doi.org/10.18632/aging.100615.

129. Nien CJ, Paugh JR, Massei S, Wahlert AJ, Kao WW, Jester JV. Age-related changes in the meibomian gland. *Exp Eye Res.* 2009;89(6):1021–1027. https://doi.org/10.1016/j.exer.2009.08.013.

130. Yoon CH, Ryu JS, Hwang HS, Kim MK. Comparative analysis of age-related changes in lacrimal glands and meibomian glands of a c57bl/6 male mouse model. *Int J Mol Sci.* 2020;21(11):1–19. https://doi.org/10.3390/ijms21114169.

131. Sun M, Moreno IY, Dang M, Coulson-Thomas VJ. Meibomian gland dysfunction: what have animal models taught us? *Int J Mol Sci.* 2020;21(22). https://doi.org/10.3390/ijms21228822.

132. Pisella PJ, Fillacier K, Elena PP, Debbasch C, Baudouin C. Comparison of the effects of preserved and unpreserved formulations of timolol on the ocular surface of albino rabbits. *Ophthalmic Res.* 2000;32(1):3–8. https://doi.org/10.1159/000055579.

133. Pisella PJ, Pouliquen P, Baudouin C. Prevalence of ocular symptoms and signs with preserved and preservative free glaucoma medication. *Br J Ophthalmol.* 2002;86(4):418–423. https://doi.org/10.1136/bjo.86.4.418.

134. Xiong C, Chen D, Liu J, et al. A rabbit dry eye model induced by topical medication of a preservative benzalkonium chloride. *Investig Ophthalmol Vis Sci.* 2008;49(5):1850–1856. https://doi.org/10.1167/iovs.07-0720.

135. Li C, Song Y, Luan S, et al. Research on the stability of a rabbit dry eye model induced by topical application of the preservative benzalkonium chloride. *PLoS One.* 2012;7(3). https://doi.org/10.1371/journal.pone.0033688.

136. Ouyang W, Wu Y, Lin X, Wang S, Yang Y, Tang L, Liu Z, Wu J, Huang C, Zhou Y, Zhang X, Liu Z. Role of CD4+ T helper cells in the development of BAC-induced dry eye syndrome in mice. *Invest Ophthalmol Vis Sci.* 2021;62(1):25. https://doi.org/10.1167/iovs.62.1.25.

137. Sullivan DA, Sullivan BD, Ullman MD, et al. Androgen influence on the meibomian gland. *Investig Ophthalmol Vis Sci.* 2000;41(12):3732–3742.

138. Peng QH, Yao XL, Wu QL, Tan HY, Zhang JR. Effects of extract of Buddleja officinalis eye drops on androgen receptors of lacrimal gland cells of castrated rats with dry eye. *Int J Ophthalmol.* 2010;3(1):43–48. https://doi.org/10.3980/j.issn.2222-3959.2010.01.10.

139. Yao XL, Peng QH, Peng J, et al. Effects of extract of Buddleja officinalis on partial inflammation of lacrimal gland in castrated rabbits with dry eye. *Int J Ophthalmol.* 2010;3(2):114–119. https://doi.org/10.3980/j.issn.2222-3959.2010.02.05.

140. Li M, Zhang X, Sun Z, et al. Relationship between dynamic changes in expression of IL-17/IL-23 in lacrimal gland and ocular surface lesions in ovariectomized mice. *Eye Contact Lens.* 2018;44(1):35–43. https://doi.org/10.1097/ICL.0000000000000289.

141. Wu Y, Wu J, Bu J, et al. High-fat diet induces dry eye-like ocular surface damages in murine. *Ocul Surf.* 2020;18(2):267–276. https://doi.org/10.1016/j.jtos.2020.02.009.

142. He X, Zhao Z, Wang S, et al. High-fat diet–induced functional and pathologic changes in lacrimal gland. *Am J Pathol.* 2020;190(12):2387–2402. https://doi.org/10.1016/j.ajpath.2020.09.002.

143. Luo L, Li DQ, Corrales RM, Pflugfelder SC. Hyperosmolar saline is a proinflammatory stress on the mouse ocular surface. *Eye Contact Lens.* 2005;31(5):186−193. https://doi.org/10.1097/01.ICL.0000162759.79740.46.

144. Li H, Li J, Hou C, Li J, Peng H, Wang Q. The effect of astaxanthin on inflammation in hyperosmolarity of experimental dry eye model in vitro and in vivo. *Exp Eye Res.* 2020;197. https://doi.org/10.1016/j.exer.2020.108113.

145. Yeh S, Song XJ, Farley W, Li DQ, Stern ME, Pflugfelder SC. Apoptosis of ocular surface cells in experimentally induced dry eye. *Investig Ophthalmol Vis Sci.* 2003;44(1):124−129. https://doi.org/10.1167/iovs.02-0581.

146. Suhalim JL, Parfitt GJ, Xie Y, et al. Effect of desiccating stress on mouse meibomian gland function. *Ocul Surf.* 2014;12(1):59−68. https://doi.org/10.1016/j.jtos.2013.08.002.

147. Bron AJ, de Paiva CS, Chauhan SK, et al. TFOS DEWS II pathophysiology report. *Ocul Surf.* 2017;15(3):438−510. https://doi.org/10.1016/j.jtos.2017.05.011.

148. Cursiefen C. Immune privilege and angiogenic privilege of the cornea. *Chem Immunol Allergy.* 2007;92:50−57. https://doi.org/10.1159/000099253.

149. Ambati BK, Nozaki M, Singh N, et al. Corneal avascularity is due to soluble VEGF receptor-1. *Nature.* 2006;443(7114):993−997. https://doi.org/10.1038/nature05249.

150. Cursiefen C, Chen L, Saint-Geniez M, et al. Nonvascular VEGF receptor 3 expression by corneal epithelium maintains avascularity and vision. *Proc Natl Acad Sci U S A.* 2006;103(30):11405−11410. https://doi.org/10.1073/pnas.0506112103.

151. Hattori T, Takahashi H, Dana R. Novel insights into the immunoregulatory function and localization of dendritic cells. *Cornea.* 2016;35(11):S49−S54. https://doi.org/10.1097/ICO.0000000000001005.

152. Lutz MB, Schuler G. Immature, semi-mature and fully mature dendritic cells: which signals induce tolerance or immunity? *Trends Immunol.* 2002;23(9):445−449. https://doi.org/10.1016/S1471-4906(02)02281-0.

153. Shen L, Jin Y, Freeman GJ, Sharpe AH, Dana MR. The function of donor versus recipient programmed death-ligand 1 in corneal allograft survival. *J Immunol.* 2007;179(6):3672−3679. https://doi.org/10.4049/jimmunol.179.6.3672.

154. Griffith TS, Brunner T, Fletcher SM, Green DR, Ferguson TA. Fas ligand-induced apoptosis as a mechanism of immune privilege. *Science.* 1995;270(5239):1189−1192. https://doi.org/10.1126/science.270.5239.1189.

155. Singh RB, Blanco T, Mittal SK, et al. Pigment Epithelium-derived Factor secreted by corneal epithelial cells regulates dendritic cell maturation in dry eye disease. *Ocul Surf.* 2020;18(3):460−469. https://doi.org/10.1016/j.jtos.2020.05.002.

156. Freeman GJ, Long AJ, Iwai Y, et al. Engagement of the PD-1 immunoinhibitory receptor by a novel B7 family member leads to negative regulation of lymphocyte activation. *J Exp Med.* 2000;192(7):1027−1034. https://doi.org/10.1084/jem.192.7.1027.

157. El-Annan J, Goyal S, Zhang Q, Freeman GJ, Sharpe AH, Dana R. Regulation of T-cell chemotaxis by programmed Death-Ligand 1 (PD-L1) in dry eye-associated corneal inflammation. *Investig Ophthalmol Vis Sci.* 2010;51(7):3418−3423. https://doi.org/10.1167/iovs.09-3684.

158. Jin Y, Chauhan SK, Annan JEI, Sage PT, Sharpe AH, Dana R. A novel function for programmed death ligand-1 regulation of angiogenesis. *Am J Pathol.* 2011;178(4):1922−1929. https://doi.org/10.1016/j.ajpath.2010.12.027.

159. Suda T, Takahashi T, Golstein P, Nagata S. Molecular cloning and expression of the fas ligand, a novel member of the tumor necrosis factor family. *Cell.* 1993;75(6):1169−1178. https://doi.org/10.1016/0092-8674(93)90326-L.

160. Ferguson TA, Griffith TS. A vision of cell death: fas ligand and immune privilege 10 years later. *Immunol Rev.* 2006;213(1):228−238. https://doi.org/10.1111/j.1600-065X.2006.00430.x.

161. Hohlbaum AM, Moe S, Marshak-Rothstein A. Opposing effects of transmembrane and soluble Fas ligand expression on inflammation and tumor cell survival. *J Exp Med.* 2000;191(7):1209−1219. https://doi.org/10.1084/jem.191.7.1209.

162. Krishnan A, Fei F, Jones A, et al. Overexpression of soluble fas ligand following adeno-associated virus gene therapy prevents retinal ganglion cell death in chronic and acute murine models of glaucoma. *J Immunol.* 2016;197(12):4626−4638. https://doi.org/10.4049/jimmunol.1601488.

163. Dawson DW, Volpert OV, Gillis P, et al. Pigment epithelium-derived factor: a potent inhibitor of angiogenesis. *Science.* 1999;285(5425):245−248. https://doi.org/10.1126/science.285.5425.245.

164. Ribeiro SMF, Poczatek M, Schultz-Cherry S, Villain M, Murphy-Ullrich JE. The activation sequence of thrombospondin-1 interacts with the latency- associated peptide to regulate activation of latent transforming growth factor-β. *J Biol Chem.* 1999;274(19):13586−13593. https://doi.org/10.1074/jbc.274.19.13586.

165. Cursiefen C, Masli S, Ng TF, et al. Roles of thrombospondin-1 and -2 in regulating corneal and iris angiogenesis. *Investig Ophthalmol Vis Sci.* 2004;45(4):1117−1124. https://doi.org/10.1167/iovs.03-0940.

166. Yabe T, Sanagi T, Yamada H. The neuroprotective role of PEDF: implication for the therapy of neurological disorders. *Curr Mol Med.* 2010;10(3):259−266. https://doi.org/10.2174/156652410791065354.

167. Dastjerdi MH, Dana R. Corneal nerve alterations in dry eye-associated ocular surface disease. *Int Ophthalmol Clin.* 2009;49(1):11−20. https://doi.org/10.1097/IIO.0b013e31819242c9.

168. Ferrari G, Chauhan SK, Ueno H, et al. A novel mouse model for neurotrophic keratopathy: trigeminal nerve stereotactic electrolysis through the brain. *Investig*

Ophthalmol Vis Sci. 2011;52(5):2532–2539. https://doi.org/10.1167/iovs.10-5688.

169. Ueno H, Ferrari G, Hattori T, et al. Dependence of corneal stem/progenitor cells on ocular surface innervation. *Investig Ophthalmol Vis Sci*. 2012;53(2):867–872. https://doi.org/10.1167/iovs.11-8438.

170. Ferrari G, Hajrasouliha AR, Sadrai Z, Ueno H, Chauhan SK, Dana R. Nerves and neovessels inhibit each other in the cornea. *Investig Ophthalmol Vis Sci*. 2013;54(1):813–820. https://doi.org/10.1167/iovs.11-8379.

171. Kheirkhah A, Dohlman TH, Amparo F, et al. Effects of corneal nerve density on the response to treatment in dry eye disease. *Ophthalmology*. 2015;122(4):662–668. https://doi.org/10.1016/j.ophtha.2014.11.006.

172. Benítez Del Castillo JM, Wasfy MAS, Fernandez C, Garcia-Sanchez J. An in vivo confocal masked study on corneal epithelium and subbasal nerves in patients with dry eye. *Investig Ophthalmol Vis Sci*. 2004;45(9):3030–3035. https://doi.org/10.1167/iovs.04-0251.

173. Szliter EA, Lighvani S, Barrett RP, Hazlett LD. Vasoactive intestinal peptide balances pro- and anti-inflammatory cytokines in the *Pseudomonas aeruginosa* -infected cornea and protects against corneal perforation. *J Immunol*. 2007;178(2):1105–1114. https://doi.org/10.4049/jimmunol.178.2.1105.

174. Luo L, Li DQ, Doshi A, Farley W, Corrales RM, Pflugfelder SC. Experimental dry eye stimulates production of inflammatory cytokines and MMP-9 and activates MAPK signaling pathways on the ocular surface. *Investig Ophthalmol Vis Sci*. 2004;45(12):4293–4301. https://doi.org/10.1167/iovs.03-1145.

175. Zheng X, de Paiva CS, Li DQ, Farley WJ, Pflugfelder SC. Desiccating stress promotion of Th17 differentiation by ocular surface tissues through a dendritic cell-mediated pathway. *Investig Ophthalmol Vis Sci*. 2010;51(6):3083–3091. https://doi.org/10.1167/iovs.09-3838.

176. Lee HS, Hattori T, Park EY, Stevenson W, Chauhan SK, Dana R. Expression of toll-like receptor 4 contributes to corneal inflammation in experimental dry eye disease. *Investig Ophthalmol Vis Sci*. 2012;53(9):5632–5640. https://doi.org/10.1167/iovs.12-9547.

177. Chen H, Gan X, Li Y, et al. NLRP12- and NLRC4-mediated corneal epithelial pyroptosis is driven by GSDMD cleavage accompanied by IL-33 processing in dry eye. *Ocul Surf*. 2020;18(4):783–794. https://doi.org/10.1016/j.jtos.2020.07.001.

178. Zheng Q, Ren Y, Reinach PS, et al. Reactive oxygen species activated NLRP3 inflammasomes prime environment-induced murine dry eye. *Exp Eye Res*. 2014;125:1–8. https://doi.org/10.1016/j.exer.2014.05.001.

179. Li DQ, Lokeshwar BL, Solomon A, Monroy D, Ji Z, Pflugfelder SC. Regulation of MMP-9 production by human corneal epithelial cells. *Exp Eye Res*. 2001;73(4):449–459. https://doi.org/10.1006/exer.2001.1054.

180. Pflugfelder SC, Farley W, Luo L, et al. Matrix metalloproteinase-9 knockout confers resistance to corneal epithelial barrier disruption in experimental dry eye. *Am J Pathol*. 2005;166(1):61–71. https://doi.org/10.1016/S0002-9440(10)62232-8.

181. Zhang Z, Yang WZ, Zhu ZZ, et al. Therapeutic effects of topical doxycycline in a benzalkonium chloride-induced mouse dry eye model. *Investig Ophthalmol Vis Sci*. 2014;55(5):2963–2974. https://doi.org/10.1167/iovs.13-13577.

182. Yoon KC, De Paiva CS, Qi H, et al. Expression of Th-1 chemokines and chemokine receptors on the ocular surface of C57BL/6 mice: effects of desiccating stress. *Investig Ophthalmol Vis Sci*. 2007;48(6):2561–2569. https://doi.org/10.1167/iovs.07-0002.

183. Mackay CR. Chemokines: immunology's high impact factors. *Nat Immunol*. 2001;2(2):95–101. https://doi.org/10.1038/84298.

184. Luster AD. Chemokines — Chemotactic Cytokines that mediate Inflammation. *N Engl J Med*. 1998;338(7):436–445. PMID: 9459648. https://doi.org/10.1056/NEJM199802123380706.

185. Goyal S, Chauhan SK, Zhang Q, Dana R. Amelioration of murine dry eye disease by topical antagonist to chemokine receptor 2. *Arch Ophthalmol*. 2009;127(7):882–887. https://doi.org/10.1001/archophthalmol.2009.125.

186. Kodati S, Chauhan SK, Chen Y, et al. CCR7 is critical for the induction and maintenance of Th17 immunity in dry eye disease. *Investig Ophthalmol Vis Sci*. 2014;55(9):5871–5877. https://doi.org/10.1167/iovs.14-14481.

187. Zhang X, Volpe EA, Gandhi NB, et al. NK cells promote Th-17 mediated corneal barrier disruption in dry eyeAshkar AA, ed. *PLoS One*. 2012;7(5):e36822. https://doi.org/10.1371/journal.pone.0036822.

188. Coursey TG, Bohat R, Barbosa FL, Pflugfelder SC, de Paiva CS. Desiccating stress–induced chemokine expression in the epithelium is dependent on upregulation of NKG2D/RAE-1 and release of IFN-γ in experimental dry eye. *J Immunol*. 2014;193(10):5264–5272. https://doi.org/10.4049/jimmunol.1400016.

189. Fan NW, Dohlman TH, Foulsham W, et al. The role of Th17 immunity in chronic ocular surface disorders. *Ocul Surf*. 2020. https://doi.org/10.1016/j.jtos.2020.05.009. Published online.

190. Verstappen GM, Corneth OBJ, Bootsma H, Kroese FGM. Th17 cells in primary Sjögren's syndrome: pathogenicity and plasticity. *J Autoimmun*. 2018;87:16–25. https://doi.org/10.1016/j.jaut.2017.11.003.

191. Dana R. Corneal antigen presentation: molecular regulation and functional implications. *Ocul Surf*. 2005;3(4):S169–S172. https://doi.org/10.1016/s1542-0124(12)70248-3.

192. Schaumburg CS, Siemasko KF, De Paiva CS, et al. Ocular surface APCs are necessary for autoreactive T cell-mediated experimental autoimmune lacrimal keratoconjunctivitis. *J Immunol*. 2011;187(7):3653–3662. https://doi.org/10.4049/jimmunol.1101442.

193. Hamrah P, Liu Y, Zhang Q, Dana MR. Alterations in corneal stromal dendritic cell phenotype and distribution in inflammation. *Arch Ophthalmol*. 2003;121(8):1132–1140. https://doi.org/10.1001/archopht.121.8.1132.

194. Takada K, Takiguchi M, Konno A, Inaba M. Autoimmunity against a tissue kallikrein in IQI/Jic mice: a model for sjögren's syndrome. *J Biol Chem.* 2005;280(5): 3982–3988. https://doi.org/10.1074/jbc.M410157200.

195. Jiang G, Ke Y, Sun D, et al. A new model of experimental autoimmune keratoconjunctivitis sicca (KCS) induced in Lewis rat by the autoantigen Klk1b22. *Investig Ophthalmol Vis Sci.* 2009;50(5):2245–2254. https://doi.org/10.1167/iovs.08-1949.

196. Stern ME, Schaumburg CS, Siemasko KF, et al. Autoantibodies contribute to the immunopathogenesis of experimental dry eye disease. *Invest Ophthalmol Vis Sci.* 2012; 53(4):2062–2075. https://doi.org/10.1167/iovs.11-9299.

197. Wang T, Li W, Cheng H, Zhong L, Deng J, Ling S. The important role of the chemokine Axis CCR7-CCL19 and CCR7-CCL21 in the pathophysiology of the immuno-inflammatory response in dry eye disease. *Ocul Immunol Inflamm.* 2019. https://doi.org/10.1080/09273948.2019.1674891. Published online.

198. Goyal S, Chauhan SK, El Annan J, Nallasamy N, Zhang Q, Dana R. Evidence of corneal lymphangiogenesis in dry eye disease: a potential link to adaptive immunity? *Arch Ophthalmol.* 2010;128(7):819–824. https://doi.org/10.1001/archophthalmol.2010.124.

199. Chauhan SK, Jin Y, Goyal S, et al. A novel prolymphangiogenic function for Th17/IL-17. *Blood.* 2011; 118(17):4630–4634. https://doi.org/10.1182/blood-2011-01-332049.

200. Goyal S, Chauhan SK, Dana R. Blockade of prolymphangiogenic vascular endothelial growth factor C in dry eye disease. *Arch Ophthalmol.* 2012;130(1):84–89. https://doi.org/10.1001/archophthalmol.2011.266.

201. Ecoiffier T, El Annan J, Rashid S, Schaumberg D, Dana R. Modulation of integrin α4 β1 (VLA-4) in dry eye disease. *Arch Ophthalmol.* 2008;126(12):1695–1699. https://doi.org/10.1001/archopht.126.12.1695.

202. Annan J El, Chauhan SK, Ecoiffier T, Zhang Q, Saban DR, Dana R. Characterization of effector T cells in dry eye disease. *Investig Ophthalmol Vis Sci.* 2009;50(8): 3802–3807. https://doi.org/10.1167/iovs.08-2417.

203. Grewal IS, Flavell RA. CD40 and CD154 in cell-mediated immunity. *Annu Rev Immunol.* 1998;16:111–135. https://doi.org/10.1146/annurev.immunol.16.1.111.

204. De Paiva CS, Villarreal AL, Corrales RM, et al. Dry eye-induced conjunctival epithelial squamous metaplasia is modulated by interferon-γ. *Investig Ophthalmol Vis Sci.* 2007;48(6):2553–2560. https://doi.org/10.1167/iovs.07-0069.

205. Chauhan SK, Dana R. Role of Th17 cells in the immunopathogenesis of dry eye disease. *Mucosal Immunol.* 2009; 2(4):375–376. https://doi.org/10.1038/mi.2009.21.

206. Stockinger B, Veldhoen M. Differentiation and function of Th17 T cells. *Curr Opin Immunol.* 2007;19(3): 281–286. https://doi.org/10.1016/j.coi.2007.04.005.

207. Bettelli E, Carrier Y, Gao W, et al. Reciprocal developmental pathways for the generation of pathogenic effector TH17 and regulatory T cells. *Nature.* 2006; 441(7090):235–238. https://doi.org/10.1038/nature04753.

208. Sadrai Z, Stevenson W, Okanobo A, et al. PDE4 inhibition suppresses IL-17-associated immunity in dry eye disease. *Investig Ophthalmol Vis Sci.* 2012;53(7): 3584–3591. https://doi.org/10.1167/iovs.11-9110.

209. Dohlman TH, Ding J, Dana R, Chauhan SK. T cell–derived granulocyte-macrophage colony-stimulating factor contributes to dry eye disease pathogenesis by promoting CD11b+ Myeloid cell maturation and migration. *Investig Ophthalmol Vis Sci.* 2017;58(2): 1330–1336. https://doi.org/10.1167/iovs.16-20789.

210. Sundrud MS, Trivigno C. Identity crisis of Th17 cells: many forms, many functions, many questions. *Semin Immunol.* 2013;25(4):263–272. https://doi.org/10.1016/j.smim.2013.10.021.

211. Piccirillo CA, Shevach EM. Naturally-occurring CD4+CD25+ immunoregulatory T cells: central players in the arena of peripheral tolerance. *Semin Immunol.* 2004;16(2):81–88. https://doi.org/10.1016/j.smim.2003.12.003.

212. Kretschmer K, Apostolou I, Hawiger D, Khazaie K, Nussenzweig MC, von Boehmer H. Inducing and expanding regulatory T cell populations by foreign antigen. *Nat Immunol.* 2005;6(12):1219–1227. https://doi.org/10.1038/ni1265.

213. Sakaguchi S, Yamaguchi T, Nomura T, Ono M. Regulatory T cells and immune tolerance. *Cell.* 2008;133(5): 775–787. https://doi.org/10.1016/j.cell.2008.05.009.

214. Foulsham W, Marmalidou A, Amouzegar A, Coco G, Chen Y, Dana R. Review: the function of regulatory T cells at the ocular surface. *Ocul Surf.* 2017;15(4): 652–659. https://doi.org/10.1016/j.jtos.2017.05.013.

215. Rubtsov YP, Niec RE, Josefowicz S, et al. Stability of the regulatory T cell lineage in vivo. *Science.* 2010; 329(5999):1667–1671. https://doi.org/10.1126/science.1191996.

216. Kimura A, Kishimoto T. IL-6: regulator of Treg/Th17 balance. *Eur J Immunol.* 2010;40(7):1830–1835. https://doi.org/10.1002/eji.201040391.

217. Noack M, Miossec P. Th17 and regulatory T cell balance in autoimmune and inflammatory diseases. *Autoimmun Rev.* 2014;13(6):668–677. https://doi.org/10.1016/j.autrev.2013.12.004.

218. Zhang X, Schaumburg CS, Coursey TG, et al. CD8+ cells regulate the T helper-17 response in an experimental murine model of sjögren syndrome. *Mucosal Immunol.* 2014; 7(2):417–427. https://doi.org/10.1038/mi.2013.61.

219. Coursey TG, Gandhi NB, Volpe EA, Pflugfelder SC, De Paiva CS. Chemokine receptors CCR6 and CXCR3 are necessary for CD4+ T cell mediated ocular surface disease in experimental dry eye disease. *PLoS One.* 2013;8(11): e78508. https://doi.org/10.1371/journal.pone.0078508. Ashour HM.

220. Dohlman TH, Chauhan SK, Kodati S, et al. The CCR6/CCL20 axis mediates Th17 cell migration to the ocular surface in dry eye disease. *Investig Ophthalmol Vis Sci.*

2013;54(6):4081−4091. https://doi.org/10.1167/iovs.1 2-11216.

221. Sato W, Aranami T, Yamamura T. Cutting edge: human Th17 cells are identified as bearing CCR2 + CCR5 − phenotype. *J Immunol.* 2007;178(12):7525−7529. https://doi.org/10.4049/jimmunol.178.12.7525.

222. Kara EE, McKenzie DR, Bastow CR, et al. CCR2 defines in vivo development and homing of IL-23-driven GM-CSF-producing Th17 cells. *Nat Commun.* 2015;6. https://doi.org/10.1038/ncomms9644.

223. Guimaraes De Souza R, Yu Z, Stern ME, Pflugfelder SC, De Paiva CS. Suppression of Th1-mediated keratoconjuncti-vitis sicca by Lifitegrast. *J Ocul Pharmacol Therapeut.* 2018; 34(7):543−549. https://doi.org/10.1089/jop.2018.0047.

224. Perez VL, Pflugfelder SC, Zhang S, Shojaei A, Haque R. Lifitegrast, a novel integrin antagonist for treatment of dry eye disease. *Ocul Surf.* 2016;14(2):207−215. https://doi.org/10.1016/j.jtos.2016.01.001.

225. McGeachy MJ, Cua DJ. Th17 cell differentiation: the long and winding road. *Immunity.* 2008;28(4):445−453. https://doi.org/10.1016/j.immuni.2008.03.001.

226. Ouyang W, Kolls JK, Zheng Y. The biological functions of T helper 17 cell effector cytokines in inflammation. *Im-munity.* 2008;28(4):454−467. https://doi.org/10.1016/j.immuni.2008.03.004.

227. Zhang X, Chen W, De Paiva CS, et al. Interferon-γ exacer-bates dry eye-induced apoptosis in conjunctiva through dual apoptotic pathways. *Investig Ophthalmol Vis Sci.* 2011;52(9):6279−6285. https://doi.org/10.1167/iovs.1 0-7081.

228. Ko BY, Xiao Y, Barbosa FL, de Paiva CS, Pflugfelder SC. Goblet cell loss abrogates ocular surface immune tolerance. *JCI Insight.* 2018;3(3). https://doi.org/10.1172/jci.insight.98222.

229. Zhang X, De Paiva CS, Su Z, Volpe EA, Li DQ, Pflugfelder SC. Topical interferon-gamma neutralization prevents conjunctival goblet cell loss in experimental mu-rine dry eye. *Exp Eye Res.* 2014;118:117−124. https://doi.org/10.1016/j.exer.2013.11.011.

230. Kryczek I, Zhao E, Liu Y, et al. Human TH17 cells are long-lived effector memory cells. *Sci Transl Med.* 2011; 3(104). https://doi.org/10.1126/scitranslmed.3002949.

231. Muranski P, Borman ZA, Kerkar SP, et al. Th17 cells are long lived and retain a stem cell-like molecular signature. *Immunity.* 2011;35(6):972−985. https://doi.org/10.1016/j.immuni.2011.09.019.

232. Fan N-W, Chen Y, Afsaneh Amouzegar RD. Contribution of effector T helper 17/1 (eTh17/1) versus effector Th17 cells (eTh17) to memory pool in dry eye disease. *Investig Ophthalmol Vis Sci.* 2019;60(9):1415.

233. Routsias JG, Tzioufas AG. Sjögren's syndrome - study of autoantigens and autoantibodies. *Clin Rev Allergy Immu-nol.* 2007;32(3):238−251. https://doi.org/10.1007/s12016-007-8003-8.

234. Yamamoto H, Sims NE, Macauley SP, Nguyen KHT, Nakagawa Y, Humphreys-Beher MG. Alterations in the secretory response of non-obese diabetic (NOD) mice to muscarinic receptor stimulation. *Clin Immunol*

Immunopathol. 1996;78(3):245−255. https://doi.org/10.1006/clin.1996.0036.

235. Bacman S, Berra A, Sterin-Borda L, Borda E. Muscarinic acetylcholine receptor antibodies as a new marker of dry eye Sjögren syndrome. *Investig Ophthalmol Vis Sci.* 2001;42(2):321−327.

236. Iizuka M, Wakamatsu E, Tsuboi H, et al. Pathogenic role of immune response to M3 muscarinic acetylcholine re-ceptor in Sjögren's syndrome-like sialoadenitis. *J Autoimmun.* 2010. https://doi.org/10.1016/j.jaut.2010.08.004. Published online.

237. Hayakawa I, Tedder TF, Zhuang Y. B-lymphocyte deple-tion ameliorates Sjögren's syndrome in Id3 knockout mice. *Immunology.* 2007;122(1):73−79. https://doi.org/10.1111/j.1365-2567.2007.02614.x.

238. Subbarayal B, Chauhan SK, Di Zazzo A, Dana R. IL-17 augments B cell activation in ocular surface autoimmunity. *J Immunol.* 2016;197(9):3464−3470. https://doi.org/10.4049/jimmunol.1502641.

239. Stern ME, Beuerman RW, Fox RI, Gao J, Mircheff AK, Pflugfelder SC. The pathology of dry eye: the interaction between the ocular surface and lacrimal glands. *Cornea.* 1998;17(6):584−589. https://doi.org/10.1097/0000322 6-199811000-00002.

240. Törnwall J, Lane TE, Fox RI, Fox HS. T cell attractant che-mokine expression initiates lacrimal gland destruction in nonobese diabetic mice. *Lab Invest.* 1999;79(12): 1719−1726.

241. Jabs DA, Lee B, Whittum-Hudson JA, Prendergast RA. Th1 versus Th2 immune responses in autoimmune lacrimal gland disease in MRL/Mp mice. *Investig Ophthalmol Vis Sci.* 2000;41(3):826−831.

242. Jabs DA, Prendergast RA. Reactive lymphocytes in lacrimal gland and vasculitic renal lesions of autoim-mune MRL/lpr mice express L3T4. *J Exp Med.* 1987. https://doi.org/10.1084/jem.166.4.1198. Published online.

243. Gao J, Morgan G, Tieu D, et al. ICAM-1 expression predis-poses ocular tissues to immune-based inflammation in dry eye patients and Sjögrens syndrome-like MRL/lpr mice. *Exp Eye Res.* 2004;78(4):823−835. https://doi.org/10.1016/j.exer.2003.10.024.

244. Voigt A, Esfandiary L, Wanchoo A, et al. Sexual dimorphic function of IL-17 in salivary gland dysfunction of the C57BL/6.NOD-Aec1Aec2 model of Sjögren's syndrome. *Sci Rep.* 2016;6. https://doi.org/10.1038/srep38717.

245. Chivasso C, Sarrand J, Perret J, Delporte C, Soyfoo MS. The involvement of innate and adaptive immunity in the initiation and perpetuation of sjögren's syndrome. *Int J Mol Sci.* 2021;22(2):1−21. https://doi.org/10.3390/ijms22020658.

246. Ortiz G, Chao C, Jamali A, et al. Effect of dry eye disease on the kinetics of lacrimal gland dendritic cells as visualized by intravital multi-photon microscopy. *Front Immunol.* 2020;11. https://doi.org/10.3389/fimmu.2020.01713.

247. Rahman M, Okamoto K, Thompson R, Katagiri A, Bereiter DA. Sensitization of trigeminal brainstem path-ways in a model for tear deficient dry eye. *Pain.* 2015;

156(5):942—950. https://doi.org/10.1097/j.pain.00000 00000000135.

248. Stepp MA, Pal-Ghosh S, Tadvalkar G, Williams AR, Pflugfelder SC, de Paiva CS. Reduced corneal innervation in the CD25 null model of Sjögren syndrome. *Int J Mol Sci.* 2018;19(12). https://doi.org/10.3390/ijms19123821.

249. Liu L, Dana R, Yin J. Sensory neurons directly promote angiogenesis in response to inflammation via substance P signaling. *FASEB J.* 2020;34(5):6229—6243. https://doi.org/10.1096/fj.201903236R.

250. Goronzy JJ, Weyand CM. Immune aging and autoimmunity. *Cell Mol Life Sci.* 2012;69(10):1615—1623. https://doi.org/10.1007/s00018-012-0970-0.

251. Farrand KF, Fridman M, Stillman IÖ, Schaumberg DA. Prevalence of diagnosed dry eye disease in the United States among adults aged 18 Years and older. *Am J Ophthalmol.* 2017;182:90—98. https://doi.org/10.1016/j.ajo.2017.06.033.

252. Tatematsu Y, Khan Q, Blanco T, et al. Thrombospondin-1 is necessary for the development and repair of corneal nerves. *Int J Mol Sci.* 2018;19(10). https://doi.org/10.3390/ijms19103191.

253. Foulsham W, Mittal SK, Taketani Y, et al. Aged mice exhibit severe exacerbations of dry eye disease with an amplified memory Th17 cell response. *Am J Pathol.* 2020;190(7):1474—1482. https://doi.org/10.1016/j.ajpath.2020.03.016.

254. Bian F, Xiao Y, Barbosa FL, et al. Age-associated antigen-presenting cell alterations promote dry-eye inducing Th1

cells. *Mucosal Immunol.* 2019;12(4):897—908. https://doi.org/10.1038/s41385-018-0127-z.

255. Wan SJ, Sullivan AB, Shieh P, et al. IL-1R and MyD88 contribute to the absence of a bacterial microbiome on the healthy murine cornea. *Front Microbiol.* 2018;9. https://doi.org/10.3389/fmicb.2018.01117. MAY.

256. Trujillo-Vargas CM, Schaefer L, Alam J, Pflugfelder SC, Britton RA, de Paiva CS. The gut-eye-lacrimal gland-microbiome axis in Sjögren Syndrome. *Ocul Surf.* 2020;18(2):335—344. https://doi.org/10.1016/j.jtos.2019.10.006.

257. Horai R, Caspi RR. Microbiome and autoimmune uveitis. *Front Immunol.* 2019;10. https://doi.org/10.3389/fimmu.2019.00232. FEB.

258. Horai R, Zárate-Bladés CR, Dillenburg-Pilla P, et al. Microbiota-dependent activation of an autoreactive T cell receptor provokes autoimmunity in an immunologically privileged site. *Immunity.* 2015;43(2):343—353. https://doi.org/10.1016/j.immuni.2015.07.014.

259. De Paiva CS, Jones DB, Stern ME, et al. Altered mucosal microbiome diversity and disease severity in sjögren syndrome. *Sci Rep.* 2016;6. https://doi.org/10.1038/srep23561.

260. Kim J, Choi SH, Kim YJ, et al. Clinical effect of IRT-5 probiotics on immune modulation of autoimmunity or alloimmunity in the eye. *Nutrients.* 2017;9(11). https://doi.org/10.3390/nu9111166.

CHAPTER 5

Pathophysiology of Dry Eye Disease Using Human Models

PENNY A. ASBELL, MD, FACS, MBA, FARVO • ÖMÜR Ö. UÇAKHAN, MD

INTRODUCTION

Dry eye disease (DED) is an umbrella term that represents a wide spectrum of disorders with different clinical presentations and variable risk factors. In 2017, in light of studies performed up to that date, the Tear Film and Ocular Surface Dry Eye Workshop II (TFOS DEWS II) defined DED as, "a multifactorial disease of the ocular surface characterized by a loss of homeostasis[1–44] of the tear film, and accompanied by ocular symptoms, in which tear film instability and hyperosmolarity, ocular surface inflammation and damage, and neurosensory abnormalities play etiological roles." This definition clearly aims to embrace the diverse pathophysiological changes underlying the disease, which may be key to early detection and new treatment development.

Studies on DED in humans have led to the classification of the disease as aqueous deficient or evaporative, however, though usually both conditions coexist as part of a continuum called "hybrid" DED. A plethora of risk factors from systemic diseases to environmental pollution can lead to tear film instability or hyperosmolarity, which in turn initiate a vicious circle involving inflammation and apoptosis of ocular surface epithelium, and neural dysfunction. The elucidation of distinct pathways underlying various clinical phenotypes by means of meticulous ophthalmic examination and appropriate testing is critical in planning treatment of individual patients with DED. However, there is currently no "pathognomonic" or "gold standard" test to diagnose DED. Further complicating the diagnosis is the discordance between signs and symptoms of the disease. Therefore, for the clinician, DED mostly remains as a diagnosis made for a variety of ocular surface problems, typically associated with symptoms of eye discomfort or eye pain, after eliminating other potential pathologies.

In this review, we cover some of the major findings related to pathophysiology of DED; tear film/ocular surface alterations, corneal morphological changes observed in neuropathic pain, aqueous versus evaporative DED and some systemic diseases, effect of age, sex, environmental factors on DED, preservative toxicity and DED, and effect of microbiome on DED. As expected, the human data is less coherent than data from animal and/or tissue culture research, but also demonstrates the heterogeneity of DED. Furthermore, outcome measures and measurement techniques may be less than reproducible from site to site, making comparison between studies difficult to analyze. Despite these shortcomings, we aim to highlight some of the major areas of research in humans with and without DED, mainly looking for tests that can be performed in humans to better diagnose DED, determine severity, and/or evaluate response to treatment.

CLINICAL FINDINGS IN HUMAN STUDIES OF DRY EYE DISEASE

Inflammatory Markers in Tears-Overview

Tear hyperosmolarity and tear film instability are recognized as important drivers of DED,[45] with tear hyperosmolarity a likely trigger of the acute immune response.[46] Stress induced by desiccation provokes epithelial activation, involving pathways by which the production of inflammatory mediators at the ocular surface is stimulated.[47–49] The subsequent activation of an adaptive immune response drives the inflammatory cascade, causing further damage to the ocular surface,[46] and this vicious cycle continues through the dysregulation of the immune system.[50] To more fully understand the inflammatory cascade in DED, tear analysis has been used to explore key mediators associated with DED. A number of molecular mediators, such as proinflammatory cytokines, chemokines, endopeptidases, and cell adhesion molecules have been studied extensively in DED patients as potential biomarkers of the disease. Sjo some mediators considered important in DED are interleukin-1b (IL-1b), IL-6, tumor necrosis factor-α (TNF-α), interferon-γ (IFN-γ), caspase 3, trans glutaminase-2 (TG-2), and matrix metalloproteinases (MMPs), such as MMP-3 and MMP-9.[51-55] It is hoped that inflammatory tear will better determine candidates for antiinflammatory therapy, more accurately determine disease activity, and provide objective therapeutic endpoints for clinical trials testing efficacy of new treatments for DED.

Matrix metalloproteinase-9

Among other cytokines, MMP-9 has a crucial role in initiation and progression of ocular surface disease. MMP-9 is a zinc and calcium ion−dependent enzyme important for tissue remodeling in normal physiological processes such as wound healing.

MMP-9 activity is regulated by epigenetic processes, cell−cell interactions, and cytokine-mediated pathways. The hyperosmolarity of the tear fluid seen in DED has been shown to trigger the stress-activated protein kinase (SAPK) signaling cascade, leading to the release of MMP-9 from corneal epithelial cells themselves, thus initiating a cycle of progressive inflammation.[55,56] MMP-9 cleaves tight junction proteins occludin and zonula occludens-1 (ZO-1), thereby disrupting the ocular surface epithelium.[57] MMP-9 also activates other inflammatory factors such as pro-IL-1 beta, pro-tumor necrosis factor (TNF)-alpha, and substance P. MMP-9 may also play role in processing molecules that initiate a positive feedback loop to increase EGFR signals to increase cell migration and upregulate MMP-9 expression.[58] Overall, T-cell recruitment, the proteolytic activity of the MMP-9 molecule itself, and activation of secretion of additional cytokines initiate a self-perpetuating cycle of inflammation, secretory dysfunction, corneal surface irregularity, and worsening eye dryness.[50,57]

The normal levels of MMP-9 (ng/mL) in human tears range from 3 to 41 ng/mL with a level less than 30 ng/mL in 90% of people.[56] The finding of elevated MMP-9 in experimental models of DED and human DED patients has led to the development of an easy-to-use point-of-care MMP-9 assay in unstimulated tear samples (InflammaDry, Rapid Pathogen Screening, Inc, Sarasota, FL, USA), to aid in the diagnosis of DED. The assay is considered positive when MMP-9 levels over 40 ng/mL are detected.[59]

In various studies, MMP-9 positivity as measured by InflammaDry ranged from 11% to 85% among patients with DED,[59-65] and 5.6−7.5% in healthy individuals in various studies.[59,66] Different diagnostic criteria for DED used in each study were suggested as a possible reason underlying the considerable variation in reported positivity. Furthermore, recently InflammaDry test results were shown to be influenced by tear volume. Low tear volume in aqueous tear-deficient DE may induce false-negative results, and reflex tearing during the test may induce false-positive results. Although not all patients with DED expressed this indicator of cell damage, in some studies, MMP-9 activity was reported to be strongly correlated with symptom scores, tear film break-up time (TBUT), conjunctival staining, corneal staining, Schirmer test, decrease in visual acuity, Schirmer test results, conjunctival staining, corneal staining, as well as the number of obstructed meibomian ducts, pathologic meibomian gland (MG) secretion, and surface area of abnormal superficial corneal epithelia,[55,59,60,66,67] whereas, in others, correlation between this test and tear osmolarity was poor in patients with mild DED,[62] and recently, Kook et al. could not demonstrate any correlation between MMP-9 test results and clinical DED indices in Sjögren's syndrome (SS) patients.[68]

In a retrospective cohort of DED patients, Soifer et al. reported that eyes with detectable MMP-9 had significantly decreased tear production over time compared to those without detectable MMP-9, suggesting a role for MMP-9 as a prognostic biomarker to predict long-term deterioration in DED.[69] Recent evidence also suggests that InflammaDry test may have predictive value for the success of antiinflammatory treatment and used to monitor treatment response. Ryu et al. reported that, following topical steroid treatment in patients with refractory DED, improvements in symptom and ocular surface staining scores were better in the MMP-9−positive subgroup of patients than in the MMP-9−negative group.[65] In another study, MMP-9−positive DED patients showed more favorable responses to topical cyclosporine A,[66] compared to MMP-9−negative patients, with decreased MMP-9 levels, improved OSDI scores, and increased TBUT, and Schirmer test results after a month of treatment. Aragona et al.[55] reported significantly higher expression of MMP-9 in SS compared to MG dysfunction patients, and SS patients with higher MMP-9 levels in the tear film showed a more favorable response to topical corticosteroid treatment. Lifitegrast 5% treatment was also reported to normalize MMP-9 levels in 38.9% of a retrospective cohort of 54 DED patient eyes with initial positive InflammaDry test.[70] Choi et al. reported statistically significantly more MMP-9 conversion rate in tears of patients who underwent botulinum toxin type A (BTX-A) injection to the medial part of the upper and lower eyelids (76.92%) compared to those who received saline injection (38.46%).[71]

Further studies regarding the reproducibility of the InflammaDry test and development of other such point-of-care diagnostics for markers of DED disease, "lab-on-a-stick" may help both diagnosis and evaluation of response to treatment would be valuable for the management of DED.

Inflammatory cytokines in tears of subpopulations of DED

Tear levels of IL-1, IL-6, and IL-8 were noted to be increased, and epidermal growth factor (EGF) decreased in SS patients; these increased concentrations were associated with the severity of DED clinical parameters, such as greater corneal staining and lower tear secretion.[72−74]

Tear inflammatory cytokine levels in dry eye with rheumatoid arthritis (RA) also correlated with corneal dendritic cell (DC) density at in vivo confocal microscopy (IVCM), and IL-1 and IL-6 concentrations decreased after the systemic treatment of RA.[75] Jackson et al. found significant correlations between tear IFN-γ concentrations, tear osmolarity, total ocular surface staining, and Schirmer's test score, all key clinical diagnostic parameters for DED, suggesting IFN-γ as a potential biomarker of tear hyperosmolarity associated with evaporative DED.[76]

Regarding changes to tears, previous studies have shown elevated IFN-γ levels in tears in patients with meibomian gland disease (MGD),[76] elevated IL-8 levels in SJS,[77] elevated levels of TNF-γ and TGF-β1 with decreased levels of EGF in trachoma,[78] elevated IL-8 and MMP-9 levels in OCP,[79] and IL-17, IL-1β, IL-6, and IL-8 levels in Graves' ophthalmopathy with exposure keratitis,[80] compared to normal controls.

Studies also reported reduced tear cytokine levels as to assess the effectiveness of topical steroid treatment in DED[81,82] or intense pulsed light therapy in treating dry eye due to MGD.[83]

Among several cytokines, interleukin-8 (IL-8) is consistently found in the tear film and conjunctiva of patients with dry eye.[84,85] It can be produced by any cell with toll-like receptors, such as epithelial cells and macrophages, and acts as a chemoattractant for neutrophils, as part of the innate immune response. A recent metaanalysis of 13 articles investigating 342 DED patients and 205 healthy controls reported significantly higher concentrations of the tear inflammatory mediators IL-1, IL-6, IL-8, IL-10, IFN-γ, TNF-α, in the tears of DED patients as compared to age-matched non-DED control subjects. Conversely, the evidence of difference was less strong for IL-17A and IL-2.[82] However, the authors cautioned against determining clinical significance, since they noted large standard deviations reported in these studies, suggesting substantial interindividual variation in cytokine concentrations that was not explained.

Tear analysis and DED

In summary, studies have pointed the association associateion of tear cytokines with DED[86] however, no consensus has been reached in regards to tear collection, methods of analysis, cut-off values, and which cytokines are best associated with ocular surface disease and/or dry eye stymptoms. Overall, although DED seems to be accompanied by release of cytokines in tears, the analysis of tear cytokines as a biomarker for DED is still an unmet need, since the variability in tear collection, sampling, storage, and analytical methods seem to have generated inconsistent data, not allowing the estimation of either a reference interval for control subjects and a cut-off value between the DED and controls.[87]

Cell Surface Markers
Major histocompatibility complex

Human leukocyte antigen D-related (HLA-DR) is a type of major histocompatibility complex class II cell surface receptor involved with antigen presentation. HLA-DR is often used as a marker of loss of immunosilencing on the ocular surface, and is one of the most commonly studied inflammatory markers in DED.[88−94] Although HLA-DR is a surface receptor that is constitutively expressed on antigen-presenting cells and immune cells,[95] under pathological conditions, it can be conditionally induced in CD45-negative conjunctival epithelial cells to regulate ocular surface immune responses.[96,97] In DED, hyperosmolarity was shown to induce HLA-DR overexpression in human conjunctival epithelial cells,[91,92,98] and this upregulation was suggested to be driven by IFN-γ as shown in Sjögren's patients.[99]

Studies investigating HLA-DR expression (HLA-DR %) in DED patients using impression cytology (IC) have generally reported elevated HLA-DR%, suggesting that antigen presentation occurs efficiently in DED.[88−94] However, in a recent study evaluating expression pattern of HLA-DR in conjunctival cell populations from 1049 samples collected from 527 patients with moderate to severe DED, almost 42% of the study patients had less than 5% of conjunctival cells expressing HLA-DR at baseline. Therefore, the authors proposed that conjunctival HLA-DR% did not appear to be a sensitive marker of DED. However, since the mean conjunctival and corneal staining scores increased with increasing levels of HLA-DR%, it was suggested that HLA-DR% levels might prove useful in defining subtypes of DED patients prone to epithelial disease, such as those with higher levels of ocular surface staining.[100] Although the differences in average HLA-DR% between various studies of DED can be attributed to variabilities in inclusion criteria, one major contributor is the lack of standardized methods for flow cytometry instrumentation, data acquisition, and analysis.

There is limited and inconsistent correlation of HLA-DR% with commonly used clinical assessments of signs and symptoms.[88,92,93] Few studies have reported on statistically significant correlation of HLA-DR% with symptoms,[93] osmolarity,[92] TBUT,[88] corneal fluorescein staining,[93,100] and Schirmer's test.[88]

Statistically significantly decreased levels of HLA-DR% were also reported following different treatment regimens such as following treatment with low-concentration clobetasone butyrate,[101] topical CsA,[89,93,102] and oral supplementation of omega-3 and omega-6 fatty acids.[103]

In summary, the validity of HLA-DR as an objectively measurable biomarker in DED seems to be limited at this time due to a lack of universal standardization of the methodology for HLA-DR detection and measurement; and due to the limited and inconsistent correlation of HLA-DR% with commonly used clinical assessments of signs and symptoms.

Fas and Fas ligand are two other human leukocyte antigen subtypes that, upon interaction, induce apoptosis. These immunomodulatory molecules have also been demonstrated in the conjunctiva and lacrimal glands of patients with DED.[104]

Cell adhesion molecules

Cell adhesion molecules are surface molecules that enhance cellular migration by binding components within the extracellular matrix and promoting immune cell infiltration onto the ocular surface. Elevated levels of intercellular adhesion molecule-1 (ICAM-1) and vascular cellular adhesion molecule-1 have been identified in the conjunctiva and lacrimal glands in DED.[105] ICAM-1 is also upregulated on the conjunctival epithelium in ocular surface inflammation and could represent a potential biomarker.[99] In one study, conjunctival inflammation was confirmed in DED patients by observing lymphocytic infiltration and immunoreactivity for HLA-DR and ICAM-1 in conjunctival biopsy specimen.[106]

Hyperosmolarity—Measurement of Tear Osmolarity

Animal studies have shown tear film hyperosmolarity to be a fundamental feature in DED irrespective of the dry eye subtype.[46,107] Tissue culture studies with human corneal epithelial cells (HCECs) exposed to hyperosmolar stress, with osmolarities ranging between 330 and 512 mOsm/kg, have reported activation of MAPK signaling pathway, leading to expression of cytokines, and initiating the inflammatory circle of DED.[46,51,108] There is also evidence of a direct cytotoxic effect of hyperosmolarity on HCECs in culture.[109] Given this research in animals and tissue culture, the measurement of tear osmolarity in DED patients is of great interest, particularly considering the limited number of minimally objective metrics available for the diagnosis of DED.[110]

In the past, various measurement techniques have been used to measure tear osmolarity, including the Clifton and vapor pressure osmometers.[111,112] Although these methods reportedly had high accuracy, sensitivity, and specificity, they were not practical, requiring significant time and specialized equipment. In 2008, the TearLab osmometer (TearLab, San Diego, CA, USA) became available as a point-of-care test device using a microchip, microelectrode technology to measure the number of charged particles in only a 0.2-µL tear sample to provide an estimate of the tear osmolarity. Today, this test is the most widely used test to measure tear osmolarity at the clinic. Normal value is considered 302 mOsm/L, with minimal intereye difference. A value of 308 mOsm/L in either eye has been used as the threshold in differentiating normal and early stages of DED, with 316 mOsm/L used a cut-off for more advanced DED. Both intereye and repeat tear osmolarity measurements in the same eye have been reported to show variability in DED patients. The worse the severity of dry eyes, the more variable tear osmolarity has been found to be (6.9 ± 5.9 mOsm/L in mild, 11.7 ± 10.9 mOsm/L in moderate, and 26.5 ± 22.7 mOsm/L in severe DES, respectively).[46] Hence, a difference of 8 mOsm/L between two eyes is also considered to be significant and compatible with an unstable tear film.[46]

Several studies have reported that DED patients had significantly elevated tear osmolarity compared to healthy controls and the hyperosmolarity increased with dry eye severity,[113–118] and some have even concluded that the TearLab osmometer is the best marker for diagnosing and classifying DED levels of severity.[115,116] Other studies have proposed that higher cut-off values (316−317 mOsm/L) demonstrated superior accuracy to other single tests for diagnosing DED.[117,119] Conversely, many recent clinical studies have raised questions on the diagnostic ability of the test[120−125] demonstrating high variability between controls and DED patients. Despite a general shift in osmolarity with DED, there was a large overlap in osmolarity values between 293 and 320 mOsm/L between normal individuals[120] and patients with dry eye.[126] Sensitivity and specificity measurements of osmolarity values for DED diagnosis using a threshold of 294 mOsm/L were 67% and 46%, respectively,[122] 40% and 100% using a threshold of >310 mOsm/L in patients with SS.[121]

Significant variability in tear osmolarity has been noted and multiple causes sited including different patient populations, variability in technique, humidity, etc.[124,125] Concerns exist particularly on what part of the tear film should be measured—tear meniscus, as measured by TearLab, or the precorneal tear film.[127,128] In fact, the precorneal tear film in DED was reported to have higher osmolarity levels, even spiking up to 800−900 mOsm/L in areas of tear film break-up,[112] Moreover, the TearLab system might have led to reflex tear production resulting in varying values, while earlier studies have suggested that pathological changes would be best obtained in basal tears rather than in reflex tears.[127−129]

In summary, although earlier studies have concluded that tear osmolarity is the best single metric for diagnosing and classifying DED, and suggested 308 mOsm/L as measured by the TearLab osmometer as the most sensitive threshold between normal and mild DED,[116] considering the high variability and overlap of values between healthy eyes and dry eyes, the tear osmolarity measurements using the TearLab osmometer still need to be interpreted cautiously as a stand-alone diagnostic tool. Further research in this area may improve our understanding as to how measurements taken by the TearLab system can be standardized or interpreted, or development of new point-of-care tests measuring tear osmolarity at the clinic may help resolve the variability issues encountered with the current system.

ANTERIOR SEGMENT IMAGING: IN VIVO CONFOCAL MICROSCOPY (IVCM)

IVCM is a currently evolving imaging and diagnostic tool, that enables real-time visualization of ocular structures in cellular detail. Optimum resolution images 500- to 800-fold magnification are acquired by focusing light onto a certain depth within a sample. There are two basic types of IVCM used in ophthalmology clinics; the slit-scanning microscope (SSCM) that uses white light source, and the laser-scanning microscope (LSCM) that uses 670 nm red wavelength diode laser as its light source. Whereas transverse and axial resolution and contrast are lower with the SSCM, the more widely used LSCM has high resolution and better contrast, but is less accurate in determining depth within the corneal tissue,[130] rendering measurements hard to standardize.

Neuropathic Pain

The cornea is the most densely innervated tissue in the body with a high density of free nerve endings, 200−300 times that of the skin[131]. The majority of nerves in the cornea have a sensory function. Sensory nerve endings termed "nociceptors" function in maintaining homeostasis, in wound healing and in sensing the environment to regulate tear secretion and distribution. IVCM allows the description of the morphology, density, and disease-induced or surgically induced alterations of corneal nerves, particularly of the sub- basal nerves, SBN.[132−134]

A challenge in DED is that symptoms of the disease are often discordant with ocular surface findings. In certain cases, DED symptoms can present without measurable abnormalities in tear film or ocular surface, thus bringing up the question of nerve damage as an underlying cause of symptoms.[135,136] Classical severe DED often occurs with appropriate nociceptive pain, that is, these nerves can appropriately transmit information from the diseased ocular surface environment (i.e., nociceptive pain). In 2017, the Tear Film and Ocular Surface Dry Eye Workshop II (TFOS DEWS II) Committee, for the first time, suggested "neurosensory abnormalities" to play role in the pathophysiology of DED.[46] Yet, a more treatment-resistant form of DED arises when they can become dysfunctional and submit signals inappropriately.[137] In these cases, there is marked disparity between the severity of symptoms and magnitude of signs and symptoms exceed the clinical signs.[138] This latter scenario is named "neuropathic pain," which is defined as "pain caused by a lesion or disease of the somatosensory nervous system, occurring in either the peripheral or central nervous system (PNS or CNS)".[139] Such patients are troubled with profound ocular surface discomfort, burning sensation, pain, hyperalgesia (increased pain sensitivity), or photoallodynia (painful sensitivity to light)[140−142] despite having a clinically unremarkable ocular surface examination, also described by the phrase "pain without stain".[143,144]

Another challenge in DED management is that individuals with "neuropathic pain" may present with comorbid ocular surface abnormalities.[145] As such, symptoms of neuropathic pain may overlap with symptoms of DED arising from ocular surface abnormalities. Individuals with both entities usually report sensations of "dryness," "discomfort," and "irritation." However, some symptoms were reported to be more suggestive of a neuropathic origin, including "burning" and evoked pain to wind, light, or extreme temperatures.[142] Therefore, identification of the instances when nerve dysfunction, including NCP, underlies patient symptoms is crucial.

Unfortunately, there are no reliable metrics to confirm the presence of NCP and diagnosis is based on assessing symptoms and clinical features of ocular surface. Absence of clinical signs despite the presence of symptoms or failure of conventional treatment for DED to relieve symptoms suggest the diagnosis of NCP. Positive medical history of a lesion or disease of the corneal nociceptive pathway such as history of corneal refractive surgery, presence of positive findings with corneal confocal microscopy (e.g., anomalies in corneal nerve morphology), presence of local or systemic disorders that may affect nociceptive processing such as fibromyalgia or migraine, and abnormal responses to topical instillation of hyperosmolar drops have been reported as additional diagnostic criteria.[137,140,146]

IVCM is the most widely studied clinical test in NCP with or without dry eye.[147–153] In few studies, subbasal nerve number and density have been reported to be significantly decreased in NOP patients compared to controls, with increased tortuosity and reflectivity.[147,149,150,154,155] Yet, the most interesting IVCM findings in patients with NOP were "microneuromas," which are sites of axonal injury with attempted nerve regeneration, viewed as "abrupt endings," "stumps," "terminal enlargements," or "relatively large, diffuse, poorly demarcated but round appearing bright areas on the nerve itself".[149,150,154,155] Such microneuroma formations along with activated keratocytes were also reported in the stromal nerves as spindle, lateral, or stump microneuromas.[147]

In two studies from the same group, corneal MNs were reported to occur in 62.5%–100% of individuals with clinically diagnosed NCP[149,154] and were proposed as a biomarker of NCP with 100% sensitivity and specificity.[150] Whereas in the latter study no microneuromas were observed in individuals with DED and

no NCP,[150] a more recent study reported MN in 11.1% of individuals with NCP versus 21.8% in patients with DED, and 6.3% of postrefractive surgery patients with DED symptoms.[155] In another study, NCP patients due to refractive surgery were reported to show similar clinical characteristics, pain levels, quality of life impact, and IVCM findings as patients with NCP due to herpetic eye disease.[156] Therefore, the significance and extent of MN presence in NCP remains poorly understood. Recently, Aggarwal et al. reported significant improvements in subbasal nerve number, length, tortuosity, and reflectivity of subbasal nerves in NOP patients, in correlation with improvements in symptoms, following treatment with autologous serum drops.[154] In a recent metaanalysis of subbasal nerve metrics in IVCM studies, Hwang et al. concluded that, at this time, no subbasal nerve metrics were consistent in differentiating between specific DED etiologies, reflecting both the heterogeneity within each etiology and the overlapping clinical features between them.[130] Prospective studies with more number of NOP patients are required to better understand IVCM findings, along with their diagnostic potential or their potential as objective metrics of response to treatment.

IVCM in SS vs non- SS DED and Inflammatory cells

IVCM has been used in a number of studies to analyze corneal, conjunctival, or MG morphology in patients with DED. Although IVCM studies have reported decreased superficial epithelial cell density,[157,158] increased[157] or decreased[158] epithelial basal cell density and presence of abnormal hyper-reflective keratocytes,[157] it has mostly been used to evaluate the morphology of subbasal nerve plexus of the cornea, and presence and morphology of immune or inflammatory cells in DED.

Subbasal nerve density is decreased in both SS and non-SS DED compared to normal subjects.[158–160] Nerves were also reported to have increased tortuosity and beaded appearance in DED patients compared to controls,[158–160] and Tepelus et al.[161] reported a significant correlation between NF density and OSDI. On the contrary, Tuisku et al.[162] and Zhang et al.[163] described an increase in the number of nerve fibers in SS. A recent metaanalysis of IVCM findings in DED populations aiming to determine the relationships between IVCM parameters and specific DED subtypes reported that comprehensive examination of number, density, and beading from all IVCM studies performed on aqueous deficiency DED showed that nerve density values overlapped considerably between

SS, non-SS, and healthy control populations when extrapolated.[75,130,157,159−169] New standardized image capturing techniques[170] and new software[153] are being developed that were reported to detect subbasal nerve alterations in DED patients with better efficacy and reproducibility.

DC infiltration is another common observation in IVCM studies in DED patients. Density of DC, which are interpreted as antigen-presenting cells, was reported to be increased in central and peripheral corneas of SS and non-SS patients compared to controls,[150,161] and in one study DC density correlated with nerve fiber density in DED patients.[161] Another recent study aiming to evaluate correlations between DC infiltration and clinical findings in DED reported differential changes in different levels of DED severity, with increased size of DC body, increased number and length of dendrites, and thus a larger DC field as the severity of DED increases.[154]

A more recent observation in DED patients was significantly high light backscattering in corneal layers in SS patients with DED compared to controls.[171] Such observation was proposed as a parameter that can be used in diagnosis and management of this disease. In few studies, the use of IVCM was also evaluated to monitor treatment response in DED. Villani et al.[172] reported that the subbasal DC density and activated keratocyte density significantly decreased after 4 weeks of treatment with topical 0.5% loteprednol etabonate. Six months of treatment with topical 0.05% cyclosporine eye drops also increased the cell density of the corneal intermediate epithelium, decreased hyperreflective keratocytes and density, tortuosity, and reflectivity of corneal nerve fibers,[166] increased corneal subbasal nerve density, and decreased DC density[173] in two studies. Autologous serum eye drops were also reported to decrease corneal basal epithelial cell density[174] and decrease the number of nerve branches and beadings in patients with DED.[175] In patients with SS-DED, NF density and morphology improved, and DC density decreased following treatment with 3% diquafosol sodium for 3 months.[167]

Meibomian Gland Disease

In few studies that investigated IVCM features of MGD, reduction of acinar unit density, increases of acinar and orifice diameters, and increased secretion reflectivity were demonstrated compared with those of SS patients[157] and healthy controls.[157,176−178] These alterations were associated with an increase in the meibum viscosity.[157] Ibrahim et al.[177] reported that MG acinar unit density showed a strong and significant

correlation with tear function, ocular surface vital staining, MG expressibility, and MG dropout grades. All parameters showed high sensitivity and specificity for MGD diagnosis, suggesting the potential of IVCM for diagnosis and determining severity of MGD and associated DED.

Fu et al.[179] analyzed nerve density, width, tortuosity, and reflectivity of subbasal nerves in mild, moderate, and severe MGD, and reported significant differences between grades of MGD in nerve density and reflectivity. Few studies reported increased inflammatory cell density in MG interstitium[176,177] and since inflammatory cell density was decreased in response to a combination of topical antibiotic, topical steroid, and oral tetracycline therapy, Matsumoto et al.[176] suggested that inflammatory cell density can be used as a new parameter for monitorization of antiinflammatory treatment response in MGD. Furthermore, Randon et al.[180] suggested an IVCM-based scoring of MGD (on the basis of meibum reflectivity, inflammation, and fibrosis) that correlated strongly with meibography scores, to better understand pathophysiology of MGD and help develop a treatment plan.

Villani et al.[157] compared corneal IVCM findings of MGD, SS, non-SS, and control patients. SS patients had the lowest nerve fiber number and highest amount of beading, followed by non-SS and MGD, than controls. SS and MGD had higher grades of nerve tortuosity compared with non-SS and controls. SS and MGD patients also had significantly increased subbasal DC density compared to normals. Following 4 weeks of treatment with topical loteprednol etabonate 0.5%, Kheirkhah et al.[152] reported no change in subbasal nerve fiber length in patients with MGD.

In a metaanalysis evaluating the value of IVCM in differential diagnosis of various DED subgroups, Hwang et al. suggested that subbasal nerve tortuosity could be used to differentiate MGD-associated DED from healthy controls, whereas neither nerve density nor morphology could be used to distinguish MGD-associated DED from other etiologies of DED.[130]

IVCM was also used effectively to disclose the demodex mites in the terminal bulbs of the eyelashes,[177,181−183] which were not observed after treatment.[177,181] Marked inflammatory infiltrates were observed around the MGs and conjunctiva of eyelids with demodicosis infestation, which also cleared with tea tree oil treatment.[181] Furthermore, Demodex-positive seborrheic blepharitis patients were reported to have significantly reduced subbasal nerve density and increased DC density compared go Demodex-negative blepharitis patients.[183] The risk of false-negative results exists in the diagnosis of Demodex infestation with both eyelash depilation and IVCM since total examination of the eyelid is not possible with either method. However, IVCM technique which allows frequent exams, and easy follow-up over time, seems to be more advantageous in the management of Demodex infestation of lids over depilation technique, which is painful and cannot be repeatedly proposed.

In summary, significant decreases in the acinar unit density and increases in the acinar unit diameter and inflammatory cell density were reported in IVCM of MGs in patients with MGD. Although it can be hypothetized that the activation of inflammatory cells may induce the morphologic changes of MG, the mechanism of enlargement of glandular acinar units in MGD patients is still not yet fully understood. IVCM seems to be useful as a supplementary diagnostic tool for the in vivo assessment of MG in patients with MGD.

Systemic Diseases Associated with DED
Graft-versus-host disease

Tepelus et al. reported decreased superficial, wing, and basal epithelial cell densities in patients with ocular graft-versus-host disease (oGVHD) compared to normals.[158] In few studies a decrease in subbasal nerve fiber density was reported in these patient eyes; however, no significant differences were reported in nerve densities between oGVHD, non-oGVHD, or healthy controls[152,158,184,185] suggesting that nerve density alone cannot be used to differentiate GVHD-associated DED from non–GVHD-associated DED or controls.[130]

In oGVHD-associated DED patients, nerve fiber densities were not reported to be different from healthy controls.[152,158,184,185] However, oGVHD-associated DED demonstrated increased tortuosity of subbasal nerves[152,158,184,185] and reduced nerve reflectivity[158,184] compared with healthy controls and HSCT patients without DED.

Interestingly, the DC density did not significantly differ from healthy controls in oGVHD.[158,184]

Sjögren's syndrome

Superficial epithelial cell density was found to be decreased,[159,160,164,167,169] whereas basal epithelial cell density was found to be decreased[159,168,174] or increased[160,169] in SS patients compared to controls.

Number and density of subbasal nerve fibers were reported to be decreased in most studies on SS patients,[159,161,167–169] with increased tortuosity and beading[159,160,164,167,169] compared to controls.

Whereas Tepelus et al.[161] and Gabriellini et al.[164] reported significantly lower nerve fiber density in SS patients compared to non-SS DED patients, Tuisku et al. observed no significant difference.[139] DC density was also reported to be significantly high in SS patients compared to controls.[150,161,167,186,187] Nerve fiber density and morphology improved, and DC density decreased following treatment with 3% diquafosol sodium for 3 months.[167] In a metaanalysis, Hwang et al.[130] concluded that DC presence was reported to be higher in individuals with SS compared with non-SS and healthy controls, and, in general, DC presence was the highest in immune-mediated diseases, lower in MGD and non–immune-mediated DED, and the lowest in individuals without DED, suggesting that elevated DC presence can be an indication of a systemic inflammatory condition. In patients with SS, MG morphology was also reported to be altered with an increase in the acinar unit density and decrease in acinar unit diameter compared to controls.[178]

IVCM was also used to study the conjunctiva in dry eye patients, focusing on confocal correlations with IC, inflammatory cells, and goblet cell evaluation. While data are conflicting about the evaluation of goblet cells (repeatability, interobserver agreement, and chances to discriminate these cells).[188,189] Inflammatory conjunctival cell density and response to treatment could be monitored with IVCM in Sjögren's patients.[187,189] Finally, IVCM was successfully applied to lacrimal gland examination in some Sjögren's patients, revealing acinar unit density, acinar unit diameter, and inflammatory cell densities of lacrimal glands were significantly worse in SS patients inflammatory cell infiltration and perilobular fibrosis.[190]

In conclusion, IVCM is a technology that has the potential to help us understand the pathophysiology of DED, improve differential diagnosis, and develop a tailored approach to treatment and also evaluate the response to treatment. Yet, there are still many issues that limit the application of IVCM findings to an individual patient with DED; the field of view is very small, for instance, HRT-II/RCM (Heidelberg Engineering GmbH, Heidelberg, Germany) that has been used in many of the published studies is only capable if imaging a 400 × 400 μm area, making it difficult to locate and serially reimage the same region of the cornea on multiple sessions, images require tiling in order to cover the entire corneal or MG area, acquisition times can be long, and the analysis is based only on reflectivity and morphology.

To better evaluate and understand the role of IVCM in DED, longitudinal studies with well-defined DED subtypes, taking sex and age into account, utilizing one type of IVCM model (white light or scanning laser) with uniform software to evaluate various parameters will be required. As such, IVCM-based imaging markers' utility can validated, confirming IVCM as a useful assessment tool supplementary to other clinical diagnostic modalities. An image-guided approach to diagnosis and treatment would provide objective parameters for evaluating disease severity and potentially monitoring treatment efficacy.

AGING AND DED

Age and female sex have been found to be the greatest risk factors for DED. Although prevalence estimates for DED vary with the definition of dry eye used and the characteristics of the population studied, in 2017, TFOS DEWS II reported that symptoms and a clinical diagnosis of dry eye show a modest change below the age of 49, with a gradual increase from age 50 and a more marked increase beyond the age of 80.[191] Large epidemiological studies have shown that after the age of 50, the prevalence of DED in women and men increases every 5 years, and the prevalence rate of women is higher than that of men.[192–198] Generally, the increase in prevalence for signs of dry eye show a greater increase than for a diagnosis based on symptoms.[191] Also reported was that, in general, females showed a higher prevalence with increased age than males, despite considerable variability among studies.

In age-related DED, a reduction in lacrimal secretion dominates the clinical picture and is the basis of tear hyperosmolarity.[46] This results chiefly from loss of secretory lacrimal tissue, but a fall in corneal sensitivity to all sensory modalities, reported in both SS and non-SS DED may contribute to the reduced secretion based on a lack of sensory drive.[199] With biological aging, the decrease of tear secretion and the increase of evaporation may be the core explanation of DED.[200,201] The function and structure of lacrimal gland is impaired with aging. The histopathologic changes such as acinar atrophy, periacinar fibrosis, periductal fibrosis can be observed in the human main lacrimal gland.[202–205] Diffuse fibrosis and diffuse atrophy in orbital lobes were more frequently observed in women than in men.[203,206] As expected, secretion of the lacrimal-derived proteins, lysozyme, lactoferrin, and peroxidase fall with age.[207–209] From about the age of 40 years, the glands are increasingly infiltrated by CD4 and CD8 T cells, which are considered to be the basis of a gradual destruction of lacrimal acinar and ductal tissue,

associated with interacinar and periductal fibrosis, paraductal blood vessel loss, and acinar cell atrophy.[46] Corneal sensitivity to mechanical[199,210–212] and chemical stimuli[199,212] falls with age, which could reduce the sensory drive to lacrimal secretion, which would be in keeping with a loss of lacrimal gland function the decrease in corneal sensitivity may explain the lack of correlation of signs and symptoms.

One of the proposed mechanisms of glandular damage over the lifespan was reported to be oxidative stress, resulting from the production of reactive oxygen species such as superoxide and hydrogen peroxide, in the process of aerobic metabolism. Free radical production occurs in the course of mitochondrial electron transfer as part of the process of energy production. In a comparison of human lacrimal tissue from young (17–48 year) versus old (76–87 year) cadavers, evidence of lipid peroxidation and of oxidative DNA damage was also found in the older group.[213]

In MGD, inspissated secretions over lifespan is thought to contribute to stasis, obstruction, and inflammation of the ductal system, leading to gland atrophy and dropout.[46,214] These pathophysiological processes result in diminished delivery of MG secretions to the tear film, compromising the integrity of the surface lipid layer and contributing to excessive aqueous tear evaporation and tear film instability. Age-related eyelid alterations like lid laxity and orifice metaplasia may also relate to dry eye.[215–219] It has been reported that Marx line, the MG orifices located anterior to the mucocutaneous junction in young healthy eyelid, migrates anteriorly with aging.[220]

Few studies have reported that aging is an important risk factor for the development of MGD.[221–226] However, since MG dropout was also reported in adolescents, hormonal and environmental factors were also hypothesized to influence the structure of MGs.[227,228]

In a recent prospective registry-based cross-sectional study aiming to understand the natural history of DED, signs of MG dysfunction emerged earlier in the natural history of disease progression, with the optimal prognostic cut-off ages for gland dropout, diminished meibum expressibility, and reduced tear film lipid layer quality occurring in the third decade of life, between 24 and 29 years of age.[229] In the aforementioned study, decreased tear meniscus height occurred relatively later in life, with the optimal predictive cut-off age being 46 years suggesting that aqueous tear deficiency predominantly affects the older population, consistent with the trends reported following the metaanalysis conducted by the TFOS DEWS II Epidemiology

Subcommittee.[191] Conjunctival and corneal staining were among the final clinical markers to emerge in the natural history of dry eye progression, with the optimal prognostic thresholds being 46 and 52 years of age.

In conclusion, advancing age was identified to be a significant risk factor for DED, and the global burden of this condition is projected to increase with the aging population. Signs of MG dysfunction emerged early in the natural history of disease progression during the third decade of life, and the brief delay prior to the development of other clinical signs of DED might indicate a window of opportunity for exploring preventative interventions in this age group.

SEX AND DED

Androgens are extremely important in the regulation of the ocular surface and adnexa.[214,230−232] They also appear to mediate many of the sex-related differences in these tissues.[233−237] Sex-related differences are evident in the anatomy, physiology, and pathophysiology of the lacrimal gland, as well as the morphological appearance, gene expression, neutral and polar lipid profiles, and secretory output of the MG.[238] Sex also effects density of goblet cells and susceptibility of the ocular surface to inflammation. Although how these variations may relate to the sex-associated prevalence of DED is unclear, androgen deficiency is associated with both aqueous-deficient and evaporative DED.[214,230,232,239−241]

Androgens influence structure and function of the lacrimal gland, including its cellular architecture, gene expression, protein synthesis, immune activity, and fluid and protein secretion[233,238,242−255]. Androgen deficiency, in turn, has been linked to lacrimal gland dysfunction and a corresponding aqueous tear deficiency.[197,230,232,256] Women with SS are androgen-deficient.[256,257−262] Researchers have also suggested that the decrease in serum androgen levels that occurs during menopause, pregnancy, lactation, or the use of estrogen-containing oral contraceptives may trigger the development of a nonimmune type of DED, termed primary lacrimal gland deficiency.[263]

Meibomian function is strongly influenced by the sex hormones, particularly androgens. In brief, androgens stimulate the synthesis and secretion of lipids by the MG and suppress the expression of genes related to keratinization.[214,264−267]

Conversely a deficiency of androgen action, such as occurs in aging, SS, antiandrogen treatment, and complete androgen insensitivity syndrome, is associated with MGD, altered meibum lipid profiles, and evidence of decreased tear film stability.[214,268−270]

The clinical evidence regarding the influence of estrogen and progesterone on dry eye is inconsistent. Although a common assumption exists in the literature that menopause is associated with increased occurrence of dry eye, a closer inspection shows that definitive evidence is lacking. The prevalence of dry eye is higher in females than males across the lifecycle and dry eye prevalence increases gradually with age in both men and women.[195,197] Such a gradual increase in both sexes is perhaps more in keeping with the gradual decrease in serum androgen levels which occurs with age rather than the abrupt decline in ovarian estrogen at menopause.

However, more dry eye symptoms were demonstrated in a study of 17- to 43-year-old women with premature ovarian failure, than in an age-matched control group,[271] alluding to a positive role for ovarian estrogen. Three reports of increased risk of dry eye in postmenopausal women undergoing aromatase inhibitor treatment for breast cancer highlight the importance of peripheral estrogen synthesis in ocular surface homeostasis.[272−274]

Assessment of pain, which is a hallmark of DED, may also be affected by gender difference. Although many studies show that men have higher pain thresholds than women, reliable evaluation of a possible sex difference in subjective reporting of pain in DED remains lacking.

Further studies are required to clarify the precise nature, extent, and mechanisms of these sex, endocrine, and gender effects on the eye in health and disease.

ENVIRONMENTAL FACTORS AND DED

Established risk factors of DED include environmental factors such as extreme temperature or reduced relative humidity,[191,275] contact lens (CL) wear, use of video display terminals, and smoking.[276−280]

Digital Display Use

Digital display (DD) use is ubiquitous and various forms of DDs, such as laptops, smartphones, tablets, or even e-readers, are being used widely in addition to desktop computers. Studies indicate a significantly higher dry eye symptom score in DD users as compared to controls,[281] as well as significantly lower fluorescein break-up time (FBUT), noninvasive break-up time, and tear meniscus height.[282−285] Additionally, oxidative stress markers in the tear film,[284] inflammatory mediators,[282] and tear osmolarity[283] have shown to be altered in DD users. Consequently, DD use has been implicated as a contributing factor to DED. The overall prevalence of DED in computer users is thought to be around 49.5%, and ranges from 9.5% to 87.5%.[286]

Abnormalities of blinking, including reduced blink rate[287–292] and incomplete eyelid closure during DD use, are considered as the main mechanisms of DD-related dry eye. Incomplete blinking, resulting from increased cognitive and task demand, was suggested to be a more pertinent issue in DD users[293–295] with a significant positive correlation with total symptom scores.[293] Incomplete blinking alters the distribution of mucin over the ocular surface, causes poor maintenance of lipid layer integrity, and reduces tear film thickness in the inferior cornea, rendering an instable tear film prone to break-up problems.[296] Since small aliquots of oil are delivered from the MGs with each blink,[46] abnormal blinking may alter MG secretion, leading in the long run to chronic changes in the gland, which may eventually cause inflammation, gland obstruction, and a further reduction of the outflow of meibum.[297] Incomplete blinking was also reported to be associated with greater levels of MG dropout, decreased tear film lipid layer thickness, tear film stability, and expressed meibum quality.[298,299]

Additionally, DD use was reported to lead to reduced tear volume and tear stability.[281,283,298,300,301] Whereas tear stability can be affected even after a few minutes of computer visualization,[300–302] it was also shown to decrease with the duration of computer use[283,298,301] Significantly increased osmolarity was measured in computer users at the end of a 9-h working day,[283] and osmolarity was negatively correlated with the duration of computer use and with FBUT and Schirmer scores.[283,303]

Contact Lens Wear

CL wear is considered a risk factor for DED. According to TFOS DEWS II report, CL wear increases the risk of developing dry eye from between 2.01 and 2.96 times.[198,304,305] Since CLs compartmentalize the tear film into two layers, namely the outer prelens and the inner postlens tear film, they lead to biophysical and biochemical alterations in the tear film. The use of CLs leads to a thinner and irregular lipid layer with poor wettability,[306] tear film instability,[307] increased tear evaporation and osmolarity,[308] lower basal tear turnover rate,[307] decreased tear volume,[309,310] and reduced levels of the mucin MUC5AC.[311] Furthermore, MGs were also reported be adversely affected by CL use, with morphological changes and increased gland dropout in time.[312]

Temperature, Humidity, Altitude, Pollution

Studies have reported strong association between low relative humidity environments and prevalence of DED.[313] Tear evaporation rate, lipid layer thickness, ocular comfort, and tear film stability and production have shown to be adversely affected by low relative humidity.[314,315] Low relative air humidity in office buildings and air-conditioned rooms negatively impact the tear film, causing symptoms of DED and leading to conjunctival and limbal hyperemia as well as a reduction in tear meniscus height.[285] Exposure of the ocular surface to low relative humidity was reported to cause conjunctival goblet cell cornification, with alterations in the delivery of mucins to the tear film.[1] High horizontal or downward air velocity can also increase tear film evaporation leading to exposure keratitis and epithelial damage.[2]

Tear film quality is also adversely affected from high temperature.[3] Lowering room temperature by 1°C (within 22–26°C) was reported to decrease dry eye symptoms by 19%.[4] Cold thermoreceptors in the cornea regulate the basal flow of tears.[5] Blinking and basal tear secretion are suppressed in warm environments, resulting in a less stable tear film lipid layer.[6,7] Dry air and cold temperatures at high altitudes are associated with the development of dry eye symptoms, hyperosmolarity, and decreased tear film stability.[8]

Another factor that may impact the tear film is air pollution.[9] Finally, glare and reflections due to improper lighting can cause discomfort and disability glare.[10]

PRESERVATIVES (BENZALKONIUM CHLORIDE, BAK) AND DED

Topical drugs may cause allergic, toxic, and/or immunoinflammatory effects on the ocular surface or may undergo chemical interaction with the tear film, either by disrupting the lipid layer through detergent effects, by reducing aqueous secretion, or by damaging goblet cells, surface epithelia, corneal nerves, or even eyelids at the skin or MG level.[11] Delayed allergic reactions can also occur, often mimicking blepharitis with low-grade inflammation.

The most studied detergent compounds are quaternary ammoniums, particularly benzalkonium chloride (BAK), which is commonly used in eye drops at concentrations ranging from 0.004% to 0.02%. In vitro or animal models have suggested that BAK has cytotoxic effects on several structures of the eye, with a threshold of toxicity found at about 0.005%, i.e., below the concentration used in most eyedrops.[12] BAK may cause or aggravate DED through various mechanisms such as toxic and proinflammatory effects; however, BAK has strong detergent properties, dissolving lipids and destroying the bacterial walls and cell membranes.

Goblet cells, which are particularly sensitive to toxic and inflammatory stress, are decreased in density in humans after short exposure to BAK or BAK-containing timolol.[13] BAK also causes disruption of the tight junctions of the corneal epithelium, and increase epithelial permeability, an effect that has led to BAK being considered an enhancer of drug penetration into the anterior chamber.[12] Hence, BAK may cause some level of toxicity in normal eyes as well as eyes that need chronic treatment such as glaucomatous eyes. Cumulative amounts of benzalkonium chloride (BAK) were shown to disrupt the tear film stability[14] and increase tear film osmolarity.[15] Tear film alterations may stimulate a series of biological changes in the ocular surface, leading to subsequent neurogenic inflammation and further impairment of the tear film, creating a vicious cycle.[16] Glaucomatous eyes undergoing treatment with BAK-containing antiglaucoma medications exhibit more lid margin abnormalities and worse MG morphology compared to those that are not treated.[17] Last, but not the least, BAK has shown neurotoxic effects to the trigeminal nerve endings,[18] density of superficial epithelial cells and the number of subbasal nerves were reduced in the preservative-containing groups, and stromal keratocyte activation and bead-like nerve shaping were higher in the glaucoma preservative therapy groups than in the control and preservative-free groups, together with a decrease in corneal sensitivity. Several studies have shown that switching from a preserved to nonpreserved formulation significantly improved the ocular surface and reduced symptoms from 54% to 65%.[19] Interestingly, in those studies, reversibility of inflammatory lesions can be obtained rapidly, as also shown with DC numbers returning to normal levels in less than 1 month.[20]

In one study, unpreserved ketotifen 0.025% eye drops were more effective and better tolerated than BAK-preserved 0.05% drops in patients with seasonal allergic conjunctivitis, a fact that was attributed to the toxic effect of BAK.[21] As allergic patients often exhibit impaired and inflammatory tear film and ocular surface, BAK-free compounds should be the first choice when treating allergic conjunctivitis or DED.

In conclusion, there is abundance of evidence that strongly supports the use of BAK-free solutions in the treatment of patients with chronic diseases, such as ocular allergy or glaucoma, to avoid ocular surface disease and findings typical of DED.

As BAK toxicity is dose-dependent, at least reducing the number of preserved eyedrops may be helpful and may reduce the burden of side effects to acceptable levels.[19,22] Low toxicity preservatives have been developed and have shown little if no adverse effects on the ocular surface.[23,24] However, their possible effects on the tear film and tolerance in dry eye patients need to be investigated.

MICROBIOME AND DED

Mucosal surfaces of the human body are associated with commensal microorganisms with a mutualistic/symbiotic relationship with the human host.[25] These microorganisms were referred to as the "normal flora"; now, commensal microorganisms are often referred to as the "microbiota" (the microbial cells), and the genetic information of the microorganisms is referred to as the "microbiome".[25]

Microbial commensal organisms can alter Th17 populations in the host organism, both in homeostasis and when perturbed.[26–28] Each individual encompasses a unique gut microbiota profile that changes over time, depending on certain variables such as lifestyle, physical exercise, body mass index (BMI), and cultural and dietary habits.[29] The gut microbiota has been reported to be interactive in maintaining balance in immune responses between regulatory T cells (Tregs) and T helper 17 (Th17) cells at mucosal surface and to act as a trigger of inducing autoimmunity.[30,31] Emerging evidences indicate that gut dysbiosis contributes to the pathophysiology or exacerbation of autoimmune diseases, including RA, SLE, systemic sclerosis, ankylosing spondylitis, and SS through the imbalance of the immune system.[31] Emerging findings also suggest the existence of a gut–eye axis, wherein gut dysbiosis may be a crucial factor influencing the onset and progression of multiple ocular diseases, including uveitis, dry eye, macular degeneration, and glaucoma.[29]

Studies have demonstrated that the gut microbiome is altered in dry eye, and there are specific bacterial classes associated with dry eye signs and symptoms.[32] Gut dysbiosis is prevalent in SS and gut dysbiosis is associated with ocular disease severity.[33,34]

Overall, studies agree on the presence of a significantly different gut microbiota of SS subjects compared to healthy controls through diversity analysis.[32,33,35,36] In most studies, in SS, greater relative abundances of *Pseudobutyrivibrio*, *Escherichia/Shigella*, and *Streptococcus* and reduced relative abundances of *Bacteroides*, *Parabacteroides*, *Faecalibacterium*, and *Prevotella* were noted compared to controls.[32] Given that gut microbiota is easily influenced by diet, ethnicity, and gender, search for a specific causal bacteria is difficult; however, some degree of gut dysbiosis seems to be present in SS subjects compared to healthy individuals. Furthermore, subjects with severe gut dysbiosis exhibited higher disease activity with hypocomplementemia and higher F-calprotectin[37]. Reduced gut microbiome diversity was also found to correlate with overall disease severity.[32,33,35] Furthermore, individuals that did not meet full Sjögren's criteria (SDE) were also found to have gut microbiome alterations compared to controls.[32]

Gut dysbiosis leads to an aberrant diversification of the B-cell repertoire and an imbalance between Treg and TH17 cell responses in adaptive immunity, subsequently triggering ocular autoimmune diseases. Both non-Sjögren and SS-related dry eyes as well as uveitis share key pathogenic features, such as an imbalance in Treg/TH17 cells, or reduced SCFAs-producing bacteria.

Recently, ocular microbiota of DED patients have also been examined.[38−42] In general, these studies mostly found *CNS, Staphylococcus epidermidis, Corynebacterium,* and *Propionibacterium acnes,* as have been described in other disease states.[38−42] Reduced microbiome diversity has been identified in OSD patients compared to healthy controls,[43,44] which also have been shown to have greater fungal diversity.[43] Further studies are warranted to uncover the role of the OSM in ocular diseases.

In summary, the beneficial or harmful effects of the gut microbiome in the pathogenesis of dry eye and other autoimmune ocular diseases are now just beginning to be understood. However, functional studies of gut microbiota are still preliminary to fully understand the pathogenesis of dry eye associated with gut dysbiosis.

Future innovation in this field may lead to a new target in ophthalmology to understand and manage ophthalmic diseases, providing alternative or adjunctive local or systemic treatments to modulate the ocular surface and gut microbiota. It remains unclear whether the OSM plays a role in the etiology of these diseases, or whether these diseases alter the OSM.

SUMMARY

In summary, DED represents an unmet medical need— a common, multifactorial, chronic disease with significant impact on quality of life. The challenge remains in the multifactorial etiology and lack of concordance between signs and symptoms of the disease limited availability of adequate questionnaires and minimallly invasive objective tests make identification of various patient subgroups difficult and therefore it is hard to determine specific mechanisms of disease and best targets for treatment. Research on DED has historically suffered from the lack of validated biomarkers and

less than objective and reproducible endpoints. Identification of biomarkers using minimally invasive methods that will lead to the development of objective metrics are hoped to improve our understanding of DED, and hence establish effective treatment strategies. Studies on various constituents of the tear film and ocular surface in health and disease, in vivo evaluation of morphological features, investigation of effects of aging, sex and environmental factors, microbiome and other risk factors on physiology and function of the ocular surface will improve our understanding of DED. Specific markers that can become validated biomarkers for DED will propel our understanding of DED and lead to better diagnosis, classification and ultimately imporved treatment efficaty.

REFERENCES

1. Corrales RM, de Paiva CS, Li D-Q, et al. Entrapment of conjunctival goblet cells by desiccation-induced cornification. *Investig Opthalmology Vis Sci.* 2011;52(6): 3492−3499. Available from: http://iovs.arvojournals. org/article.aspx?doi=10.1167/iovs.10-5782.
2. Koh S, Tung C, Kottaiyan R, Zavislan J, Yoon G, Aquavella J. Effect of airflow exposure on the tear meniscus. *J Ophthalmol.* 2012;2012:1−6. Available from: http://www.hindawi.com/journals/joph/2012/ 983182/.
3. Abusharha AA, Pearce EI, Fagehi R. Effect of ambient temperature on the human tear film. *Eye Contact Lens Sci Clin Pract.* 2016;42(5):308−312. Available from: https:// journals.lww.com/00140068-201609000-00007.
4. Mendell MJ, Fisk WJ, Petersen MR, et al. Indoor particles and symptoms among office workers: results from a double-blind cross-over study. *Epidemiology.* 2002;13(3): 296−304. Available from: http://journals.lww.com/ 00001648-200205000-00010.
5. Belmonte C, Gallar J. Cold thermoreceptors, unexpected players in tear production and ocular dryness sensations. *Investig Opthalmology Vis Sci.* 2011;52(6):3888−3892. Available from: http://iovs.arvojournals.org/article.aspx? doi=10.1167/iovs.09-5119.
6. Bron AJ, Tiffany JM, Gouveia SM, Yokoi N, Voon LW. Functional aspects of the tear film lipid layer. *Exp Eye Res.* 2004;78(3):347−360. Available from: https:// linkinghub.elsevier.com/retrieve/pii/ S0014483503003038.
7. Collins M, Seeto R, Campbell L, Ross M. Blinking and corneal sensitivity. *Acta Ophthalmol.* 2009;67(5): 525−531. Available from: http://doi.wiley.com/10. 1111/j.1755-3768.1989.tb04103.x.
8. Willmann G, Schatz A, Fischer MD, et al. Exposure to high altitude alters tear film osmolarity and breakup time. *High Alt Med Biol.* 2014;15(2):203−207. Available from: http://www.liebertpub.com/doi/10.1089/ham. 2013.1103.

9. Torricelli AAM, Novaes P, Matsuda M, Alves MR, Monteiro MLR. Ocular surface adverse effects of ambient levels of air pollution. *Arq Bras Oftalmol.* 2011;74(5): 377–381. Available from: http://www.scielo.br/scielo. php?script=sci_arttext&pid=S0004-2749201100050001 6&lng=en&nrm=iso&tlng=en.

10. Hultgren GV, Knave B. Discomfort glare and disturbances from light reflections in an office landscape with CRT display terminals. *Appl Ergon.* 1974;5(1):2–8. Available from: https://linkinghub.elsevier.com/retrieve/pii/0003 687074902518.

11. Gomes JAP, Azar DT, Baudouin C, et al. TFOS DEWS II iatrogenic report. *Ocul Surf.* 2017;15(3):511–538. Available from: https://linkinghub.elsevier.com/retrieve/pii/ S1542012417301040.

12. Baudouin C, Labbé A, Liang H, Pauly A, Brignole-Baudouin F. Preservatives in eyedrops: the good, the bad and the ugly. *Prog Retin Eye Res.* 2010;29(4): 312–334. Available from: https://linkinghub.elsevier. com/retrieve/pii/S1350946210000157.

13. Herreras JM, Pastor JC, Calonge M, Asensio VM. Ocular surface alteration after long-term treatment with an anti-glaucomatous drug. *Ophthalmology.* 1992;99(7): 1082–1088. Available from: https://linkinghub.elsevier. com/retrieve/pii/S0161642092318470.

14. Baudouin C, de Lunardo C. Short term comparative study of topical 2% carteolol with and without benzalkonium chloride in healthy volunteers. *Br J Ophthalmol.* 1998; 82(1):39–42. Available from: https://bjo.bmj.com/ lookup/doi/10.1136/bjo.82.1.39.

15. Labbé A, Terry O, Brasnu E, Van Went C, Baudouin C. Tear film osmolarity in patients treated for glaucoma or ocular hypertension. *Cornea.* 2012;31(9):994–999. Available from: https://journals.lww.com/00003226-201209000-00006.

16. Baudouin C, Aragona P, Messmer EM, et al. Role of hyperosmolarity in the pathogenesis and management of dry eye disease: proceedings of the OCEAN group meeting. *Ocul Surf.* 2013;11(4):246–258. Available from: https://linkinghub.elsevier.com/retrieve/pii/S154 2012413000906.

17. Arita R, Itoh K, Maeda S, et al. Effects of long-term topical anti-glaucoma medications on meibomian glands. *Graefe's Arch Clin Exp Ophthalmol.* 2012;250(8): 1181–1185. Available from: http://link.springer.com/ 10.1007/s00417-012-1943-6.

18. Sarkar J, Chaudhary S, Namavari A, et al. Corneal neurotoxicity due to topical benzalkonium chloride. *Investig Opthalmology Vis Sci.* 2012;53(4):1792–1802. Available from: http://iovs.arvojournals.org/article.aspx?doi=10.1 167/iovs.11-8775.

19. Jaenen N, Baudouin C, Pouliquen P, Manni G, Figueiredo A, Zeyen T. Ocular symptoms and signs with preserved and preservative-free glaucoma medications. *Eur J Ophthalmol.* 2007;17(3):341–349. Available from: http://journals.sagepub.com/doi/10.1177/11206721070 1700311.

20. Zhivov A, Kraak R, Bergter H, Kundt G, Beck R, Guthoff RF. Influence of benzalkonium chloride on langerhans cells in corneal epithelium and development of dry eye in healthy volunteers. *Curr Eye Res.* 2010;35(8): 762–769. Available from: http://www.tandfonline. com/doi/full/10.3109/02713683.2010.489181.

21. Leonardi A, Capobianco D, Benedetti N, et al. Efficacy and tolerability of ketotifen in the treatment of seasonal allergic conjunctivitis: comparison between ketotifen 0.025% and 0.05% eye drops. *Ocul Immunol Inflamm.* 2019;27(8):1352–1356. Available from: https://www. tandfonline.com/doi/full/10.1080/09273948.2018.1530 363.

22. Goldberg I, Graham SL, Crowston JG, D'Mellow G. Clinical audit examining the impact of benzalkonium chloride-free anti-glaucoma medications on patients with symptoms of ocular surface disease. *Clin Experiment Ophthalmol.* 2015;43(3):214–220. Available from: http:// doi.wiley.com/10.1111/ceo.12431.

23. Kahook MY, Noecker R. Quantitative analysis of conjunctival goblet cells after chronic application of topical drops. *Adv Ther.* 2008;25(8):743–751. Available from: http://link.springer.com/10.1007/s12325-008-0078-y.

24. Lee HJ, Jun RM, Cho MS, Choi K-R. Comparison of the ocular surface changes following the use of two different prostaglandin F2 α analogues containing benzalkonium chloride or polyquad in rabbit eyes. *Cutan Ocul Toxicol.* 2015;34(3):195–202. Available from: http://www. tandfonline.com/doi/full/10.3109/15569527.2014.944 650.

25. Okonkwo A, Rimmer V, Walkden A, et al. Next-generation sequencing of the ocular surface microbiome: in health, contact lens wear, diabetes, trachoma, and dry eye. *Eye Contact Lens Sci Clin Pract.* 2020;46(4): 254–261. Available from: https://journals.lww.com/10. 1097/ICL.0000000000000697.

26. Lee YK, Menezes JS, Umesaki Y, Mazmanian SK. Proinflammatory T-cell responses to gut microbiota promote experimental autoimmune encephalomyelitis. *Proc Natl Acad Sci India.* 2011;108(suppl. 1):4615–4622. Available from: http://www.pnas.org/cgi/doi/10.1073/pnas.1000 082107.

27. Cheng H, Guan X, Chen D, Ma W. The Th17/treg cell balance: a gut microbiota-modulated story. *Microorganisms.* 2019;7(12):583. Available from: https://www.mdpi. com/2076-2607/7/12/583.

28. Willis KA, Postnikoff CK, Freeman A, et al. The closed eye harbours a unique microbiome in dry eye disease. *Sci Rep.* 2020;10(1):12035. Available from: http://www. nature.com/articles/s41598-020-68952-w.

29. Napolitano P, Filippelli M, Davinelli S, Bartollino S, Dell'Omo R, Costagliola C. Influence of gut microbiota on eye diseases: an overview. *Ann Med Interne.* 2021; 53(1):750–761. Available from: https://www.tandfonline. com/doi/full/10.1080/07853890.2021.1925150.

30. Segre JA. Microbial growth dynamics and human disease. *Science.* 2015 4;349(6252):1058–1059. Available from:

https://www.sciencemag.org/lookup/doi/10.1126/science.aad0781.

31. Zhong D, Wu C, Zeng X, Wang Q. The role of gut microbiota in the pathogenesis of rheumatic diseases. *Clin Rheumatol.* 2018;37(1):25−34. Available from: http://link.springer.com/10.1007/s10067-017-3821-4.

32. Mendez R, Watane A, Farhangi M, et al. Gut microbial dysbiosis in individuals with Sjögren's syndrome. *Microb Cell Fact.* 2020;19(1):90. Available from: https://microbialcellfactories.biomedcentral.com/articles/10.1186/s12934-020-01348-7.

33. Moon J, Choi SH, Yoon CH, Kim MK. Gut dysbiosis is prevailing in Sjögren's syndrome and is related to dry eye severity. Appel S *PLoS One.* 2020;15(2):e0229029. Available from: https://dx.plos.org/10.1371/journal.pone.0229029.

34. Moon J, Yoon CH, Choi SH, Kim MK. Can gut microbiota affect dry eye syndrome? *Int J Mol Sci.* 2020;21(22):8443. Available from: https://www.mdpi.com/1422-0067/21/22/8443.

35. de Paiva CS, Jones DB, Stern ME, et al. Altered mucosal microbiome diversity and disease severity in Sjögren syndrome. *Sci Rep.* 2016;6(1):23561. Available from: http://www.nature.com/articles/srep23561.

36. van der Meulen TA, Harmsen HJM, Vila AV, et al. Shared gut, but distinct oral microbiota composition in primary Sjögren's syndrome and systemic lupus erythematosus. *J Autoimmun.* 2019;97:77−87. Available from: https://linkinghub.elsevier.com/retrieve/pii/S0896841118305249.

37. Mandl T, Marsal J, Olsson P, Ohlsson B, Andréasson K. Severe intestinal dysbiosis is prevalent in primary Sjögren's syndrome and is associated with systemic disease activity. *Arthritis Res Ther.* 2017;19(1):237. Available from: http://arthritis-research.biomedcentral.com/articles/10.1186/s13075-017-1446-2.

38. Seal DV, McGill JI, Mackie IA, Liakos GM, Jacobs P, Goulding NJ. Bacteriology and tear protein profiles of the dry eye. *Br J Ophthalmol.* 1986;70(2):122−125. Available from: https://bjo.bmj.com/lookup/doi/10.1136/bjo.70.2.122.

39. Graham JE, Moore JE, Jiru X, et al. Ocular pathogen or commensal: a PCR-based study of surface bacterial flora in normal and dry eyes. *Investig Opthalmology Vis Sci.* 2007;48(12):5616−5623. Available from: http://iovs.arvojournals.org/article.aspx?doi=10.1167/iovs.07-0588.

40. Hori Y, Maeda N, Sakamoto M, Koh S, Inoue T, Tano Y. Bacteriologic profile of the conjunctiva in the patients with dry eye. *Am J Ophthalmol.* 2008;146(5):729−734.e1. Available from: https://linkinghub.elsevier.com/retrieve/pii/S0002939408004388.

41. Suto C, Morinaga M, Yagi T, Tsuji C, Toshida H. Conjunctival sac bacterial flora isolated prior to cataract surgery. *Infect Drug Resist.* 2012;5:37−41. Available from: http://www.dovepress.com/conjunctival-sac-bacterial-flora-isolated-prior-to-cataract-surgery-peer-reviewed-article-IDR.

42. Zhang Y, Liu ZR, Chen H, et al. Comparison on conjunctival sac bacterial flora of the seniors with dry eye in Ganzi autonomous prefecture. *Int J Ophthalmol.* 2013;6(4):452−457.

43. Shivaji S, Jayasudha R, Sai Prashanthi G, Kalyana Chakravarthy S, Sharma S. The human ocular surface fungal microbiome. *Investig Opthalmology Vis Sci.* 2019;60(1):451−459. Available from: http://iovs.arvojournals.org/article.aspx?doi=10.1167/iovs.18-26076.

44. Zilliox MJ, Gange WS, Kuffel G, et al. Assessing the ocular surface microbiome in severe ocular surface diseases. *Ocul Surf.* 2020;18(4):706−712. Available from: https://linkinghub.elsevier.com/retrieve/pii/S1542012420301142.

45. Lemp MA, Baudouin C, Baum J, et al. The definition and classification of dry eye disease: report of the definition and classification subcommittee of the International Dry Eye Workshop (2007). *Ocul Surf.* 2007;5(2):75−92. Available from: https://linkinghub.elsevier.com/retrieve/pii/S1542012412700812.

46. Bron AJ, de Paiva CS, Chauhan SK, et al. TFOS DEWS II pathophysiology report. *Ocul Surf.* 2017;15(3):438−510. Available from: https://linkinghub.elsevier.com/retrieve/pii/S1542012417301349.

47. Rosette C, Karin M. Ultraviolet light and osmotic stress: activation of the JNK cascade through multiple growth factor and cytokine receptors. *Science.* 1996;274(5290):1194−1197. Available from: https://www.sciencemag.org/lookup/doi/10.1126/science.274.5290.1194.

48. Corrales RM, Stern ME, De Paiva CS, Welch J, Li D-Q, Pflugfelder SC. Desiccating stress stimulates expression of matrix metalloproteinases by the corneal epithelium. *Investig Opthalmology Vis Sci.* 2006;47(8):3293−3302. Available from: http://iovs.arvojournals.org/article.aspx?doi=10.1167/iovs.05-1382.

49. Pflugfelder SC, de Paiva CS, Li D-Q, Stern ME. Epithelial-immune cell interaction in dry eye. *Cornea.* 2008;27(Suppl 1):S9−S11. Available from: https://journals.lww.com/00003226-200809001-00003.

50. Stevenson W, Chauhan SK, Dana R. Dry eye disease: an immune-mediated ocular surface disorder. *Arch Ophthalmol.* 2012;130(1):90−100. Available from: http://archopht.jamanetwork.com/article.aspx?doi=10.1001/archophthalmol.2011.364.

51. Li D-Q, Chen Z, Song XJ, Luo L, Pflugfelder SC. Stimulation of matrix metalloproteinases by hyperosmolarity via a JNK pathway in human corneal epithelial cells. *Investig Opthalmology Vis Sci.* 2004;45(12):4302−4311. Available from: http://iovs.arvojournals.org/article.aspx?doi=10.1167/iovs.04-0299.

52. Luo L, Li D-Q, Corrales RM, Pflugfelder SC. Hyperosmolar saline is a proinflammatory stress on the mouse ocular surface. *Eye Contact Lens Sci Clin Pract.* 2005;31(5):186−193. Available from: https://journals.lww.com/00140068-200509000-00005.

53. De Paiva CS, Villarreal AL, Corrales RM, et al. Dry eye–induced conjunctival epithelial squamous metaplasia is modulated by interferon-γ. *Investig Opthalmology Vis Sci.* 2007;48(6):2553−2560. Available from: http://iovs.arvojournals.org/article.aspx?doi=10.1167/iovs.07-0069.

54. Chi W, Hua X, Chen X, et al. Mitochondrial DNA oxidation induces imbalanced activity of NLRP3/NLRP6 inflammasomes by activation of caspase-8 and BRCC36 in dry eye. *J Autoimmun.* 2017;80:65−76. Available from: https://linkinghub.elsevier.com/retrieve/pii/S089 684111630289X.

55. Aragona P, Aguennouz M, Rania L, et al. Matrix metalloproteinase 9 and transglutaminase 2 expression at the ocular surface in patients with different forms of dry eye disease. *Ophthalmology.* 2015;122(1):62−71. Available from: https://linkinghub.elsevier.com/retrieve/pii/S0161642014006927.

56. Lanza NL, Valenzuela F, Perez VL, Galor A. The matrix metalloproteinase 9 point-of-care test in dry eye. *Ocul Surf.* 2016;14(2):189−195. Available from: https://linkinghub.elsevier.com/retrieve/pii/S1542012416000082.

57. Pflugfelder SC, Farley W, Luo L, et al. Matrix metalloproteinase-9 knockout confers resistance to corneal epithelial barrier disruption in experimental dry eye. *Am J Pathol.* 2005;166(1):61−71. Available from: https://linkinghub.elsevier.com/retrieve/pii/S0002944010622328.

58. Lin C-C, Kuo C-T, Cheng C-Y, et al. IL-1β promotes A549 cell migration via MAPKs/AP-1- and NF-κB-dependent matrix metalloproteinase-9 expression. *Cell Signal.* 2009;21(11):1652−1662. Available from: https://linkinghub.elsevier.com/retrieve/pii/S0898656809002095.

59. Messmer EM, von Lindenfels V, Garbe A, Kampik A. Matrix metalloproteinase 9 testing in dry eye disease using a commercially available point-of-care immunoassay. *Ophthalmology.* 2016;123(11):2300−2308. Available from: https://linkinghub.elsevier.com/retrieve/pii/S0161642016307345.

60. Sambursky R, Davitt WF, Latkany R, et al. Sensitivity and specificity of a point-of-care matrix metalloproteinase 9 immunoassay for diagnosing inflammation related to dry eye. *JAMA Ophthalmol.* 2013;131(1):24−28. Available from: http://archopht.jamanetwork.com/article.aspx?doi=10.1001/jamaophthalmol.2013.561.

61. Sambursky R, Davitt WF, Friedberg M, Tauber S. Prospective, multicenter, clinical evaluation of point-of-care matrix metalloproteinase-9 test for confirming dry eye disease. *Cornea.* 2014;33(8):812−818. Available from: https://journals.lww.com/00003226-201408000-00009.

62. Schargus M, Ivanova S, Kakkassery V, Dick HB, Joachim S. Correlation of tear film osmolarity and 2 different MMP-9 tests with common dry eye tests in a cohort of non−dry eye patients. *Cornea.* 2015;34(7):739−744. Available from: https://journals.lww.com/00003226-201507000-00003.

63. Lanza NL, McClellan AL, Batawi H, et al. Dry eye profiles in patients with a positive elevated surface matrix metalloproteinase 9 point-of-care test versus negative patients. *Ocul Surf.* 2016;14(2):216−223. Available from: https://linkinghub.elsevier.com/retrieve/pii/S1542012416000094.

64. Oydanich M, Maguire MG, Pistilli M, et al. Effects of omega-3 supplementation on exploratory outcomes in the dry eye assessment and management study. *Ophthalmology.* 2020;127(1):136−138. Available from: https://linkinghub.elsevier.com/retrieve/pii/S0161642019312977.

65. Ryu KJ, Kim S, Kim MK, Paik HJ, Kim DH. Short-term therapeutic effects of topical corticosteroids on refractory dry eye disease: clinical usefulness of matrix metalloproteinase 9 testing as a response prediction marker. *Clin Ophthalmol.* 2021;15:759−767. Available from: https://www.dovepress.com/short-term-therapeutic-effects-of-topical-corticosteroids-on-refractor-peer-reviewed-article-OPTH.

66. Park JY, Kim BG, Kim JS, Hwang JH. Matrix metalloproteinase 9 point-of-care immunoassay result predicts response to topical cyclosporine treatment in dry eye disease. *Transl Vis Sci Technol.* 2018;7(5):31. Available from: http://tvst.arvojournals.org/article.aspx?doi=10.1167/tvst.7.5.31.

67. Yang S, Lee HJ, Kim D-Y, Shin S, Barabino S, Chung S-H. The use of conjunctival staining to measure ocular surface inflammation in patients with dry eye. *Cornea.* 2019;38(6):698−705. Available from: https://journals.lww.com/00003226-201906000-00006.

68. Kook KY, Jin R, Li L, Yoon HJ, Yoon KC. Tear osmolarity and matrix metallopeptidase-9 in dry eye associated with Sjögren's syndrome. *Korean J Ophthalmol.* 2020;34(3):179−186. Available from: http://ekjo.org/journal/view.php?doi=10.3341/kjo.2019.0145.

69. Soifer M, Mousa HM, Stinnett SS, Galor A, Perez VL. Matrix metalloproteinase 9 positivity predicts long term decreased tear production. *Ocul Surf.* 2021;19:270−274. Available from: https://linkinghub.elsevier.com/retrieve/pii/S1542012420301592.

70. Tong AY, Passi SF, Gupta PK. Clinical outcomes of lifitegrast 5% ophthalmic solution in the treatment of dry eye disease. *Eye Contact Lens Sci Clin Pract.* 2020;46(1):S20−S24. Available from: https://journals.lww.com/10.1097/ICL.0000000000000601.

71. Choi MG, Yeo JH, Kang JW, Chun YS, Lee JK, Kim JC. Effects of botulinum toxin type A on the treatment of dry eye disease and tear cytokines. *Graefe's Arch Clin Exp Ophthalmol.* 2019;257(2):331−338. Available from: http://link.springer.com/10.1007/s00417-018-4194-3.

72. Pflugfelder SC, Jones D, Ji Z, Afonso A, Monroy D. Altered cytokine balance in the tear fluid and conjunctiva of patients with Sjögren's syndrome keratoconjunctivitis sicca. *Curr Eye Res.* 1999;19(3):201−211. Available from: http://www.ncbi.nlm.nih.gov/pubmed/10487957.

73. Solomon A, Dursun D, Liu Z, Xie Y, Macri A, Pflugfelder SC. Pro- and anti-inflammatory forms of interleukin-1 in the tear fluid and conjunctiva of patients with dry-eye disease. *Invest Ophthalmol Vis Sci.* 2001;42(10):2283−2292. Available from: http://www.ncbi.nlm.nih.gov/pubmed/11527941.

74. Lam H, Bleiden L, de Paiva CS, Farley W, Stern ME, Pflugfelder SC. Tear cytokine profiles in dysfunctional

tear syndrome. *Am J Ophthalmol.* 2009;147(2): 198–205.e1. Available from: https://linkinghub. elsevier.com/retrieve/pii/S0002939408006909.

75. Villani E, Galimberti D, Papa N Del, Nucci P, Ratiglia R. Inflammation in dry eye associated with rheumatoid arthritis: cytokine and in vivo confocal microscopy study. *Innate Immun.* 2013;19(4):420–427. Available from: http://journals.sagepub.com/doi/10.1177/17534 25912471692.

76. Jackson DC, Zeng W, Wong CY, et al. Tear interferon-gamma as a biomarker for evaporative dry eye disease. *Investig Opthalmology Vis Sci.* 2016;57(11):4824–4830. Available from: http://iovs.arvojournals.org/article.aspx? doi=10.1167/iovs.16-19757.

77. Ang LPK, Sotozono C, Koizumi N, Suzuki T, Inatomi T, Kinoshita S. A comparison between cultivated and conventional limbal stem cell transplantation for Stevens-Johnson syndrome. *Am J Ophthalmol.* 2007;143(1): 178–180. Available from: https://linkinghub.elsevier. com/retrieve/pii/S0002939406009032.

78. Satici A, Guzey M, Dogan Z, Kilic A. Relationship between tear TNF-α, TGF-β$_1$, and EGF levels and severity of conjunctival cicatrization in patients with inactive trachoma. *Ophthalmic Res.* 2003;35(6):301–305. Available from: https://www.karger.com/Article/FullText/74067.

79. Chan MF, Sack R, Quigley DA, et al. Membrane array analysis of tear proteins in ocular cicatricial pemphigoid. *Optom Vis Sci.* 2011;88(8):1005–1009. Available from: https://journals.lww.com/00006324-201108000-00016.

80. Huang D, Xu N, Song Y, Wang P, Yang H. Inflammatory cytokine profiles in the tears of thyroid-associated ophthalmopathy. *Graefe's Arch Clin Exp Ophthalmol.* 2012;250(4):619–625. Available from: http://link. springer.com/10.1007/s00417-011-1863-x.

81. Lee H, Chung B, Kim KS, Seo KY, Choi BJ, Kim T. Effects of topical loteprednol etabonate on tear cytokines and clinical outcomes in moderate and severe meibomian gland dysfunction: randomized clinical trial. *Am J Ophthalmol.* 2014;158(6):1172–1183.e1. Available from: https://linkinghub.elsevier.com/retrieve/pii/S000293941 4004966.

82. Roda M, Corazza I, Bacchi Reggiani ML, et al. Dry eye disease and tear cytokine levels—a meta-analysis. *Int J Mol Sci.* 2020;21(9):3111. Available from: https://www. mdpi.com/1422-0067/21/9/3111.

83. Liu R, Rong B, Tu P, et al. Analysis of cytokine levels in tears and clinical correlations after intense pulsed light treating meibomian gland dysfunction. *Am J Ophthalmol.* 2017;183:81–90. Available from: https://linkinghub. elsevier.com/retrieve/pii/S0002939417303756.

84. Massingale ML, Li X, Vallabhajosyula M, Chen D, Wei Y, Asbell PA. Analysis of inflammatory cytokines in the tears of dry eye patients. *Cornea.* 2009;28(9):1023–1027.

Available from: https://journals.lww.com/00003226-200 910000-00014.

85. Enríquez-de-Salamanca A, Castellanos E, Stern ME, et al. Tear cytokine and chemokine analysis and clinical correlations in evaporative-type dry eye disease. *Mol Vis.* 2010; 16:862–873. Available from: http://www.ncbi.nlm.nih. gov/pubmed/20508732.

86. Craig JP, Nichols KK, Akpek EK, et al. TFOS DEWS II definition and classification report. *Ocul Surf.* 2017;15(3): 276–283. Available from: https://linkinghub.elsevier. com/retrieve/pii/S1542012417301192.

87. Roy NS, Wei Y, Kuklinski E, Asbell PA. The growing need for validated biomarkers and endpoints for dry eye clinical research. *Investig Opthalmology Vis Sci.* 2017;58(6): BIO1–BIO19. Available from: http://iovs.arvojournals. org/article.aspx?doi=10.1167/iovs.17-21709.

88. Pisella P-J, Brignole F, Debbasch C, et al. Flow cytometric analysis of conjunctival epithelium in ocular rosacea and keratoconjunctivitis sicca. *Ophthalmology.* 2000;107(10): 1841–1849. Available from: https://linkinghub.elsevier. com/retrieve/pii/S016164200000347X.

89. Brignole F, Pisella PJ, De Saint Jean M, Goldschild M, Goguel A, Baudouin C. Flow cytometric analysis of inflammatory markers in KCS: 6-month treatment with topical cyclosporin A. *Invest Ophthalmol Vis Sci.* 2001; 42(1):90–95. Available from: http://www.ncbi.nlm.nih. gov/pubmed/11133852.

90. Abud TB, Amparo F, Saboo US, et al. A clinical trial comparing the safety and efficacy of topical tacrolimus versus methylprednisolone in ocular graft-versus-host disease. *Ophthalmology.* 2016;123(7):1449–1457. Available from: https://linkinghub.elsevier.com/retrieve/pii/ S0161642016003316.

91. Barabino S, Montaldo E, Solignani F, Valente C, Mingari MC, Rolando M. Immune response in the conjunctival epithelium of patients with dry eye. *Exp Eye Res.* 2010;91(4):524–529. Available from: https:// linkinghub.elsevier.com/retrieve/pii/S0014483510002 198.

92. Versura P, Profazio V, Schiavi C, Campos EC. Hyperosmolar stress upregulates HLA-DR expression in human conjunctival epithelium in dry eye patients and in vitro models. *Investig Opthalmology Vis Sci.* 2011;52(8): 5488–5496. Available from: http://iovs.arvojournals. org/article.aspx?doi=10.1167/iovs.11-7215.

93. Brignole-Baudouin F, Riancho L, Ismail D, Deniaud M, Amrane M, Baudouin C. Correlation between the inflammatory marker HLA-DR and signs and symptoms in moderate to severe dry eye disease. *Investig Opthalmology Vis Sci.* 2017;58(4):2438–2448. Available from: http:// iovs.arvojournals.org/article.aspx?doi=10.1167/iovs.15-16555.

94. Baudouin C, de la Maza MS, Amrane M, et al. One-year efficacy and safety of 0.1% cyclosporine a cationic

emulsion in the treatment of severe dry eye disease. *Eur J Ophthalmol.* 2017;27(6):678–685. Available from: http://journals.sagepub.com/doi/10.5301/ejo.5001002.

95. Roche PA, Furuta K. The ins and outs of MHC class II-mediated antigen processing and presentation. *Nat Rev Immunol.* 2015;15(4):203–216. Available from: http://www.nature.com/articles/nri3818.

96. De Saint Jean M, Brignole F, Feldmann G, Goguel A, Baudouin C. Interferon-gamma induces apoptosis and expression of inflammation-related proteins in Chang conjunctival cells. *Invest Ophthalmol Vis Sci.* 1999; 40(10):2199–2212. Available from: http://www.ncbi.nlm.nih.gov/pubmed/10476784.

97. Kambayashi T, Laufer TM. Atypical MHC class II-expressing antigen-presenting cells: can anything replace a dendritic cell? *Nat Rev Immunol.* 2014;14(11):719–730. Available from: http://www.nature.com/articles/nri3754.

98. Brignole F, Pisella PJ, Goldschild M, De Saint Jean M, Goguel A, Baudouin C. Flow cytometric analysis of inflammatory markers in conjunctival epithelial cells of patients with dry eyes. *Invest Ophthalmol Vis Sci.* 2000;41(6): 1356–1363. Available from: http://www.ncbi.nlm.nih.gov/pubmed/10798650.

99. Tsubota K, Fujihara T, Saito K, Takeuchi T. Conjunctival epithelium expression of HLA-DR in dry eye patients. *Ophthalmologica.* 1999;213(1):16–19. Available from: https://www.karger.com/Article/FullText/27387.

100. Roy NS, Wei Y, Yu Y, et al. Conjunctival HLA-DR expression and its association with symptoms and signs in the DREAM study. *Transl Vis Sci Technol.* 2019;8(4):31. Available from: https://tvst.arvojournals.org/article.aspx?articleid=2748979.

101. Aragona P, Spinella R, Rania L, et al. Safety and efficacy of 0.1% clobetasone butyrate eyedrops in the treatment of dry eye in Sjögren syndrome. *Eur J Ophthalmol.* 2013; 23(3):368–376. Available from: http://journals.sagepub.com/doi/10.5301/ejo.5000229.

102. Leonardi A, Van Setten G, Amrane M, et al. Efficacy and safety of 0.1% cyclosporine a cationic emulsion in the treatment of severe dry eye disease: a multicenter randomized trial. *Eur J Ophthalmol.* 2016;26(4):287–296. Available from: http://journals.sagepub.com/doi/10.5301/ejo.5000779.

103. Brignole-Baudouin F, Baudouin C, Aragona P, et al. A multicentre, double-masked, randomized, controlled trial assessing the effect of oral supplementation of omega-3 and omega-6 fatty acids on a conjunctival inflammatory marker in dry eye patients. *Acta Ophthalmol.* 2011;89(7):e591–e597. Available from: http://doi.wiley.com/10.1111/j.1755-3768.2011.02196.x.

104. Tsubota K, Fujita H, Tsuzaka K, Takeuchi T. Quantitative analysis of lacrimal gland function, apoptotic figures, Fas and Fas ligand expression of lacrimal glands in dry eye patients. *Exp Eye Res.* 2003;76(2):233–240. Available from: https://linkinghub.elsevier.com/retrieve/pii/S0014483502002798.

105. Gao J, Morgan G, Tieu D, et al. ICAM-1 expression predisposes ocular tissues to immune-based inflammation in dry eye patients and Sjögrens syndrome-like MRL/lpr mice. *Exp Eye Res.* 2004;78(4):823–835. Available from: https://linkinghub.elsevier.com/retrieve/pii/S0014483503003609.

106. Stern ME, Gao J, Schwalb TA, et al. Conjunctival T-cell subpopulations in Sjögren's and non-Sjögren's patients with dry eye. *Invest Ophthalmol Vis Sci.* 2002;43(8): 2609–2614. Available from: http://www.ncbi.nlm.nih.gov/pubmed/12147592.

107. Baudouin C, Messmer EM, Aragona P, et al. Revisiting the vicious circle of dry eye disease: a focus on the pathophysiology of meibomian gland dysfunction. *Br J Ophthalmol.* 2016;100(3):300–306. Available from: https://bjo.bmj.com/lookup/doi/10.1136/bjophthalmol-2015-307415.

108. Higuchi A, Kawakita T, Tsubota K. IL-6 induction in desiccated corneal epithelium in vitro and in vivo. *Mol Vis.* 2011;17:2400–2406. Available from: http://www.ncbi.nlm.nih.gov/pubmed/21976951.

109. Kam W, Sullivan D, Sullivan B, Venkiteshwar M. Does hyperosmolarity induce an irreversible process leading to human corneal epithelial cell death? *Invest Ophthalmol Vis Sci.* 2016;57(12):6181.

110. Korb DR. Survey of preferred tests for diagnosis of the tear film and dry eye. *Cornea.* 2000;19(4):483–486. Available from: http://journals.lww.com/00003226-200007000-00016.

111. Tomlinson A, McCann LC, Pearce EI. Comparison of human tear film osmolarity measured by electrical impedance and freezing point depression techniques. *Cornea.* 2010;29(9):1036–1041. Available from: https://journals.lww.com/00003226-201009000-00015.

112. Gokhale M, Stahl U, Jalbert I. In situ osmometry: validation and effect of sample collection technique. *Optom Vis Sci.* 2013;90(4):359–365. Available from: https://journals.lww.com/00006324-201304000-00009.

113. Versura P, Profazio V, Campos EC. Performance of tear osmolarity compared to previous diagnostic tests for dry eye diseases. *Curr Eye Res.* 2010;35(7):553–564. Available from: http://www.tandfonline.com/doi/full/10.3109/02713683.2010.484557.

114. Suzuki M, Massingale ML, Ye F, et al. Tear osmolarity as a biomarker for dry eye disease severity. *Investig Opthalmology Vis Sci.* 2010;51(9):4557–4561. Available from: http://iovs.arvojournals.org/article.aspx?doi=10.1167/iovs.09-4596.

115. Sullivan BD, Whitmer D, Nichols KK, et al. An objective approach to dry eye disease severity. *Investig Opthalmology Vis Sci.* 2010;51(12):6125–6130. Available from: http://iovs.arvojournals.org/article.aspx?doi=10.1167/iovs.10-5390.

116. Lemp MA, Bron AJ, Baudouin C, et al. Tear osmolarity in the diagnosis and management of dry eye disease. *Am J Ophthalmol.* 2011;151(5):792–798.e1. Available from: https://linkinghub.elsevier.com/retrieve/pii/S000293941000841X.

117. Jacobi C, Jacobi A, Kruse FE, Cursiefen C. Tear film osmolarity measurements in dry eye disease using electrical

impedance technology. *Cornea.* 2011;30(12): 1289−1292. Available from: https://journals.lww.com/ 00003226-201112000-00001.

118. Masmali A, Alrabiah S, Alharbi A, El-Hiti GA, Almubrad T. Investigation of tear osmolarity using the TearLab osmolarity system in normal adults in Saudi Arabia. *Eye Contact Lens Sci Clin Pract.* 2014;40(2): 74−78. Available from: https://journals.lww.com/ 00140068-201403000-00003.

119. Khanal S, Tomlinson A, McFadyen A, Diaper C, Ramaesh K. Dry eye diagnosis. *Investig Opthalmology Vis Sci.* 2008;49(4):1407−1414. Available from: http://iovs. arvojournals.org/article.aspx?doi=10.1167/iovs.07-0635.

120. Tomlinson A, Khanal S, Ramaesh K, Diaper C, McFadyen A. Tear film osmolarity: determination of a referent for dry eye diagnosis. *Investig Opthalmology Vis Sci.* 2006;47(10):4309−4315. Available from: http:// iovs.arvojournals.org/article.aspx?doi=10.1167/iovs.05- 1504.

121. Alves M, Reinach PS, Paula JS, et al. Comparison of diagnostic tests in distinct well-defined conditions related to dry eye diseaseWedrich A, ed. *PLoS One.* 2014;9(5): e97921. Available from: https://dx.plos.org/10.1371/ journal.pone.0097921.

122. Yeh TN, Graham AD, Lin MC. Relationships among tear film stability, osmolarity, and dryness symptoms. *Optom Vis Sci.* 2015;92(9):e264−e272. Available from: https:// journals.lww.com/00006324-201509000-00020.

123. Bunya VY, Fuerst NM, Pistilli M, et al. Variability of tear osmolarity in patients with dry eye. *JAMA Ophthalmol.* 2015;133(6):662−667. Available from: http://archopht. jamanetwork.com/article.aspx?doi=10.1001/jamaophthal mol.2015.0429.

124. Baenninger PB, Voegeli S, Bachmann LM, et al. Variability of tear osmolarity measurements with a point-of-care system in healthy subjects—systematic review. *Cornea.* 2018;37(7):938−945. Available from: https://journals. lww.com/00003226-201807000-00028.

125. Tashbayev B, Utheim TP, Utheim ØA, et al. Utility of tear osmolarity measurement in diagnosis of dry eye disease. *Sci Rep.* 2020;10(1):5542. Available from: http://www. nature.com/articles/s41598-020-62583-x.

126. Willcox MDP, Argüeso P, Georgiev GA, et al. TFOS DEWS II tear film report. *Ocul Surf.* 2017;15(3):366−403. Available from: https://linkinghub.elsevier.com/retrieve/pii/ S1542012417300721.

127. Balík J. The lacrimal fluid in keratoconjunctivitis sicca. *Am J Ophthalmol.* 1952;35(6):773−782. Available from: https://linkinghub.elsevier.com/retrieve/pii/0002939452 906685.

128. Gilbard JP, Farris RL, Santamaria J. Osmolarity of tear microvolumes in keratoconjunctivitis sicca. *Arch Ophthalmol.* 1978;96(4):677−681. Available from: http://archo pht.jamanetwork.com/article.aspx?articleid=632566.

129. Messmer EM, Bulgen M, Kampik A. Hyperosmolarity of the tear film in dry eye syndrome. In: *Research Projects in Dry Eye Syndrome [Internet].* Basel: Karger Publishers;

2010:129−138. Available from: https://www.karger. com/Article/FullText/315026.

130. Hwang J, Dermer H, Galor A. Can in vivo confocal microscopy differentiate between sub-types of dry eye disease? A review. *Clin Experiment Ophthalmol.* 2021;49(4): 373−387. Available from: https://onlinelibrary.wiley. com/doi/10.1111/ceo.13924.

131. Dua HS, Said DG, Messmer EM, et al. Neurotrophic keratopathy. *Prog Retin Eye Res.* 2018;66:107−131. Available from: https://linkinghub.elsevier.com/retrieve/pii/ S1350946217301210.

132. Oliveira-Soto L, Efron N. Morphology of corneal nerves using confocal microscopy. *Cornea.* 2001;20(4): 374−384. Available from: http://journals.lww.com/ 00003226-200105000-00008.

133. Patel DV, McGhee CNJ. In vivo confocal microscopy of human corneal nerves in health, in ocular and systemic disease, and following corneal surgery: a review. *Br J Ophthalmol.* 2009;93(7):853−860. Available from: https:// bjo.bmj.com/lookup/doi/10.1136/bjo.2008.150615.

134. Villani E, Baudouin C, Efron N, et al. In vivo confocal microscopy of the ocular surface: from bench to bedside. *Curr Eye Res.* 2014;39(3):213−231. Available from: http://www.tandfonline.com/doi/full/10.3109/0271368 3.2013.842592.

135. Brooks J, Tracey I. Review: from nociception to pain perception: imaging the spinal and supraspinal pathways. *J Anat.* 2005;207(1):19−33. Available from: https://onlinelibrary.wiley.com/doi/10.1111/j.1469-758 0.2005.00428.x.

136. Belmonte C, Acosta MC, Merayo-Lloves J, Gallar J. What causes eye pain? *Curr Ophthalmol Rep.* 2015;3(2): 111−121. Available from: http://link.springer.com/10. 1007/s40135-015-0073-9.

137. Oprée A, Kress M. Involvement of the proinflammatory cytokines tumor necrosis factor-α, IL-1β, and IL-6 but not IL-8 in the development of heat hyperalgesia: effects on heat-evoked calcitonin gene-related peptide release from rat skin. *J Neurosci.* 2000;20(16):6289−6293. Available from: https://www.jneurosci.org/lookup/doi/10. 1523/JNEUROSCI.20-16-06289.2000.

138. Lee Y, Lee C-H, Oh U. Painful channels in sensory neurons. *Mol Cells.* 2005;20(3):315−324. Available from: http://www.ncbi.nlm.nih.gov/pubmed/16404144.

139. IASP terminology [Internet]. 2019. Available from: http://www.iasp-pain.org/Education/Content.aspx?%0A ItemNumber=1698 (Accessed January 2019).

140. Rosenthal P, Borsook D, Moulton EA. Oculofacial pain: corneal nerve damage leading to pain beyond the eye. *Investig Opthalmology Vis Sci.* 2016;57(13):5285−5287. Available from: http://iovs.arvojournals.org/article.aspx? doi=10.1167/iovs.16-20557.

141. Galor A, Feuer W, Lee DJ, et al. Prevalence and risk factors of dry eye syndrome in a United States Veterans affairs population. *Am J Ophthalmol.* 2011;152(3):377−384.e2. Available from: https://linkinghub.elsevier.com/retrieve/ pii/S0002939411002066.

142. Crane AM, Levitt RC, Felix ER, Sarantopoulos KD, McClellan AL, Galor A. Patients with more severe symptoms of neuropathic ocular pain report more frequent and severe chronic overlapping pain conditions and psychiatric disease. *Br J Ophthalmol.* 2017;101(2):227−231. Available from: https://bjo.bmj.com/lookup/doi/10.1136/bjophthalmol-2015-308214.

143. Rosenthal P, Baran I, Jacobs DS. Corneal pain without stain: is it real? *Ocul Surf.* 2009;7(1):28−40. Available from: https://linkinghub.elsevier.com/retrieve/pii/S1542012702902.

144. Galor A, Feuer W, Lee DJ, et al. Depression, post-traumatic stress disorder, and dry eye syndrome: a study utilizing the National United States Veterans affairs administrative database. *Am J Ophthalmol.* 2012;154(2):340−346.e2. Available from: https://linkinghub.elsevier.com/retrieve/pii/S0002939412001055.

145. Galor A, Moein H-R, Lee C, et al. Neuropathic pain and dry eye. *Ocul Surf.* 2018;16(1):31−44. Available from: https://linkinghub.elsevier.com/retrieve/pii/S154201241730068X.

146. Rosenthal P, Borsook D. Ocular neuropathic pain. *Br J Ophthalmol.* 2016;100(1):128−134. Available from: https://bjo.bmj.com/lookup/doi/10.1136/bjophthalmol-2014-306280.

147. Ross AR, Al-Aqaba MA, Almaazmi A, et al. Clinical and in vivo confocal microscopic features of neuropathic corneal pain. *Br J Ophthalmol.* 2020;104(6):768−775. Available from: https://bjo.bmj.com/lookup/doi/10.1136/bjophthalmol-2019-314799.

148. Theophanous C, Jacobs DS, Hamrah P. Corneal neuralgia after LASIK. *Optom Vis Sci.* 2015;92(9):e233−e240. Available from: https://journals.lww.com/00006324-201509000-00016.

149. Aggarwal S, Kheirkhah A, Cavalcanti BM, et al. Autologous serum tears for treatment of photoallodynia in patients with corneal neuropathy: efficacy and evaluation with in vivo confocal microscopy. *Ocul Surf.* 2015;13(3):250−262. Available from: https://linkinghub.elsevier.com/retrieve/pii/S1542012415000099.

150. Moein H-R, Akhlaq A, Dieckmann G, et al. Visualization of microneuromas by using in vivo confocal microscopy: an objective biomarker for the diagnosis of neuropathic corneal pain? *Ocul Surf.* 2020;18(4):651−656. Available from: https://linkinghub.elsevier.com/retrieve/pii/S1542012420301117.

151. Shetty R, Sethu S, Deshmukh R, et al. Corneal dendritic cell density is associated with subbasal nerve plexus features, ocular surface disease index, and serum vitamin D in evaporative dry eye disease. *Biomed Res Int.* 2016;2016:1−10. Available from: http://www.hindawi.com/journals/bmri/2016/4369750/.

152. Kheirkhah A, Qazi Y, Arnoldner MA, Suri K, Dana R. In vivo confocal microscopy in dry eye disease associated with chronic graft-versus-host disease. *Investig Opthalmology Vis Sci.* 2016;57(11):4686−4691. Available from: http://iovs.arvojournals.org/article.aspx?doi=10.1167/iovs.16-20013.

153. Giannaccare G, Pellegrini M, Sebastiani S, Moscardelli F, Versura P, Campos EC. In vivo confocal microscopy morphometric analysis of corneal subbasal nerve plexus in dry eye disease using newly developed fully automated system. *Graefe's Arch Clin Exp Ophthalmol.* 2019;257(3):583−589. Available from: http://link.springer.com/10.1007/s00417-018-04225-7.

154. Aggarwal S, Colon C, Kheirkhah A, Hamrah P. Efficacy of autologous serum tears for treatment of neuropathic corneal pain. *Ocul Surf.* 2019;17(3):532−539. Available from: https://linkinghub.elsevier.com/retrieve/pii/S1542012418302386.

155. Dermer H, Hwang J, Mittal R, Cohen AK, Galor A. Corneal sub-basal nerve plexus microneuromas in individuals with and without dry eye. *Br J Ophthalmol*; 2021. bjophthalmol-2020-317891. Available from: https://bjo.bmj.com/lookup/doi/10.1136/bjophthalmol-2020-317891.

156. Bayraktutar BN, Ozmen MC, Muzaaya N, et al. Comparison of clinical characteristics of post-refractive surgery-related and post-herpetic neuropathic corneal pain. *Ocul Surf.* 2020;18(4):641−650. Available from: https://linkinghub.elsevier.com/retrieve/pii/S1542012420301129.

157. Villani E, Magnani F, Viola F, et al. In vivo confocal evaluation of the ocular surface morpho-functional unit in dry eye. *Optom Vis Sci.* 2013;90(6):576−586. Available from: https://journals.lww.com/00006324-201306000-00009.

158. Tepelus TC, Chiu GB, Maram J, et al. Corneal features in ocular graft-versus-host disease by in vivo confocal microscopy. *Graefe's Arch Clin Exp Ophthalmol.* 2017;255(12):2389−2397. Available from: http://link.springer.com/10.1007/s00417-017-3759-x.

159. del Castillo JMB, Wasfy MAS, Fernandez C, Garcia-Sanchez J. An in vivo confocal masked study on corneal epithelium and subbasal nerves in patients with dry eye. *Investig Opthalmology Vis Sci.* 2004;45(9):3030−3035. Available from: http://iovs.arvojournals.org/article.aspx?doi=10.1167/iovs.04-0251.

160. Villani E, Galimberti D, Viola F, Mapelli C, Ratiglia R. The cornea in Sjögren's syndrome: an in vivo confocal study. *Investig Opthalmology Vis Sci.* 2007;48(5):2017−2022. Available from: http://iovs.arvojournals.org/article.aspx?doi=10.1167/iovs.06-1129.

161. Tepelus TC, Chiu GB, Huang J, et al. Correlation between corneal innervation and inflammation evaluated with confocal microscopy and symptomatology in patients with dry eye syndromes: a preliminary study. *Graefe's Arch Clin Exp Ophthalmol.* 2017;255(9):1771−1778. Available from: http://link.springer.com/10.1007/s00417-017-3680-3.

162. Tuisku IS, Konttinen YT, Konttinen LM, Tervo TM. Alterations in corneal sensitivity and nerve morphology in

patients with primary Sjögren's syndrome. *Exp Eye Res.* 2008;86(6):879–885. Available from: https://linkinghub.elsevier.com/retrieve/pii/S0014483508000882.

163. Zhang M, Chen J, Luo L, Xiao Q, Sun M, Liu Z. Altered corneal nerves in aqueous tear deficiency viewed by in vivo confocal microscopy. *Cornea.* 2005;24(7):818–824. Available from: https://journals.lww.com/00003226-200510000-00011.

164. Gabbriellini G, Baldini C, Varanini V, et al. In vivo confocal scanning laser microscopy in patients with primary Sjögren's syndrome: a monocentric experience. *Mod Rheumatol.* 2015;25(4):585–589. Available from: http://www.tandfonline.com/doi/full/10.3109/14397595.2014.979523.

165. Fea AM, Aragno V, Testa V, et al. The effect of autologous platelet lysate eye drops: an in vivo confocal microscopy study. *Biomed Res Int.* 2016;2016:1–10. Available from: http://www.hindawi.com/journals/bmri/2016/8406832/.

166. Iaccheri B, Torroni G, Cagini C, et al. Corneal confocal scanning laser microscopy in patients with dry eye disease treated with topical cyclosporine. *Eye.* 2017;31(5):788–794. Available from: http://www.nature.com/articles/eye20173.

167. Matsumoto Y, Ibrahim OMA, Kojima T, Dogru M, Shimazaki J, Tsubota K. Corneal in vivo laser-scanning confocal microscopy findings in dry eye patients with Sjögren's syndrome. *Diagnostics.* 2020;10(7):497. Available from: https://www.mdpi.com/2075-4418/10/7/497.

168. Benítez-del-Castillo JM, Acosta MC, Wassfi MA, et al. Relation between corneal innervation with confocal microscopy and corneal sensitivity with noncontact esthesiometry in patients with dry eye. *Investig Opthalmology Vis Sci.* 2007;48(1):173–181. Available from: http://iovs.arvojournals.org/article.aspx?doi=10.1167/iovs.06-0127.

169. Villani E, Galimberti D, Viola F, Mapelli C, Del Papa N, Ratiglia R. Corneal involvement in rheumatoid arthritis: an in vivo confocal study. *Investig Opthalmology Vis Sci.* 2008;49(2):560–564. Available from: http://iovs.arvojournals.org/article.aspx?doi=10.1167/iovs.07-0893.

170. Takhar JS, Joye AS, Lopez SE, et al. Validation of a novel confocal microscopy imaging protocol with assessment of reproducibility and comparison of nerve metrics in dry eye disease compared with controls. *Cornea.* 2021;40(5):603–612. Available from: https://journals.lww.com/10.1097/ICO.0000000000002549.

171. Lanza M, Iaccarino S, Varricchi G, D'Errico T, Gironi Carnevale UA, Bifani M. Corneal confocal microscopy alterations in Sjögren's syndrome dry eye. *Acta Ophthalmol.* 2017;95(5):e366–e372. Available from: https://onlinelibrary.wiley.com/doi/10.1111/aos.13194.

172. Villani E, Garoli E, Termine V, Pichi F, Ratiglia R, Nucci P. Corneal confocal microscopy in dry eye treated with corticosteroids. *Optom Vis Sci.* 2015;92(9):e290–e295. Available from: https://journals.lww.com/00006324-201509000-00023.

173. Levy O, Labbé A, Borderie V, et al. Increased corneal sub-basal nerve density in patients with Sjögren syndrome treated with topical cyclosporine A. *Clin Experiment Ophthalmol.* 2017;45(5):455–463. Available from: https://onlinelibrary.wiley.com/doi/10.1111/ceo.12898.

174. Mahelkova G, Jirsova K, Seidler stangova P, et al. Using corneal confocal microscopy to track changes in the corneal layers of dry eye patients after autologous serum treatment. *Clin Exp Optom.* 2017;100(3):243–249. Available from: https://www.tandfonline.com/doi/full/10.1111/cxo.12455.

175. Semeraro F, Forbice E, Nascimbeni G, et al. Effect of autologous serum eye drops in patients with Sjögren syndrome-related dry eye: clinical and in vivo confocal microscopy evaluation of the ocular surface. *In Vivo.* 2016;30(6):931–938. Available from: http://iv.iiarjournals.org/content/30/6/931.abstract.

176. Matsumoto Y, Shigeno Y, Sato EA, et al. The evaluation of the treatment response in obstructive meibomian gland disease by in vivo laser confocal microscopy. *Graefe's Arch Clin Exp Ophthalmol.* 2009;247(6):821–829. Available from: http://link.springer.com/10.1007/s00417-008-1017-y.

177. Ibrahim OMA, Matsumoto Y, Dogru M, et al. The efficacy, sensitivity, and specificity of in vivo laser confocal microscopy in the diagnosis of meibomian gland dysfunction. *Ophthalmology.* 2010;117(4):665–672. Available from: https://linkinghub.elsevier.com/retrieve/pii/S0161642009015048.

178. Villani E, Beretta S, De Capitani M, Galimberti D, Viola F, Ratiglia R. In vivo confocal microscopy of meibomian glands in Sjögren's syndrome. *Investig Opthalmology Vis Sci.* 2011;52(2):933–939. Available from: http://iovs.arvojournals.org/article.aspx?doi=10.1167/iovs.10-5995.

179. Fu J, Chou Y, Hao R, Jiang X, Liu Y, Li X. Evaluation of ocular surface impairment in meibomian gland dysfunction of varying severity using a comprehensive grading scale. *Medicine.* 2019;98(31):e16547. Available from: https://journals.lww.com/00005792-201908020-00016.

180. Randon M, Aragno V, Abbas R, Liang H, Labbé A, Baudouin C. In vivo confocal microscopy classification in the diagnosis of meibomian gland dysfunction. *Eye.* 2019;33(5):754–760. Available from: http://www.nature.com/articles/s41433-018-0307-9.

181. Kojima T, Ishida R, Sato EA, et al. In vivo evaluation of ocular demodicosis using laser scanning confocal microscopy. *Investig Opthalmology Vis Sci.* 2011;52(1):565–569. Available from: http://iovs.arvojournals.org/article.aspx?doi=10.1167/iovs.10-5477.

182. Randon M, Liang H, El Hamdaoui M, et al. In vivo confocal microscopy as a novel and reliable tool for the diagnosis of Demodex eyelid infestation. *Br J Ophthalmol.* 2015;99(3):336–341. Available from: https://bjo.bmj.com/lookup/doi/10.1136/bjophthalmol-2014-305671.

183. Yildiz-Tas A, Arici C, Mergen B, Sahin A. In vivo confocal microscopy in blepharitis patients with ocular demodex infestation. *Ocul Immunol Inflamm;* 2021:1–6. Available from: https://www.tandfonline.com/doi/full/10.1080/09273948.2021.1875006.

184. Steger B, Speicher L, Philipp W, Bechrakis NE. In vivo confocal microscopic characterisation of the cornea in chronic graft-versus-host disease related severe dry eye disease. *Br J Ophthalmol.* 2015;99(2):160−165. Available from: https://bjo.bmj.com/lookup/doi/10.1136/bjophthalmol-2014-305072.

185. He J, Ogawa Y, Mukai S, et al. In vivo confocal microscopy evaluation of ocular surface with graft-versus-host disease-related dry eye disease. *Sci Rep.* 2017;7(1):10720. Available from: http://www.nature.com/articles/s41598-017-10237-w.

186. Lin H, Li W, Dong N, et al. Changes in corneal epithelial layer inflammatory cells in aqueous tear−deficient dry eye. *Investig Opthalmology Vis Sci.* 2010 1;51(1):122. Available from: http://iovs.arvojournals.org/article.aspx?doi=10.1167/iovs.09-3629.

187. Wakamatsu TH, Sato EA, Matsumoto Y, et al. Conjunctival in vivo confocal scanning laser microscopy in patients with Sjögren syndrome. *Investig Opthalmology Vis Sci.* 2010;51(1):144−150. Available from: http://iovs.arvojournals.org/article.aspx?doi=10.1167/iovs.08-2722.

188. Hong J, Zhu W, Zhuang H, et al. In vivo confocal microscopy of conjunctival goblet cells in patients with Sjogren's syndrome dry eye. *Br J Ophthalmol.* 2010;94(11):1454−1458. Available from: https://bjo.bmj.com/lookup/doi/10.1136/bjo.2009.161059.

189. Villani E, Beretta S, Galimberti D, Viola F, Ratiglia R. In vivo confocal microscopy of conjunctival roundish bright objects: young, older, and Sjögren subjects. *Investig Opthalmology Vis Sci.* 2011;52(7):4829−4832. Available from: http://iovs.arvojournals.org/article.aspx?doi=10.1167/iovs.10-6215.

190. Sato EA, Matsumoto Y, Dogru M, et al. Lacrimal gland in Sjögren's syndrome. *Ophthalmology.* 2010;117(5):1055−1055.e3. Available from: https://linkinghub.elsevier.com/retrieve/pii/S016164200901392X.

191. Stapleton F, Alves M, Bunya VY, et al. TFOS DEWS II Epidemiology report. *Ocul Surf.* 2017;15(3):334−365. Available from: https://linkinghub.elsevier.com/retrieve/pii/S154201241730109X.

192. Schein OD, Muñoz B, Tielsch JM, Bandeen-Roche K, West S. Prevalence of dry eye among the elderly. *Am J Ophthalmol.* 1997;124(6):723−728. Available from: https://linkinghub.elsevier.com/retrieve/pii/S0002939414716885.

193. Schein OD, Hochberg MC, Muñoz B, et al. Dry eye and dry mouth in the elderly: a population-based assessment. *Arch Intern Med.* 1999;159(12):1359−1363. Available from: http://archinte.jamanetwork.com/article.aspx?doi=10.1001/archinte.159.12.1359.

194. Chia E-M, Mitchell P, Rochtchina E, Lee AJ, Maroun R, Wang JJ. Prevalence and associations of dry eye syndrome in an older population: the Blue Mountains Eye Study. *Clin Exp Ophthalmol.* 2003;31(3):229−232. Available from: http://doi.wiley.com/10.1046/j.1442-9071.2003.00634.x.

195. Schaumberg DA, Sullivan DA, Buring JE, Dana MR. Prevalence of dry eye syndrome among US women. *Am J Ophthalmol.* 2003;136(2):318−326. Available from: https://linkinghub.elsevier.com/retrieve/pii/S0002939403002186.

196. Moss SE. Incidence of dry eye in an older population. *Arch Ophthalmol.* 2004;122(3):369−373. Available from: http://archopht.jamanetwork.com/article.aspx?doi=10.1001/archopht.122.3.369.

197. Schaumberg DA, Dana R, Buring JE, Sullivan DA. Prevalence of dry eye disease among US men: estimates from the physicians' health studies. *Arch Ophthalmol.* 2009;127(6):763−768. Available from: http://archopht.jamanetwork.com/article.aspx?doi=10.1001/archophthalmol.2009.103.

198. Paulsen AJ, Cruickshanks KJ, Fischer ME, et al. Dry eye in the beaver dam offspring study: prevalence, risk factors, and health-related quality of life. *Am J Ophthalmol.* 2014;157(4):799−806. Available from: https://linkinghub.elsevier.com/retrieve/pii/S0002939413008131.

199. Bourcier T, Acosta MC, Borderie V, et al. Decreased corneal sensitivity in patients with dry eye. *Investig Opthalmology Vis Sci.* 2005;46(7):2341−2345. Available from: http://iovs.arvojournals.org/article.aspx?doi=10.1167/iovs.04-1426.

200. Gilbard JP. Human tear film electrolyte concentrations in health and dry-eye disease. *Int Ophthalmol Clin.* 1994;34(1):27−36. Available from: http://journals.lww.com/00004397-199403410-00005.

201. Gayton J. Etiology, prevalence, and treatment of dry eye disease. *Clin Ophthalmol.* 2009;3:405−412. Available from: http://www.dovepress.com/etiology-prevalence-and-treatment-of-dry-eye-disease-peer-reviewed-article-OPTH.

202. Nasu M, Matsubara O, Yamamoto H. Post-mortem prevalence of lymphocytic infiltration of the lacrymal gland: a comparative study in autoimmune and non-autoimmune diseases. *J Pathol.* 1984;143(1):11−15. Available from: http://doi.wiley.com/10.1002/path.1711430104.

203. Obata H, Yamamoto S, Horiuchi H, Machinami R. Histopathologic study of human lacrimal gland. *Ophthalmology.* 1995;102(4):678−686. Available from: https://linkinghub.elsevier.com/retrieve/pii/S0161642095309712.

204. Bukhari AA, Basheer NA, Joharjy HI. Age, gender, and interracial variability of normal lacrimal gland volume using MRI. *Ophthalmic Plast Reconstr Surg.* 2014;30(5):388−391. Available from: https://journals.lww.com/00002341-201409000-00007.

205. El-Fadaly AB, El-Shaarawy EAA, Rizk AA, Nasralla MM, Shuaib DMA. Age-related alterations in the lacrimal gland of adult albino rat: a light and electron microscopic study. *Ann Anat − Anat Anzeiger.* 2014;196(5):336−351. Available from: https://linkinghub.elsevier.com/retrieve/pii/S0940960214001319.

206. Obata H. Anatomy and histopathology of the human lacrimal gland. *Cornea.* 2006;25(1):S82−S89. Available from: https://journals.lww.com/00003226-200612001-00016.

207. McGill JI, Liakos GM, Goulding N, Seal DV. Normal tear protein profiles and age-related changes. *Br J Ophthalmol.* 1984;68(5):316−320. Available from: https://bjo.bmj.com/lookup/doi/10.1136/bjo.68.5.316.

208. Seal DV. The effect of ageing and disease on tear constituents. *Trans Ophthalmol Soc UK.* 1985;104(Pt 4): 355−362. Available from: http://www.ncbi.nlm.nih.gov/pubmed/3862268.

209. Mathers WD, Lane JA, Zimmerman MB. Tear film changes associated with normal aging. *Cornea.* 1996;15(3): 229−234. Available from: http://journals.lww.com/00003226-199605000-00001.

210. Boberg-Ans J. On the corneal sensitivity. *Acta Ophthalmol.* 2009;34(3):149−162. Available from: http://doi.wiley.com/10.1111/j.1755-3768.1956.tb03346.x.

211. Millodot M. The influence of age onthe sensitivity of the cornea. *Invest Ophthalmol Vis Sci.* 1977;16(3):240−242. Available from: http://www.ncbi.nlm.nih.gov/pubmed/844979.

212. Acosta MC, Alfaro ML, Borrás F, Belmonte C, Gallar J. Influence of age, gender and iris color on mechanical and chemical sensitivity of the cornea and conjunctiva. *Exp Eye Res.* 2006;83(4):932−938. Available from: https://linkinghub.elsevier.com/retrieve/pii/S001448350600 2417.

213. Kojima T, Wakamatsu TH, Dogru M, et al. Age-related dysfunction of the lacrimal gland and oxidative stress. *Am J Pathol.* 2012;180(5):1879−1896. Available from: https://linkinghub.elsevier.com/retrieve/pii/S000294401 200154X.

214. Knop E, Knop N, Millar T, Obata H, Sullivan DA. The international workshop on meibomian gland dysfunction: report of the subcommittee on anatomy, physiology, and pathophysiology of the meibomian gland. *Invest Ophthalmol Vis Sci.* 2011;52(4):1938−1978. Available from: http://www.ncbi.nlm.nih.gov/pubmed/21450915.

215. Hykin PG, Bron AJ. Age-related morphological changes in lid margin and meibomian gland anatomy. *Cornea.* 1992;11(4):334−342. Available from: http://journals.lww.com/00003226-199207000-00012.

216. Obata H. Anatomy and histopathology of human meibomian gland. *Cornea.* 2002;21(2):S70−S74. Available from: https://journals.lww.com/00003226-200210001-00005.

217. Sullivan DA, Sullivan BD, Evans JE, et al. Androgen deficiency, meibomian gland dysfunction, and evaporative dry eye. *Ann N Y acad sci.* 2002;966(1):211−222. Available from: http://doi.wiley.com/10.1111/j.1749-6632.2002.tb04217.x.

218. Chhadva P, McClellan AL, Alabiad CR, Feuer WJ, Batawi H, Galor A. Impact of eyelid laxity on symptoms and signs of dry eye disease. *Cornea.* 2016;35(4): 531−535. Available from: https://journals.lww.com/00003226-201604000-00019.

219. Alghamdi YA, Mercado C, McClellan AL, Batawi H, Karp CL, Galor A. Epidemiology of meibomian gland

220. dysfunction in an elderly population. *Cornea.* 2016; 35(6):731−735. Available from: https://journals.lww.com/00003226-201606000-00003.

220. Yamaguchi M, Kutsuna M, Uno T, Zheng X, Kodama T, Ohashi Y. Marx line: fluorescein staining line on the inner lid as indicator of meibomian gland function. *Am J Ophthalmol.* 2006;141(4):669−669.e8. Available from: https://linkinghub.elsevier.com/retrieve/pii/S000293940 5012079.

221. Arita R, Itoh K, Inoue K, Amano S. Noncontact infrared meibography to document age-related changes of the meibomian glands in a normal population. *Ophthalmology.* 2008;115(5):911−915. Available from: https://linkinghub.elsevier.com/retrieve/pii/S0161642007007282.

222. Ban Y, Shimazaki-Den S, Tsubota K, Shimazaki J. Morphological evaluation of meibomian glands using noncontact infrared meibography. *Ocul Surf.* 2013; 11(1):47−53. Available from: https://linkinghub.elsevier.com/retrieve/pii/S1542012412001711.

223. Shirakawa R, Arita R, Amano S. Meibomian gland morphology in Japanese infants, children, and adults observed using a mobile pen-shaped infrared meibography device. *Am J Ophthalmol.* 2013;155(6): 1099−1103.e1. Available from: https://linkinghub.elsevier.com/retrieve/pii/S0002939413000731.

224. Finis D, Ackermann P, Pischel N, et al. Evaluation of meibomian gland dysfunction and local distribution of meibomian gland atrophy by non-contact infrared meibography. *Curr Eye Res.* 2015;40(10):982−989. Available from: http://www.tandfonline.com/doi/full/10.3109/02713683.2014.971929.

225. Yeotikar NS, Zhu H, Markoulli M, Nichols KK, Naduvilath T, Papas EB. Functional and morphologic changes of meibomian glands in an asymptomatic adult population. *Investig Opthalmology Vis Sci.* 2016;57(10): 3996−4007. Available from: http://iovs.arvojournals.org/article.aspx?doi=10.1167/iovs.15-18467.

226. Mizoguchi T, Arita R, Fukuoka S, Morishige N. Morphology and function of meibomian glands and other tear film parameters in junior high school students. *Cornea.* 2017;36(8):922−926. Available from: https://journals.lww.com/00003226-201708000-00005.

227. Ablamowicz AF, Nichols JJ, Nichols KK. Association between serum levels of testosterone and estradiol with meibomian gland assessments in postmenopausal women. *Investig Opthalmology Vis Sci.* 2016;57(2): 295−300. Available from: http://iovs.arvojournals.org/article.aspx?doi=10.1167/iovs.15-18158.

228. Yeh TN, Lin MC. Risk factors for severe meibomian gland atrophy in a young adult population: a cross-sectional studyMadigan M, ed. *PLoS One.* 2017;12(9):e0185603. Available from: https://dx.plos.org/10.1371/journal.pone.0185603.

229. Wang MTM, Muntz A, Lim J, et al. Ageing and the natural history of dry eye disease: a prospective registry-based

cross-sectional study. *Ocul Surf.* 2020;18(4):736−741. Available from: https://linkinghub.elsevier.com/retrieve/pii/S1542012420301105.

230. Sullivan DA, Wickham LA, Krenzer KL, Rocha EM, Toda I. Aqueous tear deficiency in Sjögren's syndrome: possible causes and potential treatment. In: Pleyer U, Hartmann C, eds. *Oculodermal Diseases − Immunology of Bullous Oculo-Muco-Cutaneous Disorders.* Buren, The Netherlands: Aeolus Press; 1997:95−152.

231. Truong S, Cole N, Stapleton F, Golebiowski B. Sex hormones and the dry eye. *Clin Exp Optom.* 2014;97(4):324−336. Available from: https://www.tandfonline.com/doi/full/10.1111/cxo.12147.

232. Versura P, Giannaccare G, Campos EC. Sex-steroid imbalance in females and dry eye. *Curr Eye Res.* 2015;40(2):162−175. Available from: http://www.tandfonline.com/doi/full/10.3109/02713683.2014.966847.

233. Haendler B, Toda I, Sullivan DA, Schleuning W-D. Expression of transcripts for cysteine-rich secretory proteins (CRISPs) in the murine lacrimal gland. *J Cell Physiol.* 1999;178(3):371−378. Available from: https://onlinelibrary.wiley.com/doi/10.1002/(SICI)1097-4652(199903)178:3%3C371::AID-JCP11%3E3.0.CO;2-N.

234. Richards SM, Liu M, Jensen RV, et al. Androgen regulation of gene expression in the mouse lacrimal gland. *J Steroid Biochem Mol Biol.* 2005;96(5):401−413. Available from: https://linkinghub.elsevier.com/retrieve/pii/S0960076005002153.

235. Richards SM, Jensen RV, Liu M, et al. Influence of sex on gene expression in the mouse lacrimal gland. *Exp Eye Res.* 2006;82(1):13−23. Available from: https://linkinghub.elsevier.com/retrieve/pii/S0014483505001296.

236. Suzuki T, Schirra F, Richards SM, et al. Estrogen's and progesterone's impact on gene expression in the mouse lacrimal gland. *Investig Opthalmology Vis Sci.* 2006;47(1):158−168. Available from: http://iovs.arvojournals.org/article.aspx?doi=10.1167/iovs.05-1003.

237. Sullivan DA, Jensen RV, Suzuki T, Richards SM. Do sex steroids exert sex-specific and/or opposite effects on gene expression in lacrimal and meibomian glands? *Mol Vis.* 2009;15:1553−1572. Available from: http://www.ncbi.nlm.nih.gov/pubmed/19693291.

238. Sullivan DA, Rocha EM, Aragona P, et al. TFOS DEWS II sex, gender, and hormones report. *Ocul Surf.* 2017;15(3):284−333. Available from: https://linkinghub.elsevier.com/retrieve/pii/S1542012417300939.

239. Oprea L, Tiberghien A, Creuzot-Garcher C, Baudouin C. Influence des hormones sur le film lacrymal. *J Fr Ophtalmol.* 2004;27(8):933−941. Available from: https://linkinghub.elsevier.com/retrieve/pii/S0181551204962419.

240. Azcarate PM, Venincasa VD, Feuer W, Stanczyk F, Schally AV, Galor A. Androgen deficiency and dry eye syndrome in the aging male. *Investig Opthalmology Vis Sci.* 2014;55(8):5046−5053. Available from: http://iovs.arvojournals.org/article.aspx?doi=10.1167/iovs.14-14689.

241. Gagliano C, Caruso S, Napolitano G, et al. Low levels of 17-β-oestradiol, oestrone and testosterone correlate with severe evaporative dysfunctional tear syndrome in postmenopausal women: a case−control study. *Br J Ophthalmol.* 2014;98(3):371−376. Available from: https://bjo.bmj.com/lookup/doi/10.1136/bjophthalmol-2012-302705.

242. Toda I, Wickham LA, Sullivan DA. Gender and androgen treatment influence the expression of proto-oncogenes and apoptotic factors in lacrimal and salivary tissues of MRL/lprMice. *Clin Immunol Immunopathol.* 1998;86(1):59−71. Available from: https://linkinghub.elsevier.com/retrieve/pii/S0090122997944664.

243. Vercaeren I, Vanaken H, Van Dorpe J, Verhoeven G, Heyns W. Expression of cystatin-related protein and of the C3-component of prostatic-binding protein during postnatal development in the rat ventral prostate and lacrimal gland. *Cell Tissue Res.* 1998;292(1):115−128. Available from: http://www.ncbi.nlm.nih.gov/pubmed/9506919.

244. Toda I, Sullivan BD, Rocha EM, Da Silveira LA, Wickham LA, Sullivan DA. Impact of gender on exocrine gland inflammation in mouse models of Sjögren's syndrome. *Exp Eye Res.* 1999;69(4):355−366. Available from: https://linkinghub.elsevier.com/retrieve/pii/S0014483599907157.

245. Ranganathan V, Jana NR, De PK. Hormonal effects on hamster lacrimal gland female-specific major 20 kDa secretory protein and its immunological similarity with submandibular gland major male-specific proteins. *J Steroid Biochem Mol Biol.* 1999;70(4−6):151−158. Available from: https://linkinghub.elsevier.com/retrieve/pii/S096007609900103X.

246. Richards SM, Liu M, Sullivan BD, Sullivan DA. Gender-related differences in gene expression of the lacrimal gland. *Adv Exp Med Biol.* 2002;506:121−127. Available from: http://journals.lww.com/00003226-200011002-00152.

247. Sakulsak N, Wakayama T, Hipkaeo W, Iseki S. A novel mouse protein differentially regulated by androgens in the submandibular and lacrimal glands. *Arch Oral Biol.* 2007;52(6):507−517. Available from: https://linkinghub.elsevier.com/retrieve/pii/S0003996906003104.

248. Cavallero C. Relative effectiveness of various steroids in an androgen assay using the exorbital lacrimal gland of the castrated rat. *Acta Endocrinol.* 1967;55(1):119−130. Available from: https://eje.bioscientifica.com/view/journals/eje/55/1/acta_55_1_013.xml.

249. Ariga H, Edwards J, Sullivan DA. Androgen control of autoimmune expression in lacrimal glands of mice. *Clin Immunol Immunopathol.* 1989;53(3):499−508. Available from: https://linkinghub.elsevier.com/retrieve/pii/0090122989900111.

250. Winderickx J, Hemschoote K, De Clercq N, et al. Tissue-specific expression and androgen regulation of different genes encoding rat prostatic 22-kilodalton glycoproteins

homologous to human and rat cystatin. *Mol Endocrinol.* 1990;4(4):657–667. Available from: https://academic. oup.com/mend/article-lookup/doi/10.1210/mend-4-4-657.

251. Winderickx J, Vercaeren I, Verhoeven G, Heyns W. Androgen-dependent expression of cystatin-related protein (CRP) in the exorbital lacrimal gland of the rat. *J Steroid Biochem Mol Biol.* 1994;48(2–3):165–170. Available from: http://www.ncbi.nlm.nih.gov/pubmed/8142291.

252. Gao J, Lambert RW, Wickham LA, Banting G, Sullivan DA. Androgen control of secretory component mRNA levels in the rat lacrimal gland. *J Steroid Biochem Mol Biol.* 1995;52(3):239–249. Available from: https://linkinghub.elsevier.com/retrieve/pii/096007609400172I.

253. Ranganathan V, De PK. Androgens and estrogens markedly inhibit expression of a 20-kDa major protein in hamster exorbital lacrimal gland. *Biochem Biophys Res Commun.* 1995;208(1):412–417. Available from: https://linkinghub.elsevier.com/retrieve/pii/S0006291X85713538.

254. Huang Z, Lambert RW, Wickham LA, Sullivan DA. Analysis of cytomegalovirus infection and replication in acinar epithelial cells of the rat lacrimal gland. *Invest Ophthalmol Vis Sci.* 1996;37(6):1174–1186. Available from: http://www.ncbi.nlm.nih.gov/pubmed/8631632.

255. Sullivan DA, Block L, Pena JDO. Influence of androgens and pituitary hormones on the structural profile and secretory activity of the lacrimal gland. *Acta Ophthalmol Scand.* 1996;74(5):421–435. Available from: https://onlinelibrary.wiley.com/doi/10.1111/j.1600-0420.1996.tb00594.x.

256. Sullivan DA, Bélanger A, Cermak JM, et al. Are women with Sjögren's syndrome androgen-deficient? *J Rheumatol.* 2003;30(11):2413–2419. Available from: http://www.ncbi.nlm.nih.gov/pubmed/14677186.

257. Valtysdóttir ST, Wide L, Hällgren R. Low serum dehydroepiandrosterone sulfate in women with primary Sjögren's syndrome as an isolated sign of impaired HPA axis function. *J Rheumatol.* 2001;28(6):1259–1265. Available from: http://www.ncbi.nlm.nih.gov/pubmed/11409117.

258. Konttinen YT, Porola P, Konttinen L, Laine M, Poduval P. Immunohistopathology of Sjögren's syndrome. *Autoimmun Rev.* 2006;6(1):16–20. Available from: https://linkinghub.elsevier.com/retrieve/pii/S15689972060000346.

259. Laine M, Porola P, Udby L, et al. Low salivary dehydroepiandrosterone and androgen-regulated cysteine-rich secretory protein 3 levels in Sjögren's syndrome. *Arthritis Rheum.* 2007;56(8):2575–2584. Available from: https://onlinelibrary.wiley.com/doi/10.1002/art.22828.

260. Porola P, Virkki L, Przybyla BD, et al. Androgen deficiency and defective intracrine processing of dehydroepiandrosterone in salivary glands in Sjögren's syndrome. *J Rheumatol.* 2008;35(11):2229–2235. Available from: http://www.jrheum.org/lookup/doi/10.3899/jrheum.080220.

261. Nikolov NP, Illei GG. Pathogenesis of Sjögren's syndrome. *Curr Opin Rheumatol.* 2009;21(5):465–470. Available from: https://journals.lww.com/00002281-200909000-00005.

262. Spaan M, Porola P, Laine M, Rozman B, Azuma M, Konttinen YT. Healthy human salivary glands contain a DHEA-sulphate processing intracrine machinery, which is deranged in primary Sjögren's syndrome. *J Cell Mol Med.* 2009;13(7):1261–1270. Available from: https://onlinelibrary.wiley.com/doi/10.1111/j.1582-4934.2009.00727.x.

263. Warren DW, Azzarolo AM, Huang ZM, et al. Androgen support of lacrimal gland function in the female rabbit. *Adv Exp Med Biol.* 1998;438:89–93. Available from: http://link.springer.com/10.1007/978-1-4615-5359-5_11.

264. Sullivan DA, Sullivan BD, Ullman MD, et al. Androgen influence on the meibomian gland. *Invest Ophthalmol Vis Sci.* 2000;41(12):3732–3742. Available from: http://www.ncbi.nlm.nih.gov/pubmed/11053270.

265. Worda C, Nepp J, Huber JC, Sator MO. Treatment of keratoconjunctivitis sicca with topical androgen. *Maturitas.* 2001;37(3):209–212. Available from: https://linkinghub.elsevier.com/retrieve/pii/S037851220000181X.

266. Schiffman RM, Bradford R, Bunnell B, Lai F, Bernstein P, Whitcup SW. A multicenter, doublemasked, randomized, vehicle controlled, parallel group study to evaluate the safety and efficacy of testosterone ophthalmic solution in patients with meibomian gland dysfunction. (abstract). *Investig Ophthalmol Vis Sci.* 2006;47(13): e–5608 (ARVO e-abs).

267. Khandelwal P, Liu S, Sullivan DA. Androgen regulation of gene expression in human meibomian gland and conjunctival epithelial cells. *Mol Vis.* 2012;18:1055–1067. Available from: http://www.ncbi.nlm.nih.gov/pubmed/22605918.

268. Krenzer KL. Effect of androgen deficiency on the human meibomian gland and ocular surface. *J Clin Endocrinol Metab.* 2000;85(12):4874–4882. Available from: http://press.endocrine.org/doi/10.1210/jcem.85.12.7072.

269. Cermak JM, Krenzer KL, Sullivan RM, Dana MR, Sullivan DA. Is complete androgen insensitivity syndrome associated with alterations in the meibomian gland and ocular surface? *Cornea.* 2003;22(6):516–521. Available from: http://journals.lww.com/00003226-200308000-00006.

270. Sullivan DA, Yamagami H, Liu M, et al. Sex steroids, the meibomian gland and evaporative dry eye. *Adv Exp Med Biol.* 2002;506(Pt A):389–399. Available from: http://link.springer.com/10.1007/978-1-4615-0717-8_56.

271. Smith JA, Vitale S, Reed GF, et al. Dry eye signs and symptoms in women with premature ovarian failure. *Arch Ophthalmol.* 2004;122(2):151–156. Available from: http://archopht.jamanetwork.com/article.aspx?doi=10.1001/archopht.122.2.151.

272. Turaka K, Nottage JM, Hammersmith KM, Nagra PK, Rapuano CJ. Dry eye syndrome in aromatase inhibitor

users. *Clin Experiment Ophthalmol.* 2013;41(3):239–243. Available from: http://doi.wiley.com/10.1111/j.1442-9071.2012.02865.x.

273. Cuzick J, Sestak I, Forbes JF, et al. Anastrozole for prevention of breast cancer in high-risk postmenopausal women (IBIS-II): an international, double-blind, randomised placebo-controlled trial. *Lancet.* 2014;383(9922):1041–1048. Available from: https://linkinghub.elsevier.com/retrieve/pii/S0140673613622928.

274. Inglis H, Boyle FM, Friedlander ML, Watson SL. Dry eyes and AIs: if you don't ask you won't find out. *The Breast.* 2015;24(6):694–698. Available from: https://linkinghub.elsevier.com/retrieve/pii/S0960977615001 85X.

275. Maruyama K, Yokoi N, Takamata A, Kinoshita S. Effect of environmental conditions on tear dynamics in soft contact lens wearers. *Investig Opthalmology Vis Sci.* 2004;45(8):2563–2568. Available from: http://iovs.arvojournals.org/article.aspx?doi=10.1167/iovs.03-1185.

276. Kastelan S, Lukenda A, Salopek-Rabatić J, Pavan J, Gotovac M. Dry eye symptoms and signs in long-term contact lens wearers. *Coll Antropol.* 2013;37(1):199–203. Available from: http://www.ncbi.nlm.nih.gov/pubmed/23837244.

277. Stolz J, Astakhov S, Lisochkina A, Astakhov Y. Assessment of dry eye signs and symptoms and ocular tolerance of a preservative-free lacrimal substitute (Hylabak® reg;) versus a preserved lacrimal substitute (Systane® reg;) used for 3 months in patients after LASIK. *Clin Ophthalmol.* 2013;7:2289–2297. Available from: http://www.dovepress.com/assessment-of-dry-eye-signs-and-sympto ms-and-ocular-tolerance-of-a-pre-peer-reviewed-article-OPTH.

278. Azuma M, Yabuta C, Fraunfelder FW, Shearer TR. Dry eye in LASIK patients. *BMC Res Notes.* 2014;7:420. Available from: http://bmcresnotes.biomedcentral.com/articles/10.1186/1756-0500-7-420.

279. Sayin N, Kara N, Pekel G, Altinkaynak H. Effects of chronic smoking on central corneal thickness, endothelial cell, and dry eye parameters. *Cutan Ocul Toxicol.* 2014;33(3):201–205. Available from: http://www.tandfonline.com/doi/full/10.3109/15569527.2013.832 688.

280. Porcar E, Pons AM, Lorente A. Visual and ocular effects from the use of flat-panel displays. *Int J Ophthalmol.* 2016;9(6):881–885. Available from: http://www.ijo.cn/gjyken/ch/reader/view_abstract.aspx?file_no=20160616 &flag=1.

281. Uchino M, Yokoi N, Uchino Y, et al. Prevalence of dry eye disease and its risk factors in visual display terminal users: the osaka study. *Am J Ophthalmol.* 2013;156(4):759–766.e1. Available from: https://linkinghub.elsevier.com/retrieve/pii/S0002939413003838.

282. Ribelles A, Galbis-Estrada C, Parras MA, Vivar-Llopis B, Marco-Ramírez C, Diaz-Llopis M. Ocular surface and tear film changes in older women working with computers. *Biomed Res Int.* 2015;2015:1–10. Available from: http://www.hindawi.com/journals/bmri/2015/46 7039/.

283. Yazici A, Sari ES, Sahin G, et al. Change in tear film characteristics in visual display terminal users. *Eur J Ophthalmol.* 2015;25(2):85–89. Available from: http://journals.sagepub.com/doi/10.5301/ejo.5000525.

284. Choi JH, Li Y, Kim SH, et al. The influences of smartphone use on the status of the tear film and ocular surfaceTaylor AW, ed. *PLoS One.* 2018;13(10):e0206541. Available from: https://dx.plos.org/10.1371/journal.pone.0206541.

285. Chlasta-Twardzik E, Górecka-Nitoń A, Nowińska A, Wylęgała E. The influence of work environment factors on the ocular surface in a one-year follow-up prospective clinical study. *Diagnostics.* 2021;11(3):392. Available from: https://www.mdpi.com/2075-4418/11/3/392.

286. Courtin R, Pereira B, Naughton G, et al. Prevalence of dry eye disease in visual display terminal workers: a systematic review and meta-analysis. *BMJ Open.* 2016;6(1):e009675. Available from: https://bmjopen.bmj.com/lookup/doi/10.1136/bmjopen-2015-009675.

287. Freudenthaler N, Neuf H, Kadner G, Schlote T. Characteristics of spontaneous eyeblink activity during video display terminal use in healthy volunteers. *Graefe's Arch Clin Exp Ophthalmol.* 2003;241(11):914–920. Available from: http://link.springer.com/10.1007/s00417-003-0786-6.

288. Wong KKW. Blinking and operating: cognition versus vision. *Br J Ophthalmol.* 2002;86(4):479. Available from: https://bjo.bmj.com/lookup/doi/10.1136/bjo.86.4.479.

289. Tsubota K, Nakamori K. Dry eyes and video display terminals. *N Engl J Med.* 1993;328(8):584. Available from: http://www.nejm.org/doi/abs/10.1056/NEJM199 302253280817.

290. Patel S, Henderson R, Bradley L, Galloway B, Hunter L. Effect of visual display unit use on blink rate and tear stability. *Optom Vis Sci.* 1991;68(11):888–892. Available from: http://journals.lww.com/00006324-199111000-00010.

291. Schlote T, Kadner G, Freudenthaler N. Marked reduction and distinct patterns of eye blinking in patients with moderately dry eyes during video display terminal use. *Graefe's Arch Clin Exp Ophthalmol.* 2004;242(4):306–312. Available from: http://link.springer.com/10.1007/s00417-003-0845-z.

292. Golebiowski B, Long J, Harrison K, Lee A, Chidi-Egboka N, Asper L. Smartphone use and effects on tear film, blinking and binocular vision. *Curr Eye Res.* 2020;45(4):428–434. Available from: https://www.tandfonline.com/doi/full/10.1080/02713683.2019.1663542.

293. Portello JK, Rosenfield M, Chu CA. Blink rate, incomplete blinks and computer vision syndrome. *Optom Vis Sci.* 2013;90(5):482–487. Available from: https://journals.lww.com/00006324-201305000-00011.

294. Chu CA, Rosenfield M, Portello JK. Blink patterns. *Optom Vis Sci.* 2014;91(3):297–302. Available from: https://journals.lww.com/00006324-201403000-00009.

295. Rosenfield M, Jahan S, Nunez K, Chan K. Cognitive demand, digital screens and blink rate. *Comput Human*

Behav. 2015;51:403–406. Available from: https://link inghub.elsevier.com/retrieve/pii/S0747563215003829.

296. McMonnies CW. Incomplete blinking: exposure keratopathy, lid wiper epitheliopathy, dry eye, refractive surgery, and dry contact lenses. *Contact Lens Anterior Eye.* 2007; 30(1):37–51. Available from: https://linkinghub. elsevier.com/retrieve/pii/S1367048406001603.

297. Wan T, Jin X, Lin L, Xu Y, Zhao Y. Incomplete blinking may attribute to the development of meibomian gland dysfunction. *Curr Eye Res.* 2016;41(2):179–185. Available from: http://www.tandfonline.com/doi/full/10. 3109/02713683.2015.1007211.

298. Wu H, Wang Y, Dong N, et al. Meibomian gland dysfunction determines the severity of the dry eye conditions in visual display terminal workersSakakibara M, ed. *PLoS One.* 2014;9(8):e105575. Available from: https://dx. plos.org/10.1371/journal.pone.0105575.

299. Wang MTM, Tien L, Han A, et al. Impact of blinking on ocular surface and tear film parameters. *Ocul Surf.* 2018; 16(4):424–429. Available from: https://linkinghub. elsevier.com/retrieve/pii/S1542012418300260.

300. Cardona G, García C, Serés C, Vilaseca M, Gispets J. Blink rate, blink amplitude, and tear film integrity during dynamic visual display terminal tasks. *Curr Eye Res.* 2011; 36(3):190–197. Available from: http://www.tand fonline.com/doi/full/10.3109/02713683.2010.544442.

301. Hirota M, Uozato H, Kawamorita T, Shibata Y, Yamamoto S. Effect of incomplete blinking on tear film stability. *Optom Vis Sci.* 2013;90(7):650–657. Available from: https://journals.lww.com/00006324-201307000-00006.

302. Talens-Estarelles C, Sanchis-Jurado V, Esteve-Taboada JJ, Pons ÁM, García-Lázaro S. How do different digital displays affect the ocular surface? *Optom Vis Sci.* 2020; 97(12):1070–1079. Available from: https://journals. lww.com/10.1097/OPX.0000000000001616.

303. Fenga C, Aragona P, Di Nola C, Spinella R. Comparison of ocular surface disease index and tear osmolarity as markers of ocular surface dysfunction in video terminal display workers. *Am J Ophthalmol.* 2014;158(1): 41–48.e2. Available from: https://linkinghub.elsevier. com/retrieve/pii/S0002939414001457.

304. Tan LL, Morgan P, Cai ZQ, Straughan RA. Prevalence of and risk factors for symptomatic dry eye disease in Singapore. *Clin Exp Optom.* 2015;98(1):45–53. Available from: https://www.tandfonline.com/doi/full/10.1111/ cxo.12210.

305. Yang W-J, Yang Y-N, Cao J, et al. Risk factors for dry eye syndrome: a retrospective case-control study. *Optom Vis Sci.* 2015;92(9):e199–205. Available from: https:// journals.lww.com/00006324-201509000-00011.

306. Yokoi N, Yamada H, Mizukusa Y, et al. Rheology of tear film lipid layer spread in normal and aqueous tear–deficient dry eyes. *Investig Opthalmology Vis Sci.* 2008; 49(12):5319–5324. Available from: http://iovs.arvo journals.org/article.aspx?doi=10.1167/iovs.07-1407.

307. Santodomingo-Rubido J, Wolffsohn JS, Gilmartin B. Changes in ocular physiology, tear film characteristics, and symptomatology with 18 months silicone hydrogel contact lens wear. *Optom Vis Sci.* 2006;83(2):73–81. Available from: https://journals.lww.com/00006324-200602000-00009.

308. Hori Y. Secreted mucins on the ocular surface. *Investig Opthalmology Vis Sci.* 2018;59(14):DES151–DES156. Available from: http://iovs.arvojournals.org/article.aspx? doi=10.1167/iovs.17-23623.

309. Chen Y, Hu F, Zhou Y, Chen W, Shao H, Zhang Y. MGMT promoter methylation and glioblastoma prognosis: a systematic review and meta-analysis. *Arch Med Res.* 2013; 44(4):281–290. Available from: https://linkinghub. elsevier.com/retrieve/pii/S0188440913001045.

310. Del Águila-Carrasco AJ, Ferrer-Blasco T, García-Lázaro S, Esteve-Taboada JJ, Montés-Micó R. Assessment of corneal thickness and tear meniscus during contact-lens wear. *Contact Lens Anterior Eye.* 2015;38(3):185–193. Available from: https://linkinghub.elsevier.com/retrieve/pii/S1367 048415000120.

311. Berry M, Pult H, Purslow C, Murphy PJ. Mucins and ocular signs in symptomatic and asymptomatic contact lens wear. *Optom Vis Sci.* 2008;85(10):E930–E938. Available from: https://journals.lww.com/00006324-20081 0000-00010.

312. Uçakhan Ö, Arslanturk-Eren M. The role of soft contact lens wear on meibomian gland morphology and function. *Eye Contact Lens Sci Clin Pract.* 2019;45(5): 292–300. Available from: https://journals.lww.com/10. 1097/ICL.0000000000000572.

313. Wolkoff P. "Healthy" eye in office-like environments. *Environ Int.* 2008;34(8):1204–1214. Available from: https://linkinghub.elsevier.com/retrieve/pii/ S0160412008000676.

314. Berg EJ, Ying GS, Maguire MG, et al, DREAM Study Research Group. Climatic and Environmental Correlates of Dry Eye Disease Severity: A Report From the Dry Eye Assessment and Management (DREAM) Study. *Transl Vis Sci Technol.* 2020;9(5):25. https://doi.org/10.1167/ tvst.9.5.25. Available from: https://tvst.arvojournals.org/ article.aspx?articleid=2765460.

315. Madden LC, Tomlinson A, Simmons PA. Effect of humidity variations in a controlled environment chamber on tear evaporation after dry eye therapy. *Eye Contact Lens Sci Clin Pract.* 2013;39(2):169–174. Available from: https://journals.lww.com/00140068-201303000-00008.

CHAPTER 6

Sjögren's Syndrome Dry Eye Disease

JEREMY N. NORTEY, BS • JOHN A. GONZALES, MD

INTRODUCTION

The term *keratoconjunctivitis sicca*, introduced by the Swedish ophthalmologist Henrik Sjögren, refers to aqueous insufficient dry eye disease (DED).[1,2] Sjögren's syndrome is known for causing sicca, or dryness, of the eyes and mouth. However, Sjögren's syndrome is a complex autoimmune disease with effects on the entire body including dermatitis, pneumonitis, vasculitis, and an increased risk of developing lymphoproliferative disorders.

PATHOPHYSIOLOGY OF SJÖGREN'S SYNDROME

Sjögren's syndrome is a systemic autoimmune/autoinflammatory disorder and there is likely an immunogenetic predisposition that Sjögren's syndrome patients may share. Indeed, there are shared alleles in some major histocompatibility region of the human leukocyte antigens that have been identified in some Sjögren's syndrome patient cohorts.[3] Indeed, in the Sjögren's International Collaborative Clinical Alliance (SICCA) cohort, there were notable differences in genome wide association study analysis particularly between cohort participants with Asian and European ancestry.[4] There is also activation of interferon-based canonical pathways, which can affect innate immune factors in Sjögren's syndrome patients. There also may be differentially expressed genes in the transcriptome profile of salivary glands, peripheral blood mononuclear cells, and serum in patients with primary Sjögren's syndrome compared to Sjögren's syndrome occurring in association with other autoimmune disease.[5] While B-cells have been recognized to have a central role in the pathophysiology of Sjögren's syndrome, T-cells, particularly follicular helper T-cells, may also play an important role, which seems intuitive considering that salivary and lacrimal glands have germinal center functions.[6,7]

AN UNDERDIAGNOSED POPULATION IN THE EYE CLINIC

DED is one of the most common diagnoses made in the eye clinic.[8] Because DED is so common, general ophthalmologists are at the front line for treating DED patients.[9] While most ophthalmologists who have been previously surveyed note that DED is not difficult to diagnose, a higher proportion of cornea specialists compared to comprehensive, or general, ophthalmologists agree that there is a need for additional treatment options for moderate to severe DED.[10,11] While there is a perception that DED is not difficult to diagnose and despite the prevalence of DED and patient-reported symptoms of dry eye, Sjögren's syndrome is frequently underdiagnosed, which may start with an underreferral to appropriate specialists.[9,12]

Suspecting, let alone making a diagnosis of, Sjögren's syndrome may seem daunting to an ophthalmologist considering that the disease may present with protean manifestations and there have been numerous prior diagnostic classifications in use. None of the classification criteria prior to 2016 were accepted by both the American College of Rheumatology and European League Against Rheumatism until the ACR/EULAR diagnostic criteria were developed and validated.[13–15] The ocular tests used as part of the diagnostic classification criteria for Sjögren's syndrome can be easily performed by ophthalmologists. Additionally, ophthalmologists can further identify patients with a higher probability of being classified as Sjögren's syndrome by asking some simple yet pointed questions.

Dry Eye Disease. https://doi.org/10.1016/B978-0-323-82753-9.00003-5

DIAGNOSTIC CRITERIA FOR SJÖGREN'S SYNDROME

Prior to 2012, there were 11 classification/diagnostic criteria sets for Sjögren's syndrome, but none had ever been endorsed by the ACR or EULAR.[16–24] In 2012, new classification criteria developed using the National Institutes of Health–funded SICCA registry were provisionally approved by the ACR and subsequently published.[25] The provisional ACR criteria were based solely on objective tests (symptoms were considered as inclusion criteria for the target population to whom the criteria applied). Ultimately, an international set of classification criteria for Sjögren's syndrome was developed from a subset of participants from the SICCA registry data and from two other large cohorts (Oklahoma Medical Research Foundation and Paris-Sud Kremlin Bicêtre) and validated using approaches approved by both ACR and EULAR committees (Table 6.1).[13–15]

SYMPTOMS AND SIGNS OF DED IN SJÖGREN'S SYNDROME

Symptoms

Patient's with Sjögren's syndrome may complain of dry eye, but this is a relatively common complaint in the eye clinic in general and isn't specific for Sjögren's syndrome itself. Asking more specific questions, including "Is your mouth dry when eating a meal?" and "Can you eat a cracker without drinking a fluid or liquid?" are most helpful in distinguishing between those who

may be classified as Sjögren's syndrome and those less likely to have Sjögren's syndrome at that time.[26] Symptoms of dry eye and how they affect functional activities can be assessed by a variety of questionnaires, including the ocular surface disease index and dry eye questionnaire (such as DEQ-5, a five-item questionnaire).[27,28] Perceptions of pain can be further evaluated using the ocular pain assessment survey and neuropathic pain symptom inventory questionnaires calibrated for ocular pain.[29–31] Using questionnaires can be particularly helpful to quantify improvements in comfort and patient-reported activities in response to therapy.

Clinical Signs

Identifying patients with complaints of dry eye should proceed with testing to determine whether the patient has aqueous sufficient DED, aqueous deficient DED, a combination of aqueous sufficient and deficient DED, or neuropathic ocular pain.[2,32] Schirmer I (without anesthesia) should be performed first before procedures requiring staining of the cornea and conjunctiva are performed. A Schirmer I of ≤5 mm at 5 min is compatible with an abnormal Schirmer I test according to ACR/EULAR criteria. However, there is significant variability in the Schirmer I test, even in controls.[33,34] Nevertheless, [7]given that Schirmer I is highly specific for identifying those with keratoconjunctivitis sicca compared to those without, this test can be complimentary to another test to identify keratoconjunctivitis sicca, the ocular staining score (OSS).[35]

Staining of the cornea with fluorescein and staining of the nasal and temporal bulbar conjunctiva with lissamine green are components of the OSS (Fig. 6.1).[36] The OSS exhibits both a high specificity and sensitivity in identifying those with keratoconjunctivitis sicca compared to those without.[35] Little is known about the progression of keratoconjunctivitis sicca in Sjögren's syndrome.

SICCA 2-year follow-up showed modest progression of DED. We explored the phenotypic changes in features of Sjögren's syndrome and in Sjögren's syndrome status after 2 years.[37] There were 771 participants who returned for 2-year follow-up and had the same examinations that were originally performed at baseline. Eighty-nine percent of follow-up participants still met Sjögren's syndrome criteria. Additionally, 8% of those who did not meet Sjögren's syndrome classification at baseline had converted to Sjögren's syndrome at 2-year follow-up. An important parameter of DED, the OSS, progressed in at least 11% of those returning for follow-up, though this progression was not statistically associated with progression to Sjögren's syndrome (Table 6.1).[37] However, 2 years is a relatively short

TABLE 6.1

American College of Rheumatology/European League Against Rheumatism Diagnostic Criteria for Sjögren's Syndrome. A Score of 4 or More is Required for Classification as Sjögren's Syndrome.

Test/Sign/Item	Score/Weight
Labial salivary gland biopsy demonstrating focal lymphocytic sialadenitis with focus score ≥1 foci/4 mm²	3
Anti-SSA/Ro antibody positive	3
Unstimulated whole salivary flow rate ≤0.1 mL/min	1
Ocular staining score (OSS) ≥5 in at least one eye	1
Schirmer I ≤ 5 mm at 5 min in at least one eye	1

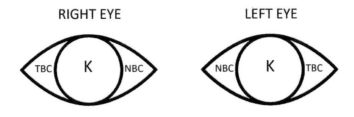

RIGHT EYE		
	Score	Number of dots
Temporal Bulbar Conjunctiva (TBC, assessed with concentrated lissamine green 1%)	0	0-9
	1	10-32
	2	33-100
	3	>100
Cornea (K, assessed with fluorescein 0.5%) For cornea only add: +1 for patches of confluent staining +1 for staining in pupillary area +1 for one or more filaments	Score	Number of dots
	0	0
	1	1-5
	2	6-30
	3	>30
	Score	Number of dots
Nasal Bulbar Conjunctiva (NBC, assessed with concentrated lissamine green 1%)	0	0-9
	1	10-32
	2	33-100
	3	>100
LEFT EYE		
	Score	Number of dots
Nasal Bulbar Conjunctiva (NBC, assessed with concentrated lissamine green 1%)	0	0-9
	1	10-32
	2	33-100
	3	>100
Cornea (K, assessed with fluorescein 0.5%) For cornea only add: +1 for patches of confluent staining +1 for staining in pupillary area +1 for one or more filaments	Score	Number of dots
	0	0
	1	1-5
	2	6-30
	3	>30
	Score	Number of dots
Temporal Bulbar Conjunctiva (TBC, assessed with concentrated lissamine green 1%)	0	0-9
	1	10-32
	2	33-100
	3	>100

FIG. 6.1 **The ocular staining score.** A score of 5 or higher in at least one eye yields a score of 1 on the diagnostic criteria for Sjögren's syndrome.

follow-up. Nevertheless, those with corneal staining have a higher odds of having a labial salivary gland biopsy with a focus score of ≥ 1.[38]

Determining if the DED in Sjögren's syndrome progresses is important because if the disease is stable over time, we can be confident that therapy instituted when DED is detected may be sufficient in a patient's long-term care. Alternatively, if DED progresses, then monitoring Schirmer I and OSS at each visit may be advisable as well and advancing therapies may be indicated.

Tear osmolarity has been suggested as biomarker to identify and categorize severity of DED.[39-41] However, tear osmolarity also exhibits significant variability in Sjögren's syndrome patients.[42,43] Additionally, in the SICCA registry cohort, tear osmolarity did not exhibit specificity or sensitivity in distinguishing between those with keratoconjunctivitis sicca and without.[35]

Ancillary Imaging in Sjögren's Syndrome Keratoconjunctivitis Sicca

Up to 30% of patients with Sjögren's syndrome have a short fiber neuropathy as evidenced on biopsy of epidermal tissues.[44] Short fiber neuropathy may also be seen elsewhere in the body, including the cornea, and offers the possibility of serving as additional biomarker in Sjögren's syndrome. Those with DED have quantifiable abnormalities in the structure and density of the corneal subbasal nerve plexus.[45-48] Longitudinal studies of patients with and without Sjögren's and how abnormalities in the subbasal nerve plexus are associated with Sjögren's syndrome are needed.

Ultrasonography of salivary glands can be helpful in identifying inflammation that correlates with histopathological features distinguishing Sjögren's syndrome from undifferentiated connective tissue diseases.[49,50] Sonography has been used to identify the presence or lack of obviously detectable lacrimal glands in Sjögren's syndrome.[51] Indeed, the lack or "invisibility" of the lacrimal glands on ultrasonography has been suggested to serve as a marker of futility in using immunosuppressive medications seeking to rehabilitate their function.[51]

TREATMENT OF SJÖGREN'S SYNDROME DRY EYE

Topical Therapy

Common and readily available options for managing DED include over-the-counter artificial tears. Their diverse formulations, relative cost-effectiveness, and lack of side effects make them the de facto first-line therapies. Artificial tears aim to supplement and replace one's own tear production. However, artificial tears are entirely palliative as they fail to address the underlying pathophysiology that drives most types of DED. A systematic review that included 43 randomized controlled trials involving the treatment of DED with artificial tears identified that the quality of evidence was low for the various formulations of artificial tears that were compared to placebo (saline or mannitol vehicle) revealing that additional research is needed to form more robust conclusions about the effectiveness of artificial tears.[52] Very few studies have compared the efficacy of different artificial tears to each other.[53] A wide variety exists with differing levels of osmolarity, viscosity, pH, viscosity enhancing agents, and lipid supplementation.[54] Additionally, preservative-free formulations are recommended when patients require frequent application of artificial tears. All of these factors play a role in patient preference.

Autologous serum tears are frequently used for patients with aqueous deficient DED (such as graft-versus-host disease and Sjögren's syndrome). However, while there have been some randomized controlled trials evaluating the use of serum tears, the lack of consistency in reporting participant-reported symptoms and objective clinical measures make declaring serum tears as a therapy that is superior to over-the-counter artificial tears challenging.[55] There is a need for "well-planned, large, high-quality RCTs … to examine participants with dry eye of different severities by using standardized questionnaires to measure participant-reported outcomes, as well as objective clinical tests and objective biomarkers to assess the benefit of AS therapy for dry eye."[55] Nevertheless, some have shown that serum tears have been associated with improvements in morphology in the corneal subbasal nerve plexus, which may be associated with symptomatic improvement in those with corneal neuropathic pain.[56]

Topical antiinflammatory therapy can be an effective strategy in mitigating the inflammation that characterizes DED. Topical corticosteroids can abrogate the inflammatory processes that lead to ocular surface damage. Dexamethasone, prednisolone acetate, prednisolone sodium phosphate, methylprednisolone, fluorometholone, and others are common examples of the wide variety of corticosteroids that can be used. Multiple reviews have shown improvements in the ocular signs of DED (including corneal fluorescein staining, tear breakup time, and Schirmer score) with the use of topical corticosteroids.[53] However, the goal with using topical corticosteroids is to use the lowest dose and lowest frequency needed to manage the signs and symptoms of DED. The side effects of topical corticosteroid use, including elevated intraocular pressure with progression to glaucoma, development of cataract, and increased risk of infectious keratitis require routine monitoring. However, when used judiciously, topical corticosteroids can be an effective therapy in the management of Sjögren's syndrome DED.

Topical cyclosporine for ocular use was developed as it offers the possibility of immunomodulation as in corticosteroids, but without their significant side effects. Topical cyclosporine is now offered in a variety of concentrations, including 0.05% (Restasis, Allergan. Irvine, CA, USA), 0.09% (Cequa, Sun Pharmaceuticals Industries, Inc. Cranbury, NJ, USA), and 0.1% (Ikervis, Santen Pharmaceuticals Co. Ltd, Osaka, Japan). As a calcineurin-inhibitor, cyclosporine inhibits calcium-dependent interleukin (IL)-2 activation of lymphocytes thereby inhibiting inflammatory responses. On the ocular surface, topical cyclosporine may offer additional properties that make it more advantageous than steroids. Cyclosporine increases the number of mucus-producing conjunctival goblet cells (which can be associated with increased lubrication) through antiapoptotic effects.[57] However, its efficacy (particularly with lower concentrations) is widely debated and multiple clinical trials have resulted in modest overall improvements in dry eye signs and symptoms compared to placebo.[57,58] Side effects of topical cyclosporine include discomfort when instilled into the eye and requirement for long-term (up to 6 months) therapy before effects may be appreciated.[54] Tacrolimus is similar drug that blocks lymphocyte activity; however, it has a higher immunosuppressive potential. One randomized controlled trial saw improvements in ocular parameters after 7 days of treatment with topical 0.03% tacrolimus and even more improvement after 90 days.[59]

Lifitegrast is an integrin antagonist that competitively binds to lymphocyte function—associated antigen-1 (LFA-1) and intercellular adhesion molecule-1 (ICAM-1) thereby inhibiting T-cell migration into tissue, reducing cytokine release, and diminishing further T-cell recruitment into sites of inflammation. A recent review found that lifitegrast had statistically significant improvements in inferior corneal staining fluorescein scores and eye dryness scores.[60] Lifitegrast seemed to exhibit a more expeditious onset of action compared to cyclosporine with symptoms improving in 14 days.[60] Side effects of lifitegrast include eye irritation, dysgeusia, and reduced visual acuity though a clinical trial comparing five RCTs determined that lifitegrast is generally safe to use and well tolerated.[61] There is currently no research that has been done directly comparing lifitegrast to cyclosporine.

Systemic Therapy

Systemic therapy for the treatment of DED in Sjögren's syndrome is not typically employed. Systemic therapy for Sjögren's syndrome is most frequently reserved when there is systemic extraglandular involvement. However, there is certainly precedent in managing other ocular inflammatory disorders with systemic immunomodulatory therapy.[62]

Given that autoantibodies, hypergammaglobulinemia, a lymphoproliferative disorders can characterize Sjögren's syndrome, B-cell targeted therapy is a logical choice. To date, there have been two larger randomized controlled trials using rituximab in Sjögren's syndrome, but both failed to meet their endpoints. In one trial there was essentially no improvement in tear production.[63] In the other there was a nonsignificant trend toward improving tear production although the clinical significance of the improvement is debatable.[64] Finally, a metaanalysis concluded that rituximab had no clinical benefit in treating primary Sjögren's syndrome.[65] Despite these findings, other B-cell—directed therapies will likely be explored for Sjögren's syndrome.

Hydroxychloroquine has been used in the treatment of Sjögren's DED. Two randomized controlled trials found no difference between hydroxychloroquine and placebo when looking at signs of dry eye, pain, and systemic inflammation.[66,67]

Muscarinic agonists are commonly used as well. Their use focuses on symptomatic treatment with efforts to increase tear production rather than target the autoimmune nature of the illness. One trial compared the use of pilocarpine oral drops with artificial saliva drops, and found pilocarpine to be more effective at enhancing salivary and lacrimal secretion.[68]

Despite the systemic treatments discussed, a major drawback to any systemic therapy is the increased risk of side effects. Rituximab use has been associated with rash development, infusion reactions, and respiratory disorders. Hydroxychloroquine has been known to cause unintentional gastrointestinal symptoms. Muscarinic overstimulation can lead to gastrointestinal disorders, blurry vision, sweating, and bradycardia. Combine the unintentional effects of these therapies with the lack of evidence for clinical benefit and these therapies become less than desired choices for treatment.

Gut Microbiome

The gut microbiome displays a remarkable ability to affect host health.[69] Perhaps modulating the gut microbiome can be used as a possible therapy in Sjögren's syndrome? Murine models of gut dysbiosis have demonstrated altered immune responses.[70] Pertaining to ocular health and disease, parenteral administration of antibiotics did not affect a murine model of autoimmune uveitis, but oral administration (with subsequent modulation of the gut microbiome) decreased intraocular inflammation.[71] In another similar model, modulation of the gut microbiome seemed to exert its effects by modulating retina-specific T-cells.[72] On the ocular surface, gut dysbiosis exerts profound influences on the conjunctiva's ability to protect itself from pathogenic microbes. For example, in dysbiotic individuals, mucosal surfaces may be affected with a relative IgA deficiency.[73–75] In a study of participants with Sjögren's syndrome DED as well as those DED, but not meeting full criteria for Sjögren's syndrome, their stool was compared to healthy controls (without DED) using 16S rRNA sequencing, there was clustering of several different bacterial classes that distinguished the DED participants from those without DED.[76] Animal models suggest that fecal transplant may decrease ocular surface inflammation in DED.[77] Modulation of the gut microbiome and its effects in murine models of DED offers exciting opportunities in treating DED in humans. Indeed, such therapy has been described in a variety of gut inflammatory conditions including in ulcerative colitis, checkpoint-inhibitor-induced colitis, and *Clostridium difficile*.[78–81] Interest in the potential for modulating systemic disease such as Sjögren's syndrome has given rise to a currently active clinical trial, the Fecal Microbial Transplant for Sjögren's Syndrome study (clinicaltrials.gov accessed February 22, 2021).

Future Considerations in Sjögren's Syndrome Dry Eye Treatment

If a systemic process is responsible for driving lymphocytic infiltration of lacrimal glands leading to fibrosis and destruction, consideration may be made for systemic immunosuppression. There is an unmet need to prevent exocrine gland destruction perhaps even if there is no significant burden of disease elsewhere in the body. Systemic immunomodulatory therapy is used, for example, in other ocular inflammatory conditions where there is no systemic rheumatologic involvement. However, there is presently an ill-define way assessing lacrimal gland inflammation and fibrosis in a noninvasive way outside of magnetic resonance imaging (MRI), which is not routinely done. MRI of the salivary glands has been performed in Sjögren's syndrome, but is not a routine procedure at most centers.[82–85] Ultrasonography of the lacrimal glands could be applied in a similar manner as is done for salivary glands to see how much fibrosis is in the glands themselves and how much can be "saved" In sarcoidosis, lacrimal gland ultrasonography has the ability to detect lacrimal gland inflammation that is not identified on clinical exam alone.[86] Currently, surrogate markers of tear production (Schirmer I and the OSS) are used to implicate lacrimal gland function, but these tests do not demonstrate the proportion of possibly functional gland that is preserved. Knowing this could stratify such patients into a category where systemic immunosuppression may have a greater impact than those with entirely fibrotic glands.

ACKNOWLEDGMENT

We wish to acknowledge Chuan Yu Wu for his asssistance in creating Fig. 6.1.

REFERENCES

1. Sjögren H. Keratoconjunctivitis sicca. *Hygiea.* 1930;82(92): 829.
2. Craig JP, Nichols KK, Akpek EK, et al. TFOS DEWS II definition and classification report. *Ocul Surf.* 2017;15(3): 276–283.
3. Cobb BL, Lessard CJ, Harley JB, Moser KL. Genes and Sjögren's syndrome. *Rheum Dis Clin N Am.* 2008;34(4): 847–868 (vii).
4. Taylor KE, Wong Q, Levine DM, et al. Genome-wide association analysis reveals genetic heterogeneity of Sjögren's syndrome according to ancestry. *Arth Rheumatol.* 2017; 69(6):1294–1305.
5. Luo J, Liao X, Zhang L, et al. Transcriptome sequencing reveals potential roles of ICOS in primary Sjögren's syndrome. *Front Cell Dev Biol.* 2020;8:592490.
6. Brokstad KA, Fredriksen M, Zhou F, et al. T follicular-like helper cells in the peripheral blood of patients with primary Sjögren's syndrome. *Scand J Immunol.* 2018:e12679.
7. Grewal JS, Pilgrim MJ, Grewal S, et al. Salivary glands act as mucosal inductive sites via the formation of ectopic germinal centers after site-restricted MCMV infection. *FASEB J.* 2011;25(5):1680–1696.
8. Liew MS, Zhang M, Kim E, Akpek EK. Prevalence and predictors of Sjogren's syndrome in a prospective cohort of patients with aqueous-deficient dry eye. *Br J Ophthalmol.* 2012;96(12):1498–1503.
9. Pflugfelder SC. Prevalence, burden, and pharmacoeconomics of dry eye disease. *Am J Manag Care.* 2008;14(3 Suppl):S102–S106.
10. Asbell PA, Spiegel S. Ophthalmologist perceptions regarding treatment of moderate to severe dry eye: results of a physician survey. *Trans Am Ophthalmol Soc.* 2009; 107:205–210.
11. Asbell PA, Spiegel S. Ophthalmologist perceptions regarding treatment of moderate-to-severe dry eye: results of a physician survey. *Eye Contact Lens.* 2010;36(1):33–38.
12. Bunya VY, Fernandez KB, Ying GS, et al. Survey of ophthalmologists regarding practice patterns for dry eye and Sjogren syndrome. *Eye Contact Lens.* 2018;44(Suppl 2): S196–s201.
13. Shiboski CH, Shiboski SC, Seror R, et al. 2016 American College of Rheumatology/European League against rheumatism classification criteria for primary Sjogren's syndrome: a consensus and data-driven methodology involving three international patient cohorts. *Arth Rheumatol.* 2016; 69(1):35–45.
14. Shiboski CH, Shiboski SC, Seror R, et al. 2016 American College of Rheumatology/European League against Rheumatism classification criteria for primary Sjogren's syndrome: a consensus and data-driven methodology involving three international patient cohorts. *Ann Rheum Dis.* 2017;76(1):9–16.
15. Shiboski CH, Shiboski SC, Seror R, et al. 2016 American College of Rheumatology/European League against rheumatism classification criteria for primary Sjogren's syndrome: a consensus and data-driven methodology involving three international patient cohorts. *Arth Rheumatol.* 2017;69(1):35–45.
16. Bloch KJ, Buchanan WW, Wohl MJ, Bunim JJ. Sjoegren's syndrome. a clinical, pathological, and serological study of sixty-two cases. *Medicine.* 1965;44:187–231.
17. Daniels TE, Silverman Jr S, Michalski JP, Greenspan JS, Sylvester RA, Talal N. The oral component of Sjögren's syndrome. *Oral Surg Oral Med Oral Pathol.* 1975;39(6): 875–885.
18. Homma M, Tojo T, Akizuki M, Yamagata H. Criteria for Sjögren's syndrome in Japan. *Scand J Rheumatol Suppl.* 1986;61:26–27.
19. Manthorpe R, Oxholm P, Prause JU, Schiødt M. The copenhagen criteria for Sjögren's syndrome. *Scand J Rheumatol Suppl.* 1986;61:19–21.
20. Skopouli FN, Drosos AA, Papaioannou T, Moutsopoulos HM. Preliminary diagnostic criteria for

Sjögren's syndrome. *Scand J Rheumatol Suppl.* 1986;61: 22–25.

21. Fox RI, Robinson CA, Curd JG, Kozin F, Howell FV. Sjögren's syndrome. Proposed criteria for classification. *Arthritis Rheum.* 1986;29(5):577–585.

22. Vitali C, Bombardieri S, Moutsopoulos HM, et al. Preliminary criteria for the classification of Sjögren's syndrome. Results of a prospective concerted action supported by the European Community. *Arthritis Rheum.* 1993;36(3): 340–347.

23. Fujibayashi T, Sugai S, Miyasaka N, Hayashi Y, Tsubota K. Revised Japanese criteria for Sjögren's syndrome (1999): availability and validity. *Mod Rheumatol.* 2004;14(6): 425–434. The Japan Rheumatism Association.

24. Vitali C, Bombardieri S, Jonsson R, et al. Classification criteria for Sjögren's syndrome: a revised version of the European criteria proposed by the American-European Consensus Group. *Ann Rheum Dis.* 2002;61(6):554–558.

25. Shiboski SC, Shiboski CH, Criswell L, et al. American College of Rheumatology classification criteria for Sjogren's syndrome: a data-driven, expert consensus approach in the Sjogren's International Collaborative Clinical Alliance cohort. *Arth Care Res.* 2012;64(4):475–487.

26. Bunya VY, Maguire MG, Akpek EK, et al. A new screening questionnaire to identify patients with dry eye with a high likelihood of having Sjögren syndrome. *Cornea.* 2021;40(2):179–187.

27. Gabbriellini G, Baldini C, Varanini V, et al. Ocular Surface Disease Index (OSDI): a potential useful instrument for the assessment of vision-targeted health-related quality of life (VT-HRQ) in primary Sjögren's syndrome (pSS) clinical trials? *Clin Exp Rheumatol.* 2012;30(5):812–813.

28. Chalmers RL, Begley CG, Caffery B. Validation of the 5-Item Dry Eye Questionnaire (DEQ-5): discrimination across self-assessed severity and aqueous tear deficient dry eye diagnoses. *Cont Lens Ant Eye.* 2010;33(2):55–60.

29. Qazi Y, Hurwitz S, Khan S, Jurkunas UV, Dana R, Hamrah P. Validity and reliability of a novel ocular pain assessment survey (OPAS) in quantifying and monitoring corneal and ocular surface pain. *Ophthalmology.* 2016; 123(7):1458–1468.

30. Bouhassira D, Attal N, Fermanian J, et al. Development and validation of the neuropathic pain symptom inventory. *Pain.* 2004;108(3):248–257.

31. Farhangi M, Feuer W, Galor A, et al. Modification of the neuropathic pain symptom inventory for use in eye pain (NPSI-eye). *Pain.* 2019;160(7):1541–1550.

32. Wolffsohn JS, Arita R, Chalmers R, et al. TFOS DEWS II diagnostic methodology report. *Ocul Surf.* 2017;15(3): 539–574.

33. van Bijsterveld OP. Diagnostic tests in the Sicca syndrome. *Arch Ophthalmol.* 1969;82(1):10–14.

34. Lemp MA. Report of the national eye institute/industry workshop on clinical trials in dry eyes. *CLAO J.* 1995; 21(4):221–232.

35. Gonzales JA, Shiboski SC, Bunya VY, et al. Ocular clinical signs and diagnostic tests most compatible with keratoconjunctivitis sicca: a latent class approach. *Cornea.* 2020; 39(8):1013–1016.

36. Whitcher JP, Shiboski CH, Shiboski SC, et al. A simplified quantitative method for assessing keratoconjunctivitis sicca from the Sjogren's Syndrome International Registry. *Am J ophthalmol.* 2010;149(3):405–415.

37. Shiboski CH, Baer AN, Shiboski SC, et al. Natural history and predictors of progression to Sjögren's syndrome among participants of the Sjögren's international collaborative clinical alliance registry. *Arth Care Res.* 2018;70(2): 284–294.

38. Bunya VY, Bhosai SJ, Heidenreich AM, et al. Association of dry eye tests with extraocular signs among 3514 participants in the Sjögren's syndrome international registry. *Am J ophthalmol.* 2016;172:87–93.

39. Lemp MA, Bron AJ, Baudouin C, et al. Tear osmolarity in the diagnosis and management of dry eye disease. *Am J ophthalmol.* 2011;151(5):792–798. e791.

40. Mathews PM, Karakus S, Agrawal D, Hindman HB, Ramulu PY, Akpek EK. Tear osmolarity and correlation with ocular surface parameters in patients with dry eye. *Cornea.* 2017;36(11):1352–1357.

41. Pepose JS, Sullivan BD, Foulks GN, Lemp MA. The value of tear osmolarity as a metric in evaluating the response to dry eye therapy in the clinic and in clinical trials. *Am J ophthalmol.* 2014;157(1):4–6.e1.

42. Bunya VY, Fuerst NM, Pistilli M, et al. Variability of tear osmolarity in patients with dry eye. *JAMA Ophthalmol.* 2015; 133(6):662–667.

43. Bunya VY, Langelier N, Chen S, Pistilli M, Vivino FB, Massaro-Giordano G. Tear osmolarity in Sjogren syndrome. *Cornea.* 2013;32(7):922–927.

44. Sène D, Authier FJ, Amoura Z, Cacoub P, Lefaucheur JP. Small fibre neuropathy: diagnostic approach and therapeutic issues, and its association with primary Sjögren's syndrome. *La Revue de medecine interne.* 2010;31(10): 677–684.

45. Alhatem A, Cavalcanti B, Hamrah P. In vivo confocal microscopy in dry eye disease and related conditions. *Semin Ophthalmol.* 2012;27(5–6):138–148.

46. Cruzat A, Qazi Y, Hamrah P. In vivo confocal microscopy of corneal nerves in health and disease. *Ocul Surf.* 2017; 15(1):15–47.

47. Hamrah P, Qazi Y, Shahatit B, et al. Corneal nerve and epithelial cell alterations in corneal allodynia: an in vivo confocal microscopy case series. *Ocul Surf.* 2017;15(1): 139–151.

48. Takhar JJ AS, Lopez SE, Marneris AG, et al. Validation of a novel confocal microscopy imaging protocol with assessment of reproducibility and comparison of nerve metrics in dry eye disease compared to controls. *Cornea.* 2021;40(5):603–612.

49. Kim JW, Lee H, Park SH, Kim SK, Choe JY, Kim JK. Salivary gland ultrasonography findings are associated with

clinical, histological, and serologic features of Sjögren's syndrome. *Scand J Rheumatol.* 2018;47(4):303–310.

50. Luciano N, Baldini C, Tarantini G, et al. Ultrasonography of major salivary glands: a highly specific tool for distinguishing primary Sjögren's syndrome from undifferentiated connective tissue diseases. *Rheumatology.* 2015;54(12):2198–2204.

51. Giovagnorio F, Pace F, Giorgi A. Sonography of lacrimal glands in Sjögren syndrome. *J Ultrasound Med.* 2000;19(8):505–509.

52. Pucker AD, Ng SM, Nichols JJ. Over the counter (OTC) artificial tear drops for dry eye syndrome. *Cochrane Database Syst Rev.* 2016;2:Cd009729.

53. Jones L, Downie LE, Korb D, et al. TFOS DEWS II management and therapy report. *Ocul Surf.* 2017;15(3):575–628.

54. Vehof J, Utheim TP, Bootsma H, Hammond CJ. Advances, limitations and future perspectives in the diagnosis and management of dry eye in Sjögren's syndrome. *Clin Exp Rheumatol.* 2020;38(Suppl 126(4)):301–309.

55. Pan Q, Angelina A, Marrone M, Stark WJ, Akpek EK. Autologous serum eye drops for dry eye. *Cochrane Database Syst Rev.* 2017;2(2):Cd009327.

56. Aggarwal S, Colon C, Kheirkhah A, Hamrah P. Efficacy of autologous serum tears for treatment of neuropathic corneal pain. *Ocul Surf.* 2019;17(3):532–539.

57. de Paiva CS, Pflugfelder SC, Ng SM, Akpek EK. Topical cyclosporine A therapy for dry eye syndrome. *Cochrane Database Syst Rev.* 2019;9(9):Cd010051.

58. Schwartz LM, Woloshin S. A clear-eyed view of restasis and chronic dry eye disease. *JAMA Int Med.* 2018;178(2):181–182.

59. Moscovici BK, Holzchuh R, Sakassegawa-Naves FE, et al. Treatment of Sjögren's syndrome dry eye using 0.03% tacrolimus eye drop: prospective double-blind randomized study. *Cont Lens Ant Eye.* 2015;38(5):373–378.

60. Haber SL, Benson V, Buckway CJ, Gonzales JM, Romanet D, Scholes B. Lifitegrast: a novel drug for patients with dry eye disease. *Ther Adv Ophthalmol.* 2019;11, 2515841419870366.

61. Nichols KK, Donnenfeld ED, Karpecki PM, et al. Safety and tolerability of lifitegrast ophthalmic solution 5.0%: pooled analysis of five randomized controlled trials in dry eye disease. *Eur J Ophthalmol.* 2019;29(4):394–401.

62. Jabs DA, Rosenbaum JT, Foster CS, et al. Guidelines for the use of immunosuppressive drugs in patients with ocular inflammatory disorders: recommendations of an expert panel. *Am J ophthalmol.* 2000;130(4):492–513.

63. Bowman SJ, Everett CC, O'Dwyer JL, et al. Randomized controlled trial of rituximab and cost-effectiveness analysis in treating fatigue and oral dryness in primary Sjögren's syndrome. *Arth Rheumatol.* 2017;69(7):1440–1450.

64. Devauchelle-Pensec V, Mariette X, Jousse-Joulin S, et al. Treatment of primary Sjögren syndrome with rituximab: a randomized trial. *Ann Intern Med.* 2014;160(4):233–242.

65. Letaief H, Lukas C, Barnetche T, Gaujoux-Viala C, Combe B, Morel J. Efficacy and safety of biological DMARDs modulating B cells in primary Sjögren's syndrome: systematic review and meta-analysis. *Joint Bone Spine.* 2018;85(1):15–22.

66. Yoon CH, Lee HJ, Lee EY, et al. Effect of hydroxychloroquine treatment on dry eyes in subjects with primary sjogren's syndrome: a double-blind randomized control study. *J Kor Med Sci.* 2016;31(7):1127–1135.

67. Gottenberg JE, Ravaud P, Puéchal X, et al. Effects of hydroxychloroquine on symptomatic improvement in primary Sjögren syndrome: the JOQUER randomized clinical trial. *JAMA.* 2014;312(3):249–258.

68. Cifuentes M, Del Barrio-Díaz P, Vera-Kellet C. Pilocarpine and artificial saliva for the treatment of xerostomia and xerophthalmia in Sjögren syndrome: a double-blind randomized controlled trial. *Br J Dermatol.* 2018;179(5):1056–1061.

69. Peterson CT, Sharma V, Elmén L, Peterson SN. Immune homeostasis, dysbiosis and therapeutic modulation of the gut microbiota. *Clin Exp Immunol.* 2015;179(3):363–377.

70. Wang C, Schaefer L, Bian F, et al. Dysbiosis modulates ocular surface inflammatory response to liposaccharide. *Invest Ophthalmol Vis Sci.* 2019;60(13):4224–4233.

71. Nakamura YK, Metea C, Karstens L, et al. Gut microbial alterations associated with protection from autoimmune uveitis. *Invest Ophthalmol Vis Sci.* 2016;57(8):3747–3758.

72. Horai R, Zárate-Bladés CR, Dillenburg-Pilla P, et al. Microbiota-dependent activation of an autoreactive T cell receptor provokes autoimmunity in an immunologically privileged site. *Immunity.* 2015;43(2):343–353.

73. Strugnell RA, Wijburg OL. The role of secretory antibodies in infection immunity. *Nat Rev Microbiol.* 2010;8(9):656–667.

74. Perdigón G, Fuller R, Raya R. Lactic acid bacteria and their effect on the immune system. *Curr Issues Intest Microbiol.* 2001;2(1):27–42.

75. Kugadas A, Wright Q, Geddes-McAlister J, Gadjeva M. Role of microbiota in strengthening ocular mucosal barrier function through secretory IgA. *Invest Ophthalmol Vis Sci.* 2017;58(11):4593–4600.

76. Mendez R, Watane A, Farhangi M, et al. Gut microbial dysbiosis in individuals with Sjögren's syndrome. *Microb Cell Factories.* 2020;19(1):90.

77. Zaheer M, Wang C, Bian F, et al. Protective role of commensal bacteria in Sjögren Syndrome. *J Autoimmun.* 2018;93:45–56.

78. Fang H, Fu L, Wang J. Protocol for fecal microbiota transplantation in inflammatory bowel disease: a systematic review and meta-analysis. *BioMed Res Int.* 2018;2018:8941340.

79. Wang Y, Wiesnoski DH, Helmink BA, et al. Fecal microbiota transplantation for refractory immune checkpoint inhibitor-associated colitis. *Nat Med.* 2018;24(12):1804–1808.

80. Kleger A, Schnell J, Essig A, et al. Fecal transplant in refractory *Clostridium difficile* colitis. *Deutsches Arzteblatt Int.* 2013;110(7):108–115.

81. Costello SP, Chung A, Andrews JM, Fraser RJ. Fecal microbiota transplant for *Clostridium difficile* colitis-induced toxic megacolon. *Am J Gastroenterol.* 2015;110(5):775–777.

82. Izumi M, Eguchi K, Ohki M, et al. MR imaging of the parotid gland in Sjögren's syndrome: a proposal for new diagnostic criteria. *Am J Roentgenol.* 1996;166(6): 1483–1487.

83. Izumi M, Eguchi K, Nakamura H, Nagataki S, Nakamura T. Premature fat deposition in the salivary glands associated with Sjögren syndrome: MR and CT evidence. *Am J Neuroradiol.* 1997;18(5):951–958.

84. Kojima I, Sakamoto M, Iikubo M, Shimada Y, Nishioka T, Sasano T. Relationship of MR imaging of submandibular glands to hyposalivation in Sjögren's syndrome. *Oral Dis.* 2019;25(1):117–125.

85. Hammenfors DS, Brun JG, Jonsson R, Jonsson MV. Diagnostic utility of major salivary gland ultrasonography in primary Sjögren's syndrome. *Clin Exp Rheumatol.* 2015; 33(1):56–62.

86. Éksarenko OV, Kharlap SI, Safonova TN, Vashkulatova É A. Lacrimal gland changes in sarcoidosis according to the results of spatial digital ultrasonography. *Vestn Oftalmol.* 2013;129(1):10–15.

CHAPTER 7

Graft Versus Host Disease and Dry Eye Disease

DANIELA ROCA, MD • JESSICA MUN, BA • BAYASGALAN SURENKHUU, MD, MS • MURUGESAN VANATHI, MD • SANDEEP JAIN, MD

INTRODUCTION

Graft-versus-host disease (GVHD) is a potentially life-threatening multiorgan systemic disease affecting patients treated with hematopoietic stem cell transplantation (SCT). GVHD is characterized by immune dysregulation and tissue inflammation with single- or multisystem involvement resulting in tissue fibrosis and organ dysfunction.[1] Characteristic diagnostic features involving skin, mouth, gastrointestinal (GI) tract, lung, fascia, genitalia, eyes, nails, scalp, or hair are seen.[2] Chronic GVHD (cGVHD) is a complex immune-mediated disorder that can target multiple organs, usually manifesting in the first year after HSCT and may occur in up to 30%–70% of the patients undergoing HSCT.[3] Ocular GVHD (oGVHD), the most common long-term complication, affects 40%–60% of patients treated with allo-HSCT.[4−7] Typically, oGVHD involves ocular surface, including the cornea, conjunctiva, lacrimal glands, meibomian glands, and eyelids.[5,6] Risk factors for oGVHD include male recipients of female donors[8] skin,[8,9] oral mucosa,[7,9] liver,[10] or GI tract involvement during acute or chronic stages of GVHD and lung involvement in cGVHD.[11] Preexisting diabetes,[11] recipients of transplants from Epstein−Barr Virus−positive donors, Asian and other ethnicities compared to Caucasian ethnicity were more likely to develop oGVHD.[10]

DEFINITION OF OGVHD DIAGNOSTIC CRITERIA

As of now there are no molecular biomarkers that are pathognomonic or diagnostic for oGVHD, therefore the classifications are based on clinical tests. There are two widely acknowledged diagnostic classification criteria for oGVHD. The first one is the 2014 National Institute of Health Consensus conference (NIH) criteria. According to the NIH classification criteria, the diagnosis of chronic GVHD requires at least one diagnostic manifestation or one distinctive manifestation confirmed by biopsy or testing of the same or other involved organ. "Diagnostic" manifestations sufficient by themselves to establish the diagnosis of chronic GVHD may be found in the skin, mouth, GI tract, lung, fascia, and genitalia (for example, lichen planus or lichen sclerosis, poikiloderma, sclerosis, or esophageal webs). There are no diagnostic features of the nails, eyes, liver, or other organs.[12] Distinctive manifestation of chronic GVHD include new onset of dry, "gritty" or painful eyes, cicatricial conjunctivitis, KCS, and confluent areas of punctate keratopathy. New ocular sicca documented by low Schirmer's test with a mean value of ≤5 mm at 5 min or a new onset of KSC by slit lamp exam with mean Schirmer's test values of 6−10 mm not due to other causes is sufficient for the diagnosis of ocular chronic GVHD.[12] The International Chronic oGVHD consensus group (ICCGVHD) diagnostic criteria is based on scores derived from Ocular Surface Disease Index (OSDI), Schirmer's test without anesthesia, corneal fluorescein staining (CFS), conjunctival injection and presence of systemic GVHD. The diagnostic categories included no oGVHD, probable oGVHD and definite oGVHD.[13] While a comparative study of the newer NIH 2014 criteria and ICCGVHD criteria found moderate agreement between the two, ICCGVHD criteria was noted to be better at differentiating oGVHD patients from non-oGVHD DED (dry eye disease).[6] Pre-allo-HSCT evaluation for DED is now widely recommended to help differentiate between preexisting dry eye and the new onset DED diagnosed as oGVHD post-allo-HSCT.

Dry Eye Disease. https://doi.org/10.1016/B978-0-323-82753-9.00015-1

CLINICAL FEATURES

Clinical Symptoms

Eye pain and tearing are the main complaints in acute oGVHD.[14] The clinical symptoms of chronic oGVHD usually resemble those seen in DED or KCS syndrome. The distinctive manifestations of chronic oGVHD as per the NIH consensus criteria comprise new onset of dry, "gritty," or painful eyes.[2] Other symptoms may include irritation, watering, photophobia, redness, and blurring.[4]

Clinical Signs

Acute oGVHD commonly presents as pseudomembranous or hemorrhagic conjunctivitis.[14,15] A less severe form with conjunctival injection or chemosis may also be seen.[16] Corneal signs include epithelial sloughing,[16,17] corneal epithelial keratitis, or filamentary keratitis which may be secondary to the conjunctival cicatrization due to the disease.[18] Some patients may present with lagophthalmos.[19] Ocular involvement in aGVHD is considered an extremely poor prognostic sign associated with a higher GVHD-related mortality.[14] Chronic oGVHD primarily is a result of inflammatory and fibrotic changes in the ocular surface comprising the cornea, conjunctiva, lacrimal glands, meibomian glands, and eyelids (Fig. 7.1). It should be noted that other factors such as conditioning regimens, irradiative therapy, and immunosuppression might also impact the clinical manifestations in addition to the GVHD disease process itself. Corneal signs due to the KCS syndrome include punctate keratitis, epithelial erosions, and epithelial defects (Fig. 7.2) which may progressively worsen to keratinization, stromal thinning, melt, and perforation. Recurrent corneal perforation, sometimes bilaterally, is not uncommon with calcareous degeneration or lipid

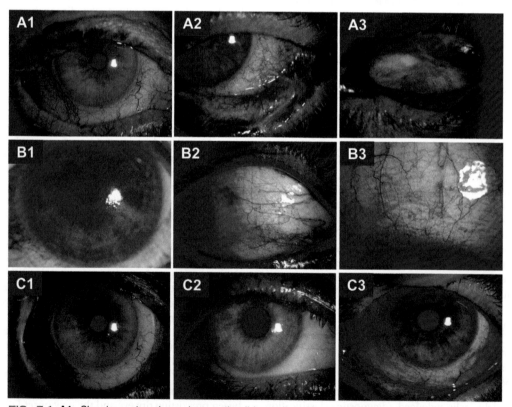

FIG. 7.1 **A1:** Showing external eye image, the lid margin with telangiectasia. **A2:** Fornix shortening, subconjunctival fibrosis, and extensive redness. **A3:** Conjunctival subepithelial fibrosis (CSEF) in the upper lid. **B1:** Lissamine green staining showing severe corneal Superficial Punctate Keratitis (SPKs). **B2:** Severe conjunctival staining with lissamine green. **B3:** Superior bulbar staining (SLK type) with lissamine green. **C1:** Scleral lens that is commonly used for treating oGVHD. **C2:** A soft bandage contact lens used for treating oGVHD. **C3:** shows that the cornea and conjunctiva that is covered with contact lens does not stain with lissamine green dye, however conjunctival areas outside contact lens show severe staining.

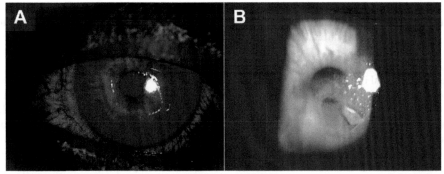

FIG. 7.2 **(A)** Persistent epithelial defect in oGVHD patient. **(B)** Inflammatory mucus cellular aggregates (MCA) sticking to the epithelial defect area. These MCA are composed of neutrophil extracellular traps (NETS) that contain bioactive molecules and cytokines that may cause cytotoxicity.

keratopathy being seen rarely. The progression from the stage of epithelial ulceration to perforation tends to be rapid and is often refractory to standard medical or surgical treatment modalities.[20–22] Progressive ocular surface inflammation leads to corneal neovascularization, conjunctivalization, and less commonly limbal stem cell deficiency (LSCD), which will adversely affect visual acuity.[22–24] Decreased corneal sensation tends to predispose development of neurotrophic ulceration.[25] Conjunctival involvement is a distinctive aspect of chronic oGVHD, seen in about half of the chronic oGVHD and is a marker for severe systemic involvement of GVHD.[16,26] Less severe cases manifest as a conjunctival hyperemia or chronic conjunctivitis involving both palpebral and bulbar conjunctiva. Other less common features include cicatricial conjunctivitis with obliteration of fornices, cicatricial entropion, symblepharon, ankyloblepharon, and lagophthalmos, which could progress to conjunctival keratinization and punctal occlusion.[16,26,27] Conjunctival subepithelial fibrosis seen as fine white lines under intact conjunctival epithelium are indicative of a past insult.[28] Pseudomembranous and serosanguineous conjunctivitis are less frequently seen forms of conjunctival involvement which though more characteristic of acute oGVHD, have been seen in chronic oGVHD too.[16] Subtarsal fibrosis in upper tarsus noted in 40% chronic oGVHD cases along with worsening of ocular surface epitheliopathy in these patients was suggested to be of diagnostic value in oGVHD.[29] Decreased conjunctival goblet cell density and increased squamous cell metaplasia and surface keratinization of the ocular surface have also been noted.[25] Superior limbal keratoconjunctivitis like inflammation has been reported as a manifestation of oGVHD, which can worsen to LSCD and corneal pannus formation. This has been attributed to

soft tissue microtrauma from increased frictional forces compounded by tear mucin deficiency due to goblet cell loss.[30] Meibomian glands are severely affected with rapid and aggressive destruction over time in chronic oGVHD[31] resulting in unstable tear film aggravating the DED. T-cell–mediated damage to the MG epithelial cells is primarily responsible for the gland dysfunction with hyperkeratinization of duct epithelium and subepithelial stromal fibrosis contributing to obstructive Meibomian Gland Dysfunction (MGD) in chronic GVHD.[32] The prevalence of MGD ranges about 47.8%–68.4% in oGVHD.[33,34] The MG loss and damage in oGVHD is often more severe than that seen in other DED such as Sjögren's syndrome.[35] Early detection and aggressive management can perhaps help in minimizing damage in oGVHD as few studies have shown some reversibility of MG damage in the initial stages.[31,36,37] Meibography revealed loss of about 80% MG function in oGVHD patients evaluated over a 1-year period with over 25% being refractory to treatment.[31] Lid margin irregularity, vascular engorgement, plugging of MG, and displacement of mucocutaneous junction due to duct outlet obstruction is also seen.[31,38] In vivo confocal microscopy (IVCM) imaging has documented morphological changes like inflammatory cell infiltration, gland atrophy, and fibrosis.[38] MG loss does seem to be more with increasing severity of oGVHD.[34] Prevalence of posterior blepharitis associated with MGD has been reported in 47%–63% of chronic GVHD patients, with significant correlation with the severity of KCS symptoms.[33,39]

Lacrimal gland involvement is responsible for the tear aqueous deficiency in oGVHD with the resultant DED or KCS being the most characteristic feature in up to 69%–77% of oGVHD cases.[40] Fibrosis and inflammation caused by stromal fibroblasts with

T-cell infiltration, around the periductal area of lacrimal gland, leads to the destruction of the tubuloalveolar secretory units.[41,42] Bilateral nasolacrimal duct obstruction (NLDO) leading to dacryocystitis has been reported in oGVHD.[43,44] NLDO induced by epithelial and subepithelial inflammation and punctal occlusion—both inflammatory and spontaneous have also been observed.[45,46] Eyelids abnormalities (lagophthalmos, trichiasis, poliosis, entropion, and, less commonly, ectropion) occur due to chronic tarsal conjunctival inflammation, atrophic eyelid alterations, keratinization, and cicatricial changes.[47] True cicatricial ectropion due to mechanical shortening of the anterior lamella caused by cutaneous involvement of GVHD has also been reported.[48] Increased eyelid laxity in oGVHD, resulting from higher elastolytic enzyme (like MMP-9) activity mediated by the chronic inflammatory process both due to GVHD and systemic malignancy, compounds the ocular discomfort symptoms and ocular surface signs.[49] Eyelid skin may exhibit scleroderma like skin lesions, pigmentary discolorations, vitiligo, and dermatitis.[7] The other less commonly seen signs which may be seen in chronic oGVHD include cataract, episcleritis, scleritis, posterior scleritis, anterior uveitis, vitritis, serous choroidal detachment,[50] and reduced corneal subbasal nerve plexus densities, herpetic keratitis, and cytomegalovirus retinitis.[51]

NEWER DIAGNOSTIC MODALITIES

Though a number of new diagnostic methods have been added to the armamentarium of DED diagnostics, there is no single adequate test for oGVHD diagnosis with a combination of clinical parameters and investigational modalities being recommended.

Meibography is the technique of in vivo observation of meibomian glands. Meibography in oGVHD shows complete or partial Meibomian gland loss/atrophy, structural alteration such as distortion or dilation of ducts.[31,35,37] Occasional finding of slender MG either pre- and early post-HSCT has been attributed to long-term immunosuppression causing sebaceous hyperplasia which results in obstruction MGD and can be reversed in some cases.[36] As MG loss seen prior to the allo-HSCT can progress rapidly following oGVHD onset, noninvasive meibography for routine evaluation of hematological malignancies patients prior to and at regular follow-up posttransplant has been recommended.[37] A cut-off value of 40% of MG area calculated using image analysis software has been adopted for diagnosing MGD in oGVHD patients.[34] Consensus on correlation of MG area loss on meibography to oGVHD severity is not conclusive with some in agreement[34,35] and few others[28,38] not concurring. The same also applies to correlation between ocular surface clinical parameters and MG loss on meibography.[31,34,37] Hence, besides local inflammation there seems to exist a multifactorial etiology for MGD in oGVHD (Fig. 7.3). **Noncontact tear interferometry** visualizes the interferometric pattern of the lipid layer of tear film and measures its thickness, thereby providing a functional MG assessment.[52] A higher grade of severity of lipid layer interferometric pattern changes has been seen in oGVHD patients,[38] with greater instability of the lipid layer in oGVHD patients as compared to Sjögren's syndrome.[53] While different tear interferometric patterns have been described to correlate with different subtypes of DED, inadequate tear volume makes it difficult to observe a typical interference pattern in severe aqueous-deficient (AD) Sjögren's syndrome, oGVHD or Stevens–Johnson Syndrome.[54] oGVHD with afflictions of lacrimal gland and MG manifests a combined AD-evaporative DED and shows a reduced lipid layer thickness in tear interferometry in comparison to non-oGVHD and healthy eyes.[55]

In Vivo Confocal Microscopy changes in oGVHD include decreased corneal epithelial cell density,[56] epithelial dendritic cell, conjunctival epithelial immune

A.   Healthy subject

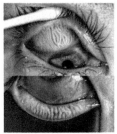 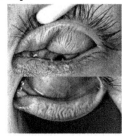

B.   oGVHD

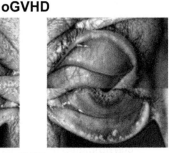

FIG. 7.3 Meibomian Gland Dropout—Lipiview in a healthy subject **(A)** and oGVHD patient **(B)**. Infrared meibography: Infrared meibography shows normal Meibomian gland architecture rather in oGVHD patients there is severe truncation and dropout of the Meibomian glands.

cell, increased goblet immune cell,[57,58] anterior stromal cell density, anterior stromal extracellular matrix accumulation (reflective of engraftment of donor fibroblasts or altered fibroblast cell populations in the host cornea),[59] reduced subbasal nerve number and density, altered branching, reflectivity and increased tortuosity,[57–59] and altered conjunctival epithelial and stromal immune cell density.[57] IVCM changes seem to correlate well with disease severity scores (Japanese Dry Eye score, ICCGVHD).[58] IVCM can be a useful tool to study the cellular structural changes in DED with and without GVHD.[56] (Fig. 7.4).

In-Vivo Confocal microscopy (HRT3)

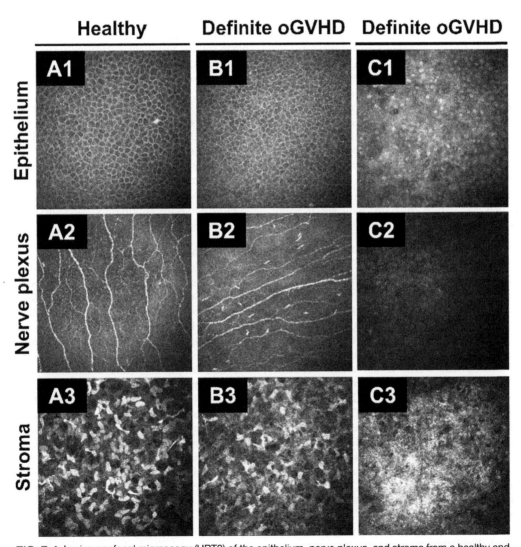

FIG. 7.4 In vivo confocal microscopy (HRT3) of the epithelium, nerve plexus, and stroma from a healthy and definite oGVHD patient. In the healthy subject the nerves appear as solid lines with no interspersed cells (A1, A2, and A3). The epithelium shows "honeycomb" appearance without any central reflectance. In definite oGVHD two abnormal patterns are seen on confocal microscopy (B1, B2, B3, C1, C2, and C3). In the first pattern, numerous inflammatory cells are present alongside corneal nerves. In the second pattern, there is absence of corneal nerves and the surface epithelium shows a central reflectance within the honeycomb area. In the second pattern, the stroma also shows increased reflectance.

Tear film osmolarity is a global indicator of DED irrespective of the subtype or etiology and is considered its best single predictor[60] with a cut-off value of >310 mOsm/L for diagnosing oGVHD (98.4% sensitivity and 60.7% specificity).[61] A cut-off value of 312 mOsm/L has been recommended for differentiating definite oGVHD (as per ICCGVHD criteria) from non-oGVHD (sensitivity of 91% and specificity of 82%).[62] There is a significantly raised tear osmolarity in oGVHD with good correlation with severity of clinical parameters (Schirmer's, TBUT, OSDI, and staining scores) and increasing disease severity.[36,60,62] Currently, tear osmolarity in isolation is not recommended to diagnose oGVHD but is a useful supplement to clinical dry eye tests used in oGVHD diagnosis in post-allo-HSCT.[61,62] A novel digital imaging analysis technique for quantification and morphological characterization of CFS which may help distinguish DED due to Sjögren's and oGVHD has been recently proposed by Pelligrini et al.[63] Shimizu et al. evaluated corneal higher-order aberrations (HOAs) using Zernike analysis in anterior segment optical coherence tomography (CASIA system, SS-1000, Tomey, Japan) and found higher corneal HOAs in chronic oGVHD eyes than the non-GVHD and normal eyes, which correlated with visual acuity and severity scores.[64]

ROLE OF TEAR BIOMARKERS, INFLAMMATORY MEDIATORS, AND PROTEIN IN DIAGNOSTICS

The immune reaction in GVHD comprises donor T-cells trigger of host antigen-presenting cells, which activate the donor effector T-cells to mediate the target tissue damage. The precise role of the various subtypes of T-cells, cytokines, and B-cells is not clear.[65] Though CD4+ and CD8+ T-cells are the predominant infiltrates in ocular surface tissues in chronic oGVHD.[66] Studies evaluating tear cytokines in oGVHD found raised ICAM-1 (intercellular adhesion molecule 1), IL (interleukin)-1Ra, IL-2, IL-1 β, IL-6, IL-8, IL-10, IL-2AP70, IL-17A, IFN (interferon)-γ, TNF (tumor necrosis factor)-α, MMP (matrix metalloproteinase)-9, and VEGF (vascular endothelial growth factor).[55,67–71] Recent reports of increased conjunctival neutrophil infiltration and tear inflammatory mediators[72] produced by neutrophil elastase, MMP-9, MMP-8, and MPO (myeloperoxidase) highlights the role of neutrophils in oGVHD immunopathogenesis with these neutrophils releasing nuclear chromatin complexes as extracellular DNA (eDNA) webs that are termed neutrophil extracellular traps (NETs).[73] oGVHD is associated with excessive accumulation of NETs which are recognized to be contributory to pathologic changes (corneal epitheliopathy, conjunctival fibrosis, ocular surface inflammation, and MGD) seen.[55] Neutrophil secreted biomarkers [eDNA, neutrophil gelatinase-associated lipocalin (NGAL), Oncostatin M (OSM) and TNF superfamily member14 (TNFSF14)] could be useful in differentiating DED due to oGVHD from other etiologies.

TREATMENT

A multidisciplinary approach and coordination with the HSCT team is imperative in management of oGVHD. In recent times, with greater emphasis on organ-specific treatment, increasing systemic immunosuppression is no longer considered an optimal treatment approach for organ-specific GVHD.

Because oGVHD can progress rapidly to irreversible functional loss and scarring, it is imperative to start effective treatment early and then taper medication down. The preferred approach is a rapidly control of the disease and step-down approach. The three-pronged treatment approach, as adopted in other ocular surface immune-mediated inflammatory diseases, comprises lubrication, prevention, and control of tear evaporation, and most importantly, reducing ocular surface inflammation.[74]

Medical Management
Lubrication
In both acute and chronic oGVHD with severe aqueous deficiency dry eye, topical lubrication with nonpreserved phosphate-free artificial tears is the first-line treatment. Frequent use of tear substitutes throughout the day supplemented with viscous ointment before bedtime helps not only in preserving the ocular surface but also in diluting tears inflammatory mediators. Topical mucolytics [acetylcysteine (5%–10%)] is beneficial in DED with filamentary keratitis. Though oral secretagogues, such as pilocarpine or cevimeline (selective muscarinic agonists), may be beneficial in stimulating aqueous tear flow in chronic oGVHD induced sicca symptoms, their use is limited by adverse drug reactions and toxicity. Dual treatment with topical secretagogues rebamipide and diquafosol have been used in oGVHD patients with beneficial effects.[75]

Prevention of tear evaporation
Tear film instability and evaporative dry eye due to MGD should be treated on usual lines with warm compresses, lid scrubs, and maintenance of lid hygiene. Topical erythromycin ointment and systemic tetracycline antibiotics, mainly doxycycline and minocycline, and macrolide antibiotics, azithromycin, help to reduce

inflammation of the meibomian glands and subsequently meibum secretion and tear film quality. Further, nutritional supplements such as fish oil (omega-3 fatty acids) and flaxseed oil (2000 mg/d) may be helpful owing to their antiinflammatory properties. Use of moist chamber goggles to increase the periocular humidity has been employed to alleviate discomfort in DED patients, though the effects may be transient.[76]

Reducing ocular surface inflammation
Topical steroids are used in both acute and chronic oGVHD, although their role in the former remains controversial. While some studies did not find a role for topical steroid therapy in altering the disease course of pseudomembranous conjunctivitis,[16,77] Kim et al. suggested that the use of aggressive topical steroid therapy along with pseudomembrane removal may help improve epithelial healing and reduce cicatricial changes in these patients.[78] In chronic oGVHD, they are helpful in patients presenting with cicatricial changes.[79] Topical steroids are contraindicated in patients with corneal epithelial defects, stromal thinning, or infection. Adverse effects of long-term steroid use (glaucoma, cataracts, corneal thinning, and secondary infectious keratitis) are common comorbidities in these eyes. Hence, use of topical immunosuppressants, [cyclosporine (CsA) eye drops, and tacrolimus ointment] has been advocated.

Topical CsA eye drops have been used with some success in patients with chronic oGVHD and KCS refractory to conventional lubrication and steroid drops. Increase in goblet cell density and epithelial cell turnover in the conjunctiva along with improvement in symptoms, CFS, and basal tear secretion has been noted. Tacrolimus is similar to CsA but with greater immunosuppressive potency, and its systemic use has also shown to be beneficial in oGVHD.[80]

Topical IL-1 receptor antagonist or Anakinra 2.5% (FDA-approved immunomodulator drug for rheumatoid arthritis treatment) has shown some promise in a double-masked randomized control trial with improvement in symptoms and reduction in corneal epitheliopathy after 12 weeks instillation in oGVHD.[81] Tranilast (n-[3,4-anthoranilic acid]) is a known antiallergic drug which has been used to treat condition such as allergic rhinitis and atopic dermatitis. It also has an inhibitory effect on the transforming growth factor-β (TGF-β) induced extracellular matrix production. Topical Tranilast acts by inhibiting the production and/or release of ocular inflammatory mediators and cytokines and in collagen synthesis as well as TGF-β–

induced matrix production and has been found to effective in treating mild dry eye associated with cGVHD.[82]

Subanticoagulant dose heparin (100 IU/mL) by diminishing the effects of NETs has been shown to have a therapeutic effect in oGVHD.[58] Deoxyribonuclease I (DNase), a major extracellular endonuclease, selectively targets extracellular DNA and thus degrades NET. Early clinical trials have demonstrated the therapeutic potential of topical recombinant human deoxyribonuclease I (0.1% DNase), pulmozyme (Genentech) in patients with oGVHD DED without severe adverse effects.[83] Intravenous immunoglobulin (IVIG) through its immunomodulatory activity may reduce autoimmune-mediated inflammation in DED.[84] Topical IVIG drops application for oGVHD DED is currently being investigated in Phase1/ll clinical trials.

Biological tear substitutes
Appropriate management of corneal epithelial erosions, corneal ulcers, and perforations is required to maintain the health and integrity of the corneal surface. Biological tear substitutes such as autologous serum acts like preservative-free tears being rich in nutrients such as epithelial and nerve growth factors, cytokines, vitamin A, fibronectin, and transforming growth factor A. It acts by providing lubrication and improving corneal sensitivity, thereby contributing to enhanced integrity.[85] However, their use is not recommended in presence of active inflammation, systemic infections, extremes of age (infant or elderly), or overall poor health such as malnutrition. Umbilical cord serum eye drops or allogeneic serum eye drops have been tried as alternatives but are limited by risk of transmission of serious blood-borne diseases.[86] Topical therapy with autologous platelet lysate drops rich in platelet-derived growth factors, known to improve wound healing and corneal reepithelization, have been found to be a safe and effective option for oGVHD patients refractory to conventional therapy.[87,88]

Contact lenses have also been used to provide ocular surface protection in oGVHD, as in other ocular surface disorders. Soft silicone hydrogel bandage contact lenses and rigid gas-permeable scleral lenses have been tried. However, they should be used with caution, especially in the acute setting, keeping in mind the increased risk of infection and ischemia. Scleral lenses require also more training to use, and hence not all patients can handle them appropriately.[89]

Surgical management
Surgical intervention is mostly reserved as the last resort and may be necessary for severe cases. Superficial

epithelial debridement and removal of filaments is helpful in cases of filamentary keratitis. Amniotic membrane transplantation may be required in cases of persistent epithelial defects, superior limbic keratoconjunctivitis, and symblepharon formation.[90] Punctual occlusion in the setting of the severe ocular surface is controversial. Severe cases of DED may even warrant a temporary tarsorrhaphy[91] to decrease ocular surface exposure. Mucous membrane grafts and skin grafts may be required for management of cicatricial lid disease. Allogenic limbal SCT from the same hematopoietic stem cell donor,[22,23] lamellar keratoplasty,[92] tectonic patch grafts, and penetrating keratoplasty[91] are performed in a limited capacity and only as final effort, in view of poor prognosis for graft survival because of severe preexisting ocular surface inflammation. Ocular surface stem cell transplantation using conjunctival and limbal allografts obtained from the patient's HSCT donor has been reported to be a promising treatment modality associated with good long-term survival of graft.[22,23] Keratoprosthesis may also be considered in severe cases for visual rehabilitation with bilateral blindness; osteo-odonto keratoprosthesis has been successfully performed in a few cases.[93]

CONCLUSION

GVHD is the major cause of morbidity and mortality in patients after allogeneic hematopoietic cell transplantation. oGVHD is not just another dry eye disease. It is a rapidly progressive immunological disease that can lead to severe and irreversible ocular disease. It could involve the whole ocular surface, requiring a multipronged approach of treatment. There is no single treatment that can work but a combination of eye drops (serum tears and tear substitutes). There is a window of opportunity where a step-down treatment can reduce symptoms. The best approach is to have a baseline examination before BMT and in intervals after the BMT to detect any early ocular surface disease that may cause irreversible damage.

REFERENCES

1. Lee SJ. Classification systems for chronic graft-versus-host disease. *Blood.* 2017;129(1):30−37.
2. Jagasia MH, Greinix HT, Arora M, et al. National Institutes of Health Consensus Development Project on criteria for clinical trials in chronic graft-versus-host disease: I. The 2014 diagnosis and staging working group report. *Biol Blood Marrow Transplant.* 2015;21(3):389−401.e1.
3. Aki SZ, Inamoto Y, Carpenter PA, et al. Confounding factors affecting the National Institutes of Health (NIH) chronic graft-versus-host disease organ-specific score and global severity. *Bone Marrow Transplant.* 2016;51(10):1350−1353.
4. Espana EM, Shah S, Santhiago MR, Singh AD. Graft versus host disease: clinical evaluation, diagnosis and management. *Graefes Arch Clin Exp Ophthalmol.* 2013;251(5):1257−1266.
5. Munir SZ, Aylward J. A review of ocular graft-versus-host disease. *Optom Vis Sci.* 2017;94(5):545−555.
6. Pathak M, Diep PP, Lai X, Brinch L, Ruud E, Drolsum L. Ocular findings and ocular graft-versus-host disease after allogeneic stem cell transplantation without total body irradiation. *Bone Marrow Transplant.* 2018;53(7):863−872.
7. Westeneng AC, Hettinga Y, Lokhorst H, Verdonck L, Van Dorp S, Rothova A. Ocular graft-versus-host disease after allogeneic stem cell transplantation. *Cornea.* 2010;29(7):758−763.
8. Jacobs R, Tran U, Chen H, et al. Prevalence and risk factors associated with development of ocular GVHD defined by NIH consensus criteria. *Bone Marrow Transplant.* 2012;47(11):1470−1473.
9. Khan R, Nair S, Seth T, et al. Ocular graft versus host disease in allogenic haematopoetic stem cell transplantation in a tertiary care centre in India. *Indian J Med Res.* 2015;142:543−548. NOVEMBER.
10. Wang JCC, Teichman JC, Mustafa M, O'Donnell H, Broady R, Yeung SN. Risk factors for the development of ocular graft-versus-host disease (GVHD) dry eye syndrome in patients with chronic GVHD. *Br J Ophthalmol.* 2015;99(11):1514−1518.
11. Na KS, Yoo YS, Mok JW, Lee JW, Joo CK. Incidence and risk factors for ocular GVHD after allogeneic hematopoietic stem cell transplantation. *Bone Marrow Transplant.* 2015;50(11):1459−1464.
12. Pavletic SZ, Vogelsang GB, Lee SJ. 2014 National Institutes of Health Consensus Development Project on criteria for clinical trials in chronic graft-versus-host disease: preface to the series. *Biol Blood Marrow Transplant.* 2015;21(3):387−388.
13. Ogawa Y, Kim SK, Dana R, et al. International chronic ocular graft-vs-host-disease (GVHD) consensus group: proposed diagnostic criteria for chronic GVHD (Part I). *Sci Rep.* 2013;3.
14. Saito T, Shinagawa K, Takenaka K, et al. Ocular manifestation of acute graft-versus-host disease after allogeneic peripheral blood stem cell transplantation. *Int J Hematol.* 2002;75(3):332−334.
15. Janin A, Facon T, Castier P, Mancel E, Jouet JP, Gosselin B. Pseudomembranous conjunctivitis following bone marrow transplantation: immunopathological and ultrastructural study of one case. *Hum Pathol.* 1996;27(3):307−309.
16. Jabs D. The eye in bone marrow transplantation. III. Conjunctival graft-vs-host disease. *Arch Ophthalmol.* 1989;107(9):1343−1348.
17. Uchino M, Ogawa Y, Kawai M, et al. Ocular complications in a child with acute graft-versus-host disease following

cord blood stem cell transplantation: therapeutic challenges. *Acta Ophthalmol Scand.* 2006;84(4):545–548.

18. Nassar A, Tabbara KF, Aljurf M. Ocular manifestations of graft-versus-host disease. *Saudi J Ophthalmol.* 2013;27(3): 215–222.

19. Sung AD, Chao NJ. Concise review: acute graft-versus-host disease: immunobiology, prevention, and treatment. *Stem Cells Transl Med.* 2013;2(1):25–32.

20. Stevenson W, Shikari H, Saboo US, Amparo F, Dana R. Bilateral corneal ulceration in ocular graft-versus-host disease. *Clin Ophthalmol.* 2013;7:2153–2158.

21. Mohammadpour M, Maleki S, Hashemi H, Beheshtnejad AH. Recurrent corneal perforation due to chronic graft versus host disease. *Clin Report J Ophthalmic Vis Res.* 2016;11(1): 108–111.

22. Jarade EF, El Rami H, Abdelmassih Y, Amro M. Chronic ocular GVHD: limbal and conjunctival stem cell allografts from the same hematopoietic stem cell donor. *Int J Ophthalmol.* 2018;11(9):1569–1572.

23. Cheung AY, Genereux BM, Auteri NJ, Sarnicola E, Govil A, Holland EJ. Conjunctival-limbal allografts in graft-versus-host disease using same HLA-identical bone marrow transplantation donor. *Can J Ophthalmol.* 2018;53(3): e120–e122.

24. Busin M, Giannaccare G, Sapigni L, et al. Conjunctival and limbal transplantation from the same living-related bone marrow donor to patients with severe ocular graft-vs-host disease. *JAMA Ophthalmol Am Med Assoc.* 2017; 135(10):1123–1125.

25. Wang Y, Ogawa Y, Dogru M, et al. Baseline profiles of ocular surface and tear dynamics after allogeneic hematopoietic stem cell transplantation in patients with or without chronic GVHD-related dry eye. *Bone Marrow Transplant.* 2010;45(6):1077–1083.

26. Balaram M, Rashid S, Dana R. Chronic ocular surface disease after allogeneic bone marrow transplantation. *Ocul Surf.* 2005;3(4):203–210.

27. Tabbara KF, Al-Ghamdi A, Al-Mohareb F, et al. Ocular findings after allogeneic hematopoietic stem cell transplantation. *Ophthalmology.* 2009;116(9):1624–1629.

28. Kusne Y, Temkit M, Khera N, Patel DR, Shen JF. Conjunctival subepithelial fibrosis and meibomian gland atrophy in ocular graft-versus-host disease. *Ocul Surf.* 2017;15(4): 784–788.

29. Kheirkhah A, Coco G, Satitpitakul V, Dana R. Subtarsal fibrosis is associated with ocular surface epitheliopathy in graft-versus-host disease [Internet] *Am J Ophthalmol.* 2018;189:102–110. Available from: https://doi.org/10.1016/j.ajo.2018.02.020.

30. Sivaraman KR, Jivrajka RV, Soin K, et al. Superior limbic keratoconjunctivitis-like inflammation in patients with chronic graft-versus-host disease. *Ocul Surf.* 2016;14(3): 393–400.

31. Hwang HS, Ha M, Kim HS, Na KS. Longitudinal analysis of meibomian gland dropout in patients with ocular graft-versus-host disease. *Ocul Surf.* 2019;17(3):464–469.

32. Ogawa Y, Shimmura S, Dogru M, Tsubota K. Immune processes and pathogenic fibrosis in ocular chronic graft-versus-host disease and clinical manifestations after allogeneic hematopoietic stem cell transplantation. *Cornea.* 2010;29(SUPPL. 1):68–77.

33. Ogawa Y, Okamoto S, Wakui M, et al. Dry eye after haematopoietic stem cell transplantation. *Br J Ophthalmol.* 1999; 83(10):1125–1130.

34. Que L, Zhang X, Li M. Single-center retrospective study on meibomian gland loss in patients with ocular chronic graft-versus-host disease. *Eye Contact Lens.* 2018;44(June 2016):S169–S175.

35. Choi W, Ha JY, Li Y, Choi JH, Ji YS, Yoon KC. Comparison of the meibomian gland dysfunction in patients with chronic ocular graft-versus-host disease and Sjögren's syndrome. *Int J Ophthalmol.* 2019;12(3):393–400.

36. Kim S, Yoo YS, Kim HS, Joo CK, Na KS. Changes of meibomian glands in the early stage of post hematopoietic stem cell transplantation. *Exp Eye Res.* 2017;163:85–90.

37. Engel LA, Wittig S, Bock F, et al. Meibography and meibomian gland measurements in ocular graft-versus-host disease. *Bone Marrow Transplant.* 2015;50(7):961–967.

38. Ban Y, Ogawa Y, Ibrahim OMA, et al. Morphologic evaluation of meibomian glands in chronic graft-versus-host disease using in vivo laser confocal microscopy. *Mol Vis.* 2011;17:2533–2543.

39. Ogawa YKM. Dry eye as a major complication associated with chronic graft-versus-host disease after hematopoietic stem cell transplantation. *Cornea.* 2003;7:19–27.

40. Tung CI. Graft versus host disease: what should the oculoplastic surgeon know? *Curr Opin Ophthalmol.* 2017;28(5): 499–504.

41. Ogawa Y, Kuwana M, Yamazaki K, Mashima Y, Yamada M, Mori T, Okamoto S, Oguchi Y, Kawakami Y. Periductal area as the primary site for T-cell activation in lacrimal gland chronic graft-versus-host disease. *Investig Ophthalmol Vis Sci.* 2003;44(5).

42. Ogawa Y, Yamazaki K, Kuwana M, et al. A significant role of stromal fibroblasts in rapidly progressive dry eye in patients with chronic GVHD. *Invest Ophthalmol Vis Sci.* 2001; 42(1).

43. Campbell AA, Jakobiec FA, Rashid A, Dana R, Yoon MK. Bilateral sequential dacryocystitis in a patient with graft-versus-host disease. *Ophthalmic Plast Reconstr Surg.* 2016; 32(4):e89–92.

44. Hanada R, Ueoka Y. Obstruction of nasolacrimal ducts closely related to graft-versus-host disease after bone marrow transplantation. *Bone Marrow Transplant.* 1989; 4(1):125–126. Stock Press.

45. Satchi K, McNab AA. Conjunctival cicatrizing disease presenting with lacrimal obstruction. *Orbit.* 2016;35(6): 321–323.

46. Kamoi M, Ogawa Y, Dogru M, et al. Spontaneous lacrimal punctal occlusion associated with ocular chronic graft-versus-host disease. *Curr Eye Res.* 2007;32(10):837–842.

47. Dulz S, Wagenfeld L, Richard G, Schrum J, Muschol N, Keserü M. A case of a bilateral cicatricial upper eyelid entropion after hematopoietic stem cell transplantation in mucopolysaccharidosis type i. *Ophthalmic Plast Reconstr Surg.* 2017;33(3S):S75–S77.

48. Powell MR, Davies BW. Cicatricial ectropion secondary to graft-versus-host disease. *Ophthalmic Plast Reconstr Surg.* 2018;34(1):e22−e23.

49. Giannaccare G, Bernabei F, Pellegrini M, et al. Eyelid metrics assessment in patients with chronic ocular graft versus-host disease. *Ocul Surf.* 2019;17(1):98−103.

50. Dietrich-Ntoukas T, Steven P. Okuläre graft-versus-host-disease. *Ophthalmologe.* 2015;112(12):1027−1040.

51. Dikmetas O, Kocabeyoglu SMM. The association between meibomian gland atrophy and corneal subbasal nerve loss in patients with chronic ocular graft-versus-host disease. *Curr Eye Res.* 2021;11:1−6.

52. Arita R, Fukuoka S, Morishige N. Functional morphology of the lipid layer of the tear film. *Cornea.* 2017;36(11):S60−S66.

53. Khanal STA. Tear physiology in dry eye associated with chronic GVHD. *Bone Marrow Transplant.* 2012;47(1):115−119.

54. Arita R, Morishige N, Fujii T, Fukuoka S, Chung JL, Seo KYIK. Tear interferometric patterns reflect clinical tear dynamics in dry eye patients. *Invest Ophthalmol Vis Sci.* 2016;57(8):3928−3934.

55. An S, Raju I, Surenkhuu B, et al. Neutrophil extracellular traps (NETs) contribute to pathological changes of ocular graft-vs.-host disease (oGVHD) dry eye: implications for novel biomarkers and therapeutic strategies. *Ocul Surf.* 2019;17(3):589−614.

56. Tepelus TC, Chiu GB, Maram J, Huang J, Chopra V, Sadda SRLO. Corneal features in ocular graft-versus-host disease by in vivo confocal microscopy. *Graefes Arch Clin Exp Ophthalmol.* 2017;255(12):2389−2397.

57. Kheirkhah A, Qazi Y, Arnoldner MA, Suri KDR. In vivo confocal microscopy in dry eye disease associated with chronic graft-versus-host disease. *Invest Ophthalmol Vis Sci.* 2016;57(11):4686−4691.

58. He J, Ogawa Y, Mukai S, et al. In vivo confocal microscopy evaluation of ocular surface with graft-versus-host disease-related dry eye disease. *Sci Rep.* 2017;7(1):10720.

59. Steger B, Speicher L, Philipp WBN. In vivo confocal microscopic characterisation of the cornea in chronic graft-versus-host disease related severe dry eye disease. *Br J Ophthalmol.* 2015;99(2):160−165.

60. Berchicci L, Iuliano L, Miserocchi E, Bandello FMG. Tear osmolarity in ocular graft-versus-host disease. *Cornea.* 2014;33(12):1252−1256.

61. Na KS, Yoo YS, Hwang KY, Mok JW, Joo CK. Tear osmolarity and ocular surface parameters as diagnostic markers of ocular graft-versus-host disease. *Am J Ophthalmol.* 2015;160(1):143−149.e1.

62. Schargus M, Meyer-ter-Vehn T, Menrath J, Grigoleit GUGG. Correlation between tear film osmolarity and the disease score of the international chronic ocular graft-versus-host-disease consensus group in hematopoietic stem cell transplantation patients. *Cornea.* 2015;34(8):911−916.

63. Pellegrini M, Bernabei F, Moscardelli F, et al. Assessment of corneal fluorescein staining in different dry eye subtypes using digital image analysis. *Transl Vis Sci Technol.* 2019;8(6):34.

64. Shimizu E, Aketa N, Yazu H, et al. Corneal higher-order aberrations in eyes with chronic ocular graft-versus-host disease. *Ocul Surf.* 2020;18(1):98−107.

65. Biology RBP. Of chronic graft-vs-host disease: immune mechanisms and progress in biomarker discovery. *World J Transplant.* 2016;6(4):608−619.

66. Herretes S, Ross DB, Duffort S, et al. Recruitment of donor T cells to the eyes during ocular GVHD in recipients of MHC-matched allogeneic hematopoietic stem cell transplants. *Invest Ophthalmol Vis Sci.* 2015;56(4):2348−2357.

67. Nair S, Vanathi M, Mahapatra M, et al. Tear inflammatory mediators and protein in eyes of post allogenic hematopoeitic stem cell transplant patients. *Ocul Surf.* 2018;16(3):352−367.

68. Cocho L, Fernández I, Calonge M, et al. Biomarkers in ocular chronic graft versus host disease: tear cytokine- and chemokine-based predictive model. *Invest Ophthalmol Vis Sci.* 2016;57(2):746−758.

69. Hu B, Qiu YHJ. Tear cytokine levels in the diagnosis and severity assessment of ocular chronic graft-versus-host disease(GVHD). *Ocul Surf.* 2020;18(2):298−304.

70. Jung JW, Han SJ, Song MK, et al. Tear cytokines as biomarkers for chronic graft-versus-host disease. *Biol Blood Marrow Transplant.* 2015;21(12):2079−2085.

71. Riemens A, Stoyanova E, Rothova AKJ. Cytokines in tear fluid of patients with ocular graft-versus-host disease after allogeneic stem cell transplantation. *Mol Vis.* 2012;18:797−802.

72. Arafat SN, Robert MC, Abud T, et al. Elevated neutrophil elastase in tears of ocular graft-versus-host disease patients. *Am J Ophthalmol.* 2017;176:46−52.

73. Sonawane S, Khanolkar V, Namavari A, et al. Ocular surface extracellular DNA and nuclease activity imbalance: a new paradigm for inflammation in dry eye disease. *Invest Ophthalmol Vis Sci.* 2012;53(13):8253−8263.

74. CI T. Current approaches to treatment of ocular graft-versus-host disease. *Int Ophthalmol Clin.* 2017;57(2):65−88.

75. Yamane M, Ogawa Y, Fukui M, et al. Long-term rebamipide and diquafosol in two cases of immune-mediated dry eye. *Optom Vis Sci.* 2015;92(4):S25−S32.

76. Nassiri N. Ocular graft versus host disease following allogeneic stem cell transplantation: a review of current knowledge and recommendations. *J Ophthalmic Vis Res.* 2013;8(4):351−358.

77. Hirst LW, Jabs DA, Tutschka PJ, Green WRSG. The eye in bone marrow transplantation. I. Clinical study. *Arch Ophthalmol.* 1983;101(4):580−584.

78. Couriel DR, Hosing C, Saliba R, et al. Extracorporeal photochemotherapy for the treatment of steroid-resistant chronic GVHD. *Blood.* 2006;107(8):3074−3080.

79. Robinson MR, Lee SS, Rubin BI, et al. Topical corticosteroid therapy for cicatricial conjunctivitis associated with chronic graft-versus-host disease. *Bone Marrow Transplant.* 2004;33(10):1031−1035.

80. Wang Y, Ogawa Y, Dogru M, et al. Ocular surface and tear functions after topical cyclosporine treatment in dry eye patients with chronic graft-versus-host disease. *Bone Marrow Transplant.* 2008;41(3):293—302.

81. Amparo F, Dastjerdi MH, Okanobo A, et al. Topical interleukin 1 receptor antagonist for treatment of dry eye disease: a randomized clinical trial. *JAMA Ophthalmol.* 2013; 131(6):715—723.

82. Ogawa Y, Dogru M, Uchino M, et al. Topical tranilast for treatment of the early stage of mild dry eye associated with chronic GVHD. *Bone Marrow Transplant.* 2010; 45(3):565—569.

83. Mun C, Gulati S, Tibrewal S, et al. A Phase I/II placebo-controlled randomized pilot clinical trial of recombinant deoxyribonuclease (DNase) eye drops use in patients with dry eye disease. *Transl Vis Sci Technol.* 2019;8(3):10.

84. Kwon J, Surenkhuu B, Raju I, et al. Pathological consequences of anti-citrullinated protein antibodies in tear fluid and therapeutic potential of pooled human immune globulin-eye drops in dry eye disease. *Ocul Surf.* 2020; 18(1):80—97.

85. Pan Q, Angelina A, Marrone M, Stark WJAE. Autologous serum eye drops for dry eye. *Cochrane Database Syst Rev.* 2017;2(2).

86. Yoon KC, Jeong IY, Im SK, Park YG, Kim HJCJ. Therapeutic effect of umbilical cord serum eyedrops for the treatment of dry eye associated with graft-versus-host disease. *Bone Marrow Transplant.* 2007;39(4):231—235.

87. Pezzotta S, Del Fante C, Scudeller L, Cervio M, Antoniazzi ERPC. Autologous platelet lysate for treatment of refractory ocular GVHD. *Bone Marrow Transplant.* 2012; 47(12):558—563.

88. Pezzotta S, Del Fante C, Scudeller L, Rossi GC, Perotti C, Bianchi PEAE. Long-term safety and efficacy of autologous platelet lysate drops for treatment of ocular GvHD. *Bone Marrow Transplant.* 2017;52(1):101—106.

89. Thulasi P, Djalilian AR. Update in current diagnostics and therapeutics of dry eye disease. *Ophthalmology.* 2017; 124(11):S27—S33. Available from: https://doi.org/10.1016/j.ophtha.2017.07.022.

90. Peric Z, Skegro I, Durakovic N, et al. Amniotic membrane transplantation-a new approach to crossing the HLA barriers in the treatment of refractory ocular graft-versus-host disease. *Bone Marrow Transplant.* 2018;53(11): 1466—1469.

91. Tarnawska DWE. Corneal grafting and aggressive medication for corneal defects in graft-versus-host disease following bone marrow transplantation. *Eye.* 2007; 21(12):1493—1500.

92. Inagaki E, Ogawa Y, Matsumoto Y, Kawakita T, Shimmura STK. Four cases of corneal perforation in patients with chronic graft-versus-host disease. *Mol Vis.* 2011;25(17):598—606.

93. Plattner K, Goldblum D, Halter J, Kunz C, Koeppl RG-HN. Osteo-odonto-keratoprosthesis in severe ocular graft versus host disease. *Klin Monbl Augenheilkd.* 2017;234(4): 455—456.

CHAPTER 8

Meibomian Gland Dysfunction and Dry Eye Disease

JENNIFER P. CRAIG, PHD, FCOPTOM, FAAO, FBCLA, FCLS •
MICHAEL T.M. WANG, MBCHB

INTRODUCTION

Meibomian gland dysfunction (MGD) is among the most commonly encountered chronic ocular conditions in clinical practice, and is acknowledged to be a leading contributor of evaporative dry eye disease.[1] The condition is characterized by chronic and diffuse abnormality of the meibomian glands, including terminal duct obstruction and/or qualitative and quantitative changes in glandular secretions. This culminates in alteration of the tear film, clinically apparent inflammation, and ocular surface disease.[2] The associated symptoms of ocular dryness, irritation, and visual disturbance are recognized to have profound impacts on quality of life, visual function, and work productivity.[3]

ANATOMY AND PHYSIOLOGY

The meibomian glands are sebaceous glands, arranged in a parallel fashion within the tarsal plates and perpendicular to the eyelid margin (Fig. 8.1).[4] There are upwards of 30 glands situated in the upper eyelid and around 25 glands in the lower eyelid.[5]

Each meibomian gland consists of a central duct which is connected to smaller ductules, and multiple acini that are separated from the tarsal tissue by a fine basement membrane. The contents of the acini are released via a holocrine mechanism into the ductules, and then travel through the central duct which opens directly onto the posterior lid margin. Epithelial cells of the meibomian glands or meibocytes are continually produced and migrate toward the center of the acini during maturation, before they degenerate and shed the entirety of their cell contents into the lumen of the ductules. The cell contents comprise lipids, proteins, and nucleic acids, which contribute to the final product secreted by the glands, known as meibum.[4] The

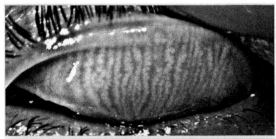
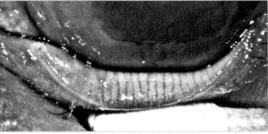

FIG. 8.1 Distribution of meibomian glands illustrated via noncontact infrared meibography imaging of the everted upper and lower eyelids. The meibomian glands appear white against a darker background.

secretory force which facilitates the delivery of lipids to the posterior lid margin is driven primarily by the continuous production and migration of meibocytes toward the center of the acnini.[6] The mechanical forces generated by the *orbicularis oculi* and the muscles of Riolan during blinking compress the tarsal plate and meibomian glands, which further supplements the secretory drive for the delivery of meibomian lipids to the lid margin.[7] In addition, the blinking mechanism also facilitates the distribution of meibum across the ocular surface, where it forms the superficial lipid layer of the precorneal tear film.[8] In contrast to other

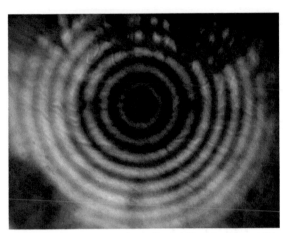

FIG. 8.2 Grade 3 ("wave") tear film lipid layer pattern, visible by interferometry with the Oculus Keratograph 5M.

sebaceous glands distributed throughout the body, which are regulated primarily via hormonal mechanisms, the meibomian glands also receive parasympathetic innervation. This is consistent with the neural supply to other components of the lacrimal functional unit, including the lacrimal and accessory glands and the conjunctival goblet cells.[9]

The surface lipid layer of the precorneal tear film (Fig. 8.2) is formed by the meibomian secretions and fulfills a number of key functions, including inhibition of aqueous tear evaporation, maintenance of a smooth optical refracting surface, and it confers protection to the underlying ocular surface tissues from external debris and pathogens.[10,11] The superficial lipids of the tear film comprise two distinct components. An outer hydrophobic layer exposed to the air consists primarily of nonpolar wax and cholesteryl esters, while an aqueous-facing, inner hydrophilic layer contains water-soluble polar lipids, including short-chain and hydroxylated fatty acids, glycosylated lipids, and phospholipids. These are intercalated by lipid-binding proteins, and facilitate the spreading of the nonpolar lipids of the hydrophobic layer over the underlying muco-aqueous phase of the tear film.[10]

PATHOGENESIS

MGD is a multifactorial condition, which involves complex interactions between a myriad of host, microbial, hormonal, metabolic, and environmental factors.[4,12] The current understanding is that MGD and dry eye disease are intricately linked, forming a self-perpetuating double vicious circle (Fig. 8.3).[13]

Obstruction of the meibomian glands is understood to be driven by two key mechanisms, including excess epithelial keratinization of the ductal system and increased viscosity of the meibomian lipid secretions.[4] The susceptibility of the meibomian gland ductal epithelium to excess keratinization is thought to be attributable to the similar embryological origins to the eyelash follicles. In addition, the pathophysiological effects associated with aging, hormonal imbalance, medication use, and other exogenous factors are also believed to contribute to the release of intrinsic physiological inhibition of keratinization and the aberrant differentiation of progenitor cells.[4] Concurrent changes in lipid composition of meibum can lead to increased melting points and greater viscosity of the gland secretions, thereby further contributing to blockage of the ductal system.[4] Overall, these pathophysiological changes culminate in diminished delivery of meibum to the lid margin and tear film, leading to excessive aqueous tear evaporation, and initiation of a vicious circle of tear film instability, hyperosmolarity, ocular surface epithelial damage.[12] The subsequent loss of tear film and ocular surface homeostasis and the resulting inflammatory responses can then trigger further excess keratinization of the meibomian gland orifices.[4,13]

Ductal obstruction and meibum stasis can also lead to intrinsic changes to the meibomian glands that further perpetuate the double vicious circle of MGD and dry eye disease.[4,13] Stasis of the meibomian lipids within the ductal system can lead directly to increased viscosity, thereby exacerbating pre-existing obstruction of the ductal system. Blockage of the meibomian gland orifices in combination with continuous secretory activity within the acini culminates in progressive increase in the intraluminal pressure of the meibomian glands.[4] The prolonged exposure to higher intraluminal pressure can, in turn, induce activation of the ductal epithelium which exacerbates keratinization. In addition, chronic elevation of pressure can also lead to ductal system dilation, structural atrophy of the acini, and ultimately meibomian gland dropout, which further diminishes the secretion and delivery of meibum to the tear film.[4,13] Meibum stasis also predisposes toward the overcolonization of commensal bacteria, present on the lid margin and in the meibomian glands, that secrete a variety of lipid-degrading enzymes, including lipases and esterases. The resulting degradation of meibomian lipids and release of toxic mediators and free fatty acids induces further destabilization of the tear film. Ensuing inflammatory responses involving the ocular surface, lid margin, and meibomian glands then further exacerbate excess keratinization.[4,12,13]

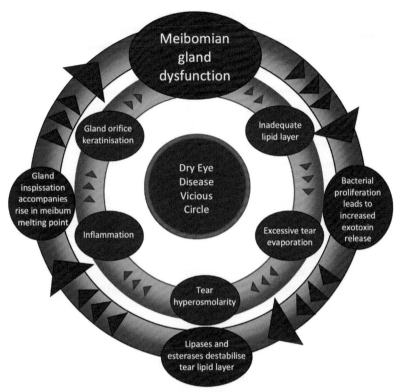

FIG. 8.3 The pathophysiology of dry eye disease and meibomian gland dysfunction are intricately linked in a double vicious circle. (Adapted from Baudouin C, Messmer EM, Aragona P, et al. Revisiting the vicious circle of dry eye disease: a focus on the pathophysiology of meibomian gland dysfunction. *Br J Ophthalmol*. 2016; 100(3):300–306.)

EPIDEMIOLOGY

There is considerable variation in the prevalence estimates for MGD reported in the current literature, which is likely attributed in part to the methodological heterogeneity and differences in disease definition used in existing epidemiological studies.[3,14] The global consensus Tear Film and Ocular Surface Society (TFOS) International Workshop on Meibomian Gland Dysfunction reported that the prevalence of MGD varies from 3.5% to 70% in different parts of the world,[14] while another meta-analysis reported a pooled prevalence estimate of 36% among population-based studies.[15] A summary of population-based studies assessing the prevalence of MGD is presented in Table 8.1.

In recent decades, there has been a growing interest in the epidemiology of MGD, on account of the potential to inform targeted screening and risk factor modification strategies in clinical practice. Systemic and ocular risk factors of MGD that have been identified to date are summarized in Table 8.2.[3,14]

Aging is one of the most consistently identified risk factors for MGD.[3,14] Indeed, advancing age is associated with an increased frequency and severity of anatomical changes in lid margin architecture, keratinization, vascularization, and telangiectasia being reported. This is accompanied by a clinically apparent decline in the quality and quantity of gland secretions, as well as alterations in the lipid profile on laboratory analysis.[14,28–31] Nevertheless, the etiological drivers underlying the association between aging and MGD remain yet to be fully understood, and are thought to involve cumulative lifetime exposure to a combination of environmental and physiological factors, that lead to changes in hormonal regulation, neurosensory pathways, and ocular surface homeostasis.[3,14] The higher prevalence of MGD in postmenopausal women, as well as patients with androgen deficiency, would also appear to corroborate the role of hormonal regulation in the development of MGD.[14,32]

The increased prevalence of MGD among the East Asian ethnic group has also been consistently

TABLE 8.1
Population-Based Studies Assessing the Prevalence of Meibomian Gland Dysfunction (MGD).

Study	Location	Age Group, Years	Sample Size	Prevalence (95% CI), %
Craig et al., 2020[16]	Dunedin, New Zealand	45	885	7.3 (5.8–9.3)
Han et al., 2011[17]	Yongin, South Korea	≥65	139	51.8 (43.6–59.9)
Hashemi et al., 2017[18]	Shahroud, Iran	≥45	4700	26.3 (24.5–28.1)
Hashemi et al., 2021[19]	Tehran, Iran	≥60	3284	71.2 (68.3–74.1)
Jie et al., 2009[20]	Beijing, China	≥40	1957	68.0 (65.6–70.4)
Lekhanont et al., 2006[21]	Bangkok, Thailand	≥40	550	46.2 (42–51)
Lin et al., 2003[22]	Taipei, Taiwan	≥65	1361	60.8 (59.5–62.1)
McCarty et al., 1998[23]	Melbourne, Australia	≥40	926	19.9 (17.4–22.7)
Schein et al., 1997[24]	Salisbury, Maryland, US	≥65	2482	3.5 (2.8–4.4)
Siak et al., 2012[25]	Singapore	40–80	3271	56.3 (53.3–59.4)
Uchino et al., 2006[26]	Chiba, Japan	≥60	113	61.9 (52.1–70.9)
Viso et al., 2012[27]	O Salnés, Spain	>40	619	30.5 (27.0–34.3)

highlighted by a large number of epidemiological studies.[3,14,26,33–35] The propensity of the East Asian ethnic group to the development of MGD is thought to be partially attributed to anatomical differences, including greater axial length and the more inferior attachment point of the *levator palpebrae superioris* aponeurosis, which contributes to increased eyelid tension and incomplete blinking.[36] These factors, in turn, appear to promote stasis of the meibomian secretions and lead to accelerated gland dropout.[8]

Contact lens wear is also a common risk factor for the development of MGD and evaporative dry eye disease.[3,14] Meibomian gland dropout and atrophy have been reported to occur with greater frequency and severity among contact lens wearers, although the underlying pathophysiological mechanisms remain yet to be established.[4,14] In addition, contact lens wear can also destabilize the structural integrity of the superficial lipid layer, predisposing toward excessive aqueous evaporation from the precorneal tear film.[14,37,38]

DIAGNOSIS AND ASSESSMENT

Evaluation of MGD involves two main components, including assessment of meibomian gland morphology and function, as well as clinical signs and symptoms of secondary dry eye disease.[39] The recent global consensus Tear Film and Ocular Surface Society Dry Eye Disease Workshop II (TFOS DEWS II) recommends that diagnostic assessment for dry eye disease occurs prior to the subtype classification testing for potential underlying etiological drivers, such as aqueous tear deficiency and MGD.[40]

Dry Eye Disease Diagnosis

The global consensus TFOS DEWS II criteria for dry eye disease is summarized in Table 8.3, and mandates the presence of both subjective symptoms and clinical signs before a diagnosis of dry eye disease can be confirmed.[40] The validated symptomology questionnaires of choice includes the 5-item Dry Eye Questionnaire (DEQ-5) and the Ocular Surface Disease Index (OSDI), with a positive symptom score requiring either a DEQ-5 score ≥6, or an OSDI score ≥13.[40,41] Clinical signs of ocular surface homeostatic disturbance can be confirmed by positive scores in noninvasive tear film stability (breakup time <10s), tear osmolarity (absolute measurement in either eye ≥308 mOsm/L, or interocular difference of >8 mOsm/L), or ocular surface staining (corneal staining >5 spots, conjunctival staining >9 spots, lid margin staining ≥ 2 mm length and ≥25% width).[40] Automated objective noninvasive measurements of tear film break-up time are preferred, such as those obtained from the Oculus Keratograph 5M (Fig. 8.4) or Medmont E300, although subjective measurements using clinical devices such as the EasyTearView +, Polaris, and Tearscope, can be used

TABLE 8.2

Summary of Systemic and Ocular Risk Factors of Meibomian Gland Dysfunction (MGD).[3,14]

Systemic Risk Factors	Ocular Risk Factors
Aging	Aniridia
Antidepressant therapy	Anterior or posterior
Antihistamine therapy	blepharitis
East Asian ethnicity	Contact lens wear
Androgen deficiency	Eyelid tattooing
Atopy	Floppy eyelid syndrome
Benign prostate hyperplasia	Giant papillary
Cicatricial pemphigoid	conjunctivitis
Complete androgen-insensitivity syndrome	Ichthyosis
	Incomplete blinking
Discoid lupus erythematosus	Salzmann nodular
Ectodermal dysplasia syndrome	degeneration
	Ocular *Demodex*
Hematopoietic stem cell transplantation	infestation
	Trachoma
Hormone replacement and contraceptive therapy	
Hypertension	
Isotretinoin therapy	
Menopause	
Migraine headaches	
Parkinson's disease	
Pemphigoid	
Polycystic ovarian syndrome	
Psoriasis	
Rosacea	
Sjögren's syndrome	
Stevens–Johnson syndrome	
Thyroid disease	
Toxic epidermal necrolysis	
Turner syndrome	

TABLE 8.3

Summary of the Global Consensus Tear Film and Ocular Surface Society Dry Eye Disease Workshop II (TFOS DEWS II) Diagnostic Criteria for Dry Eye Disease.

Component	Criteria
Dry eye symptoms	One of the following: • 5-item dry eye questionnaire (DEQ-5) score ≥ 6 • Ocular surface disease index (OSDI) score ≥ 13
	And
Dry eye signs	One of the following: • Noninvasive tear film break-up time <10s (fluorescein break-up time should only be used if noninvasive methods are unavailable) • Tear osmolarity in either eye ≥ 308 mOsm/L • Interocular difference in tear osmolarity >8 mOsm/L • Corneal staining >5 spots • Conjunctival staining >9 spots • Lid margin staining ≥ 2 mm in length and $\geq 25\%$ width

as an alternative.[40] The instillation of aqueous sodium fluorescein is recognized to destabilize the tear film and artificially shorten break-up time measurements, and should therefore be considered only when noninvasive instruments are unavailable. Excess fluid should be shaken off wetted fluorescein strips prior to application to ensure that minimal amounts are instilled.[42,43]

Tear osmolarity is most commonly assessed using the TearLab osmometer in the clinical setting, and measurements from both eyes are required to provide absolute measurements and calculate interocular variability.[44] Following instillation of both sodium fluorescein and lissamine green dyes, corneal, conjunctival, and lid margin staining (Fig. 8.5) are assessed by slit lamp biomicroscopy, ideally with use of a yellow barrier filter to optimize visibility of the fluorescein staining.[40,45]

Aqueous Tear Production Assessment

Following confirmation of a diagnosis of dry eye disease, as described, subtype classification testing to evaluate the underlying etiological drivers, including aqueous tear deficiency and MGD, can be helpful for guiding subsequent management. The rate of tear flow is not typically affected in MGD, and therefore assessment of tear production can be helpful in differentiating purely aqueous deficient dry eye disease, from evaporative or mixed etiology dry eye disease.[40]

Noninvasive tear meniscus height measurement (Fig. 8.6), with a diagnostic threshold of <0.2 mm, is the recommended diagnostic test for aqueous tear deficiency, while invasive methods such as the Schirmer and phenol red thread test are less preferable and exhibit poorer reliability and repeatability.[40]

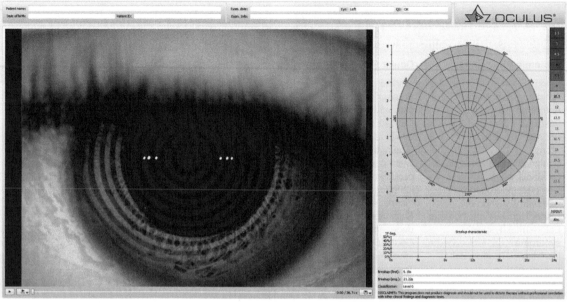

FIG. 8.4 Automated and objective noninvasive tear break-up time measurement with the Oculus Keratograph 5M. A first break-up time of less than 10 s is a clinical sign of dry eye disease.

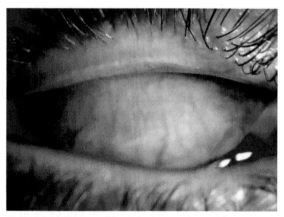

FIG. 8.5 Upper lid margin staining ("lid wiper epitheliopathy") with lissamine green is an early sign of ocular surface epithelial damage.

Meibomian Gland Dysfunction Workup

Assessment of lid margin morphology, meibography, and gland expression is integral for the diagnostic workup for MGD, while the evaluation of the tear film lipid layer interferometry is also recommended, where possible, as a sensitive marker of meibomian gland function.[39,40,46]

Lid margin morphology can be assessed by slit lamp biomicroscopy (Fig. 8.7), and signs typically associated with MGD are summarized in Table 8.4.[39] Lid margin irregularity and notching occur secondary to meibomian gland dropout and loss of tissue, and can be accompanied by a scalloped appearance of the tear meniscus. Hyperkeratinization can also be detected, where keratinized tissue encroaches on the normally smooth and nonkeratinized lid margin mucous membrane.

Retroplacement or a posterior shift of the mucocutaneous junction can also be observed in some cases (Fig. 8.8). Less commonly, the positions of the meibomian gland orifices can shift with squamous metaplasia or become obscured by keratinized epithelium, while anteroplacement is a relatively rare finding. A reduction in the number of meibomian gland orifices, or the formation of hard-surfaced oil domes capping the orifices are also common signs. Chronic cicatrization of the surrounding submucosal tissue can lead to distortion of the gland orifice shape from round to oval, while narrowing and loss of definition of the orifices and the development of surrounding telangiectasia are also frequently observed.[39]

In vivo visualization of meibomian gland morphology can be achieved through noncontact infrared meibography (Figs. 8.1 and 8.9), following eversion of the superior and inferior eyelids in turn, using instruments such as the Oculus Keratograph 5M or Johnson & Johnson Vision TearScience LipiView.[39,40]

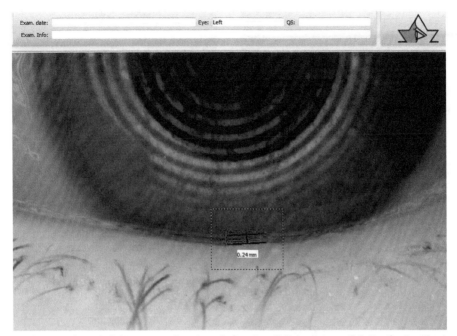

FIG. 8.6 Tear meniscus height measured noninvasively using digital calipers within the Oculus Keratograph 5M software.

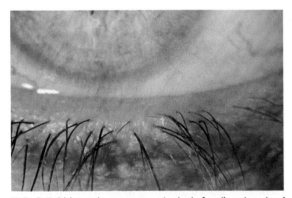

FIG. 8.7 Lid margin appearance typical of meibomian gland dysfunction, showing irregularity of the lower eyelid margin surface due to keratinization and gland blockage, together with mild surface telangiectasia and madarosis.

TABLE 8.4
Summary of Lid Margin Signs Associated With Meibomian Gland Dysfunction (MGD).[39]
Lid Margin Signs
• Lid margin irregularity and notching • Lid margin hyperkeratinization • Retroplacement or anteroplacement of the mucocutaneous junction • Reduction in number of meibomian gland orifices • Meibomian gland orifice capping • Lid margin telangiectasia

A number of morphological features, including gland dropout (Fig. 8.9), shortening, dilation, and tortuosity can be assessed. Meibomian gland dropout is commonly graded subjectively using the qualitative meiboscore (Table 8.5),[47] or using objective quantification methods by image analysis software that calculates the proportion of the area of tarsal conjunctiva devoid of visible glands relative to the total area.[48]

Meibomian gland function can be assessed directly by the diagnostic expression of the glands with a dedicated calibrated device, such as the Johnson & Johnson Vision TearScience Meibomian Gland Evaluator which delivers a repeatable pressure of 1.2 g/mm^2, or by application of gentle digital pressure.[40] Commonly used subjective grading schemes described by Bron et al. are summarized in Table 8.6.[49]

In vivo tear film lipid layer evaluation is a very valuable method facilitating indirect assessment of meibomian gland function, and demonstrates high

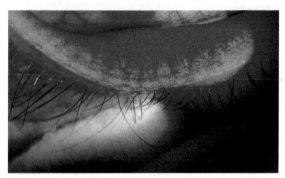

FIG. 8.8 Mucocutaneous junction (MCJ) retroplacement in meibomian gland dysfunction, highlighted by the interruption of the normally lissamine green–stained junction by meibomian gland orifices.

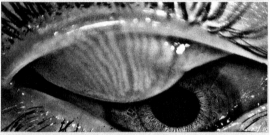

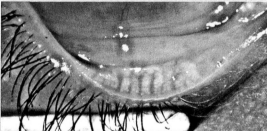

FIG. 8.9 Meibomian gland drop out visible on noncontact infrared meibography.

TABLE 8.5
Summary of the Meiboscale Criteria for Grading Meibomian Gland Dropout.[47]

Grade	Description
0	No gland dropout
1	1%–25% gland dropout
2	26%–50% gland dropout
3	51%–75% gland dropout
4	76%–100% gland dropout

TABLE 8.6
Summarized Grading Scale Criteria for Meibomian Gland Expressibility, as Described by Bron et al.[49]

Grade	Description
NUMBER OF MEIBOMIAN ORIFICES YIELDING LIQUID SECRETIONS	
0	76%–100% orifices yielding liquid secretions
1	51%–75% orifices yielding liquid secretions
2	26%–50% orifices yielding liquid secretions
3	1%–25% orifices yielding liquid secretions
4	0% orifices yielding liquid secretions
EXPRESSED MEIBUM QUALITY	
0	Clear fluid
1	Slightly turbid
2	Thick opaque
3	Toothpaste like
4	Complete orifice blockage

diagnostic sensitivity for MGD.[39,40,46] It can be evaluated qualitatively through the subjective review of lipid layer interferometric patterns generated by instruments such as the EasyTearView +, Bon Polaris, Kowa DR1-α, or Oculus Keratograph (Fig. 8.2), by automated comparison to a subjectively defined grading scale, as with the Simovision SBM Sistemi System, or quantitatively measured using the Johnson & Johnson Vision Tear-Science LipiView.[39,40] Lipid layer interferometry is commonly graded according to the modified Guillon-Keeler system, as summarized in Table 8.7.[35,50]

MANAGEMENT
Where careful diagnostic testing has elucidated MGD as the likely source of a patient's dry eye symptoms or as a risk factor for iatrogenic dry eye,[37] for example prior to contact lens fitting or pre-surgery, adopting a logical stepwise approach to the management of MGD is recommended.

Patient engagement in managing MGD is critical, and a proactive attitude toward educating patients, in order to explain the chronic nature of the disease and

TABLE 8.7
Summary of the Modified Guillon–Keeler Grading Scale for Tear Film Lipid Layer Interferometry.[35,50]

Grade	Description
0	Noncontinuous layer: nonvisible or abnormal colored fringes
1	Open meshwork pattern
2	Closed meshwork pattern
3	Wave or flow pattern
4	Amorphous appearance
5	Normal colored fringes

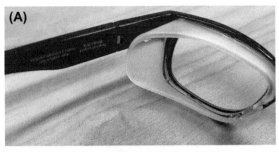

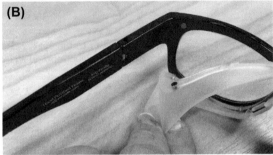

FIG. 8.10 Moisture retention spectacles, **(A)**: silicone inserts attached to a spectacle frame help to reduce the tear evaporation rate by creating a humidified local environment; **(B)**: the inserts, held in place by tiny magnets, are easily detached and reattached as required.

the need for long-term management, is important. Topical anti-inflammatory therapy as a first-line treatment for MGD is not recommended as this frequently fails to address the problem at its source. Offering patients transient symptomatic relief as a "quick fix," risks promotion of unrealistic expectations that make longer term solutions seem less attractive to patients. It can further encourage an unhealthy dependence on a largely palliative therapy which, due to its undesirable safety profile[51] that includes premature cataract development, risk of intraocular pressure rise, and increased susceptibility to infection, is unsuitable for long-term application.

Irrespective of the source of the dry eye, restoration of homeostasis is key to "breaking" the vicious circle of instability, hyperosmolarity, inflammation, and ocular surface damage. Directly addressing the source problem(s) would be expected to lessen the downstream impacts of this self-perpetuating cycle, in turn reducing ocular surface inflammation and the risk of cellular damage.

Evaporative dry eye secondary to MGD typically arises from a poor quantity or quality of meibum. This results in a suboptimal tear lipid layer that permits excessive evaporation of underlying aqueous tears.[11] Tips to help reduce the rate of evaporation from the eye's surface can offer some symptomatic improvement for patients. This may be achieved by increasing the relative humidity around the exposed ocular surface, by avoiding air-conditioned environments or introducing local humidifiers,[52] or by wearing moisture-retaining goggles[53] or spectacles with foam or silicone inserts, (Fig. 8.10A and B) which have the added benefit of reducing air flow across the ocular surface.

Lowering the relative height of computer screens can reduce the exposed ocular surface area during use, and patients should be cautioned against irregular and incomplete blinking which commonly accompany digital device use,[54] and are associated with signs and symptoms of dry eye disease.[8] Blinking exercises show some potential to improve blink quality in symptomatic individuals.[55,56] Recommendations regarding cosmetic product and face cream use might also be warranted, due to their potential impact on the ocular surface from migration across the lid margins and into the tear film.[37,57]

A key aim of MGD treatment is to achieve a thicker and more stable lipid layer to restore its otherwise compromised ability to inhibit aqueous tear evaporation. Improving gland function and encouraging increased meibum flow and quality should therefore be a primary objective of MGD therapy, and may be tackled logically, by adopting a 3-step approach as described below to (1) prepare the lid margin at the site of the gland orifices, (2) encourage increased meibum flow, and (3) optimize the lipid layer quality.

Preparing the Lid Margin
Patient-applied lid hygiene
Given the close association between anterior blepharitis and MGD, an important first step in optimizing the

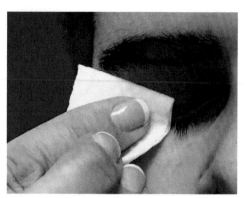

FIG. 8.11 Lid cleansing wipes applied to the eyelids and lashes are an important component of patient-applied lid hygiene.

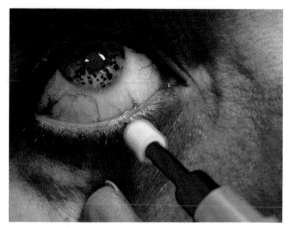

FIG. 8.12 Microblepharoexfoliation is applied as an in-office eyelid hygiene practice.

health of the lid margins is to manage any anterior blepharitis and prepare the gland orifices to facilitate the release of meibum. With careful instruction, lid hygiene to reduce crusting around the lashes and decrease the local bioburden can be performed at home by patients using a wide range of commercial lid cleansers, available as single use wipes, foams, or solutions for application to the lids using cotton pads (Fig. 8.11).[58] Lid wipes containing tea tree oil or its active ingredient terpinen-4-ol may be indicated where cylindrical dandruff, encircling the lash bases has been noted, signifying the presence of *Demodex*.[59,60] Okra-based products have demonstrated similar efficacy to TTO and may be less toxic to the ocular surface.[61,62] While there exists limited high-quality evidence comparing the relative efficacy of commercial lid cleansing products, caution has been raised about the risks of increased inflammation and goblet cell damage from the application of diluted baby shampoo for lid cleansing.[63]

In-office lid hygiene strategies

In more advanced cases, there may be benefit in preceding patient-applied hygiene advice with a thorough in-office lid hygiene visit. This might include treatments such as biofilm removal by microblepharoexfoliation, performed with a spinning fluid-soaked foam-tipped applicator[64] (Fig. 8.12), application of higher concentration solutions such as weekly 50% tea tree oil application for several weeks[60] to manage severe *Demodex* infestation, or lid margin debridement scaling to remove excess keratinization that can obstruct MG orifices.[65]

Simple debridement can be performed with a golf club spud (epithelial debrider) following application of lissamine green to highlight the excess keratinized

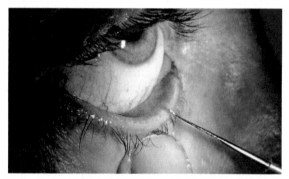

FIG. 8.13 Lower lid margin debridement of excess keratinized tissue with a golf club spud.

epithelium and topical anesthesia to help loosen the keratinized tissue (Fig. 8.13), in order to increase meibomian gland function in affected patients.[65,66] Bacterial overcolonization in blepharitis might be brought under control with a course of topical antibiotics, effective against the gram-positive bacteria of the periocular flora, as a short-term option, and an increasing literature shows ocular benefits from applying natural products such as manuka honey[67–69] and castor oil[70] with purported mild antibacterial and antiinflammatory properties. Severe cases of *Demodex* infestation, or where patient compliance is poor, may respond to treatment with oral ivermectin.[71]

Improving Meibum Outflow

Patient applied gland warming and expression strategies

The application of heat to melt the inspissated meibum can encourage outflow of the oils from the glands in

MGD, to thicken the tear lipid layer,[72] stabilize the tear film,[73] and reduce dry eye symptoms.[74] A temperature of over 40°C for 10 min is recommended as optimal.[75] A range of devices that heat the eyelids externally is available, with little evidence of superiority of one over the other. Microwaveable compresses show better heat retention than portable masks containing pouches heated by a thermochemical reaction, although demonstrate similar efficacy in treating mild disease,[76,77] but washcloths fail to retain sufficient heat over the required period to be effective.[78] Comparable efficacy in improving tear quality has been demonstrated with a latent heat device that allows unrestricted visibility during regulated moist heat application to the eyelids.[73,79]

Recommendations for patient-applied heat therapy are most often accompanied by advice to massage the glands to encourage expression of the melted oils.[80-82] This can be performed manually, or with a dedicated silicone device.[83]

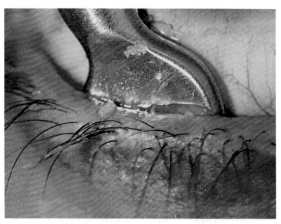

FIG. 8.14 Therapeutic meibomian gland expression performed by applying pressure on the warmed external eyelid surface, against a rigid paddle.

In-office lid warming and expression strategies
A number of thermal in-office treatments for MGD have become available in recent years. These may be designed for application to the external eyelids with subsequent manual expression recommended,[84] or they may be designed to heat the inner eyelid and incorporate gland expression as an integral part of the procedure.[85,86] Treatments that maintain temperatures of above 40°C immediately adjacent to the meibomian glands, combined with gland expression, show potential to confer long-term benefits following a single application,[85-87] but are more costly, thus limiting their widespread adoption.

Manual therapeutic expression increases tear film stability,[88] and can improve treatment outcomes in MGD.[89] The aim is to express thickened meibum from within the gland, and this can be performed effectively with the aid of rigid paddle(s) and/or cotton tipped applicators (Fig. 8.14), to allow the necessary pressure to be applied to the glands without simultaneously applying pressure to the globe.

Alternative strategies
Intense pulsed light therapy has demonstrated efficacy in treating MGD, with a treatment profile that displays cumulative improvements in the tear lipid and tear film stability over a course of treatment,[90-92] reflecting more than simply heat application, and may be particularly suited to patients with MGD associated with rosacea.[93] The application of IPL is most commonly accompanied by therapeutic expression for maximal clinical benefit,[94] and may contribute to reducing ocular surface inflammation,[95] and *Demodex* load.[96,97]

Intraductal probing is an invasive therapeutic strategy for MGD that seeks to physically unblock individual meibomian glands using a fine probe.[98] Inconsistent outcomes in controlled trials and failure to demonstrate benefit relative to control in a recent placebo-controlled trial, question the merit of this technique.[99,100]

Emerging strategies
Treatment options for MGD are constantly evolving and expanding and a number of novel therapies that employ different mechanistic approaches, such as high frequency electrotherapy,[101] radiofrequency,[102] and keratolysis,[103] are currently under investigation in clinical trials.

Improving Lipid Layer Quality
For patients in whom the strategies above have failed to improve symptoms and signs adequately, or for whom the meibum released following treatment is of suboptimal quality, further options can be considered.

Oral antibiotics
Oral tetracycline antibiotics have recognized antiinflammatory properties when prescribed in low dose over an extended period for MGD.[104,105] They possess an ability to reduce bacterial exotoxin levels at the ocular surface, most specifically bacterial lipases, which disrupt the tear film lipid layer. Doxycycline, a tetracycline derivative, shows benefits when prescribed in low-dose over an extended period,[104,106] but its use is contraindicated in children or in pregnant or lactating women.[107] Similar ocular surface benefits have been reported with use of the macrolide, azithromycin,

prescribed topically,[108,109] or orally.[110–112] Azithromycin has a generally superior safety profile to the tetracyclines, with fewer contraindications.[111,113]

Dietary supplementation

Essential fatty acids (EFAs), ingested within the diet or as a dietary supplement, play a role in modulating inflammatory levels within the body. On the basis of systematic review and metaanalysis, it has been suggested that Omega-3 EFAs, in moderate daily dose, may be therapeutically beneficial for MGD.[114]

Artificial tear supplementation

Conventional aqueous tear supplements have a limited and largely palliative role in managing evaporative dry eye secondary to MGD, typically offering only transient relief of symptoms due to rapid evaporation in the absence of an adequate lipid layer. In such cases homeostasis may be restored with the application of lipid-containing supplements, available in the form of liposomal sprays,[115] combination lipid-aqueous drops,[116,117] and lipid-only drops.[118] Mixed dry eye, with elements of aqueous and lipid deficiency, may benefit from the application of combination supplements, or sequentially applied aqueous and lipid supplements. Lipid-based drops applied prior to exposure to an adverse environment offer prophylactic benefits,[119,120] and restoration of homeostasis from regular application over several months shows potential for improved tear film and ocular surface signs, beyond the immediate palliative symptomatic benefits that typically occur within the first month of commencing treatment.[116]

SUMMARY/CONCLUSION

MGD is a key chronic trigger of the vicious circle of dry eye disease, which can lead to debilitating symptoms and ocular surface sequelae. Understanding the risk factors and identifying deficiencies with clear evidence-based diagnostic criteria and then targeting identified deficiencies with appropriate management strategies is important in restoring ocular surface homeostasis. Patient-applied therapies play an important role in managing this chronic condition, but success relies on good patient compliance. Educating patients about their condition and relevant modifiable risk factors, as well as providing justification and thorough training in the application of selected management strategies increases patient engagement, compliance and the chance of success. Testing for dry eye subtypes using appropriate diagnostic procedures and evidence-based diagnostic criteria enables source(s) of the problem to be confidently and consistently identified, therapeutic strategies to be tailored, and tear film and ocular surface changes over time, and with treatment, to be monitored. Patients should be reviewed regularly to revise treatment plans as necessary, and help maintain patient engagement. A trial period of 1 month with any new treatment allows benefits to be elicited before considering the introduction of alternative or supplementary treatments.[116] The multifactorial nature of dry eye disease and MGD demands a multifaceted approach. For efficiency, specialist practices may consider a delegated role for an "ocular hygienist" to assist with performing diagnostic procedures and delivering patient education and basic treatments. As the availability of novel therapeutic strategies for managing MGD rises exponentially, informing clinical practice on the basis of high-quality scientific evidence remains of paramount importance in seeking to maximize patient outcomes.

REFERENCES

1. Craig JP, Nichols KK, Akpek EK, et al. TFOS DEWS II definition and classification report. *Ocul Surf.* 2017;15(3):276–283.
2. Nelson JD, Shimazaki J, Benitez-del-Castillo JM, et al. The international workshop on meibomian gland dysfunction: report of the definition and classification sub committee. *Invest Ophthalmol Vis Sci.* 2011;52(4):1930–1937.
3. Stapleton F, Alves M, Bunya VY, et al. TFOS DEWS II epidemiology report. *Ocul Surf.* 2017;15(3):334–365.
4. Knop E, Knop N, Millar T, Obata H, Sullivan DA. The international workshop on meibomian gland dysfunction: report of the subcommittee on anatomy, physiology, and pathophysiology of the meibomian gland. *Invest Ophthalmol Vis Sci.* 2011;52(4):1938–1978.
5. Greiner JV, Glonek T, Korb DR, et al. Volume of the human and rabbit meibomian gland system. *Adv Exp Med Biol.* 1998;438:339–343.
6. Olami Y, Zajicek G, Cogan M, Gnessin H, Pe'er J. Turnover and migration of meibomian gland cells in rats' eyelids. *Ophthalmic Res.* 2001;33(3):170–175.
7. Linton RG, Curnow DH, Riley WJ. The meibomian glands: an investigation into the secretion and some aspects of the physiology. *Br J Ophthalmol.* 1961;45(11):718–723.
8. Wang MTM, Tien L, Han A, et al. Impact of blinking on ocular surface and tear film parameters. *Ocul Surf.* 2018;16(4):424–429.
9. Perra MT, Serra A, Sirigu P, Turno F. Histochemical demonstration of acetylcholinesterase activity in human Meibomian glands. *Eur J Histochem.* 1996;40(1):39–44.
10. Willcox MDP, Argüeso P, Georgiev GA, et al. TFOS DEWS II tear film report. *Ocul Surf.* 2017;15(3):366–403.

11. Craig JP, Tomlinson A. Importance of the lipid layer in human tear film stability and evaporation. *Optom Vis Sci.* 1997;74(1):8−13.
12. Bron AJ, de Paiva CS, Chauhan SK, et al. TFOS DEWS II pathophysiology report. *Ocul Surf.* 2017;15(3):438−510.
13. Baudouin C, Messmer EM, Aragona P, et al. Revisiting the vicious circle of dry eye disease: a focus on the pathophysiology of meibomian gland dysfunction. *Br J Ophthalmol.* 2016;100(3):300−306.
14. Schaumberg DA, Nichols JJ, Papas EB, Tong L, Uchino M, Nichols KK. The international workshop on meibomian gland dysfunction: report of the subcommittee on the epidemiology of, and associated risk factors for, MGD. *Invest Ophthalmol Vis Sci.* 2011;52(4):1994−2005.
15. Hassanzadeh S, Varmaghani M, Zarei-Ghanavati S, Heravian Shandiz J, Azimi Khorasani A. Global prevalence of meibomian gland dysfunction: a systematic review and meta-analysis. *Ocul Immunol Inflamm.* 2021;29(1):66−75.
16. Craig JP, Wang MTM, Ambler A, Cheyne K, Wilson GA. Characterising the ocular surface and tear film in a population-based birth cohort of 45-year old New Zealand men and women. *Ocul Surf.* 2020;18(4):808−813.
17. Han SB, Hyon JY, Woo SJ, Lee JJ, Kim TH, Kim KW. Prevalence of dry eye disease in an elderly Korean population. *Arch Ophthalmol.* 2011;129(5):633−638.
18. Hashemi H, Rastad H, Emamian MH, Fotouhi A. Meibomian gland dysfunction and its determinants in Iranian adults: a population-based study. *Contact Lens Anterior Eye.* 2017;40(4):213−216.
19. Hashemi H, Asharlous A, Aghamirsalim M, et al. Meibomian gland dysfunction in geriatric population: tehran geriatric eye study. *Int Ophthalmol.* 2021;41(7):2539−2546.
20. Jie Y, Xu L, Wu YY, Jonas JB. Prevalence of dry eye among adult Chinese in the Beijing Eye Study. *Eye.* 2009;23(3):688−693.
21. Lekhanont K, Rojanaporn D, Chuck RS, Vongthongsri A. Prevalence of dry eye in Bangkok, Thailand. *Cornea.* 2006;25(10):1162−1167.
22. Lin PY, Tsai SY, Cheng CY, Liu JH, Chou P, Hsu WM. Prevalence of dry eye among an elderly Chinese population in Taiwan: the Shihpai Eye Study. *Ophthalmology.* 2003;110(6):1096−1101.
23. McCarty CA, Bansal AK, Livingston PM, Stanislavsky YL, Taylor HR. The epidemiology of dry eye in Melbourne, Australia. *Ophthalmology.* 1998;105(6):1114−1119.
24. Schein OD, Muñoz B, Tielsch JM, Bandeen-Roche K, West S. Prevalence of dry eye among the elderly. *Am J Ophthalmol.* 1997;124(6):723−728.
25. Siak JJ, Tong L, Wong WL, et al. Prevalence and risk factors of meibomian gland dysfunction: the Singapore Malay eye study. *Cornea.* 2012;31(11):1223−1228.
26. Uchino M, Dogru M, Yagi Y, et al. The features of dry eye disease in a Japanese elderly population. *Optom Vis Sci.* 2006;83(11):797−802.
27. Viso E, Rodríguez-Ares MT, Abelenda D, Oubiña B, Gude F. Prevalence of asymptomatic and symptomatic meibomian gland dysfunction in the general population of Spain. *Invest Ophthalmol Vis Sci.* 2012;53(6):2601−2606.
28. Wang MTM, Muntz A, Lim J, et al. Ageing and the natural history of dry eye disease: a prospective registry-based cross-sectional study. *Ocul Surf.* 2020;18(4):736−741.
29. Hykin PG, Bron AJ. Age-related morphological changes in lid margin and meibomian gland anatomy. *Cornea.* 1992;11(4):334−342.
30. Wang MTM, Vidal-Rohr M, Muntz A, et al. Systemic risk factors of dry eye disease subtypes: a New Zealand cross-sectional study. *Ocul Surf.* 2020;18(3):374−380.
31. Sullivan BD, Evans JE, Dana MR, Sullivan DA. Influence of aging on the polar and neutral lipid profiles in human meibomian gland secretions. *Arch Ophthalmol.* 2006;124(9):1286−1292.
32. Sullivan DA, Rocha EM, Aragona P, et al. TFOS DEWS II sex, gender, and hormones report. *Ocul Surf.* 2017;15(3):284−333.
33. Craig JP, Lim J, Han A, Tien L, Xue AL, Wang MTM. Ethnic differences between the Asian and Caucasian ocular surface: a co-located adult migrant population cohort study. *Ocul Surf.* 2019;17(1):83−88.
34. Kim JS, Wang MTM, Craig JP. Exploring the Asian ethnic predisposition to dry eye disease in a pediatric population. *Ocul Surf.* 2019;17(1):70−77.
35. Craig JP, Wang MT, Kim D, Lee JM. Exploring the predisposition of the asian eye to development of dry eye. *Ocul Surf.* 2016;14(3):385−392.
36. Wang MTM, Craig JP. Natural history of dry eye disease: perspectives from inter-ethnic comparison studies. *Ocul Surf.* 2019;17(3):424−433.
37. Gomes JAP, Azar DT, Baudouin C, et al. TFOS DEWS II iatrogenic report. *Ocul Surf.* 2017;15(3):511−538.
38. Craig JP, Willcox MD, Argueso P, et al. The TFOS International Workshop on Contact Lens Discomfort: report of the contact lens interactions with the tear film subcommittee. *Invest Ophthalmol Vis Sci.* 2013;54(11):TFOS123−156.
39. Tomlinson A, Bron AJ, Korb DR, et al. The international workshop on meibomian gland dysfunction: report of the diagnosis subcommittee. *Invest Ophthalmol Vis Sci.* 2011;52(4):2006−2049.
40. Wolffsohn JS, Arita R, Chalmers R, et al. TFOS DEWS II diagnostic methodology report. *Ocul Surf.* 2017;15(3):539−574.
41. Wang MTM, Xue AL, Craig JP. Comparative evaluation of 5 validated symptom questionnaires as screening instruments for dry eye disease. *JAMA Ophthalmol.* 2019;137(2):228−229.
42. Wang MTM, Craig JP. Comparative evaluation of clinical methods of tear film stability assessment: a randomized crossover trial. *JAMA Ophthalmol.* 2018;136(3):291−294.
43. Mooi JK, Wang MTM, Lim J, Müller A, Craig JP. Minimising instilled volume reduces the impact of fluorescein on clinical measurements of tear film stability. *Contact Lens Anterior Eye.* 2017;40(3):170−174.

44. Wang MTM, Ormonde SE, Muntz A, Craig JP. Diagnostic profile of tear osmolarity and inter-ocular variability for dry eye disease. *Clin Exp Ophthalmol.* 2020;48(2): 255–257.

45. Wang MTM, Dean SJ, Xue AL, Craig JP. Comparative performance of lid wiper epitheliopathy and corneal staining in detecting dry eye disease. *Clin Exp Ophthalmol.* 2019;47(4):546–548.

46. Wang MTM, Dean SJ, Muntz A, Craig JP. Evaluating the diagnostic utility of evaporative dry eye disease markers. *Clin Exp Ophthalmol.* 2020;48(2):267–270.

47. Pult H, Riede-Pult B. Comparison of subjective grading and objective assessment in meibography. *Contact Lens Anterio.* 2013;36(1):22–27.

48. Srinivasan S, Menzies K, Sorbara L, Jones L. Infrared imaging of meibomian gland structure using a novel keratograph. *Optom Vis Sci.* 2012;89(5):788–794.

49. Bron AJ, Benjamin L, Snibson GR. Meibomian gland disease. Classification and grading of lid changes. *Eye.* 1991; 5(Pt 4):395–411.

50. Guillon JP. Use of the tearscope plus and attachments in the routine examination of the marginal dry eye contact lens patient. *Adv Exp Med Biol.* 1998;438:859–867.

51. McGhee CN, Dean S, Danesh-Meyer H. Locally administered ocular corticosteroids: benefits and risks. *Drug Saf.* 2002;25(1):33–55.

52. Wang MTM, Chan E, Ea L, et al. Randomized trial of desktop humidifier for dry eye relief in computer users. *Optom Vis Sci.* 2017;94(11):1052–1057.

53. Korb DR, Blackie CA. Using goggles to increase periocular humidity and reduce dry eye symptoms. *Eye Contact Lens.* 2013;39(4):273–276.

54. Golebiowski B, Long J, Harrison K, Lee A, Chidi-Egboka N, Asper L. Smartphone use and effects on tear film, blinking and binocular vision. *Curr Eye Res.* 2020; 45(4):428–434.

55. Kim AD, Muntz A, Lee J, Wang MTM, Craig JP. Therapeutic benefits of blinking exercises in dry eye disease. *Contact Lens Anterior Eye.* 2020;44(3):101329.

56. Murakami D, Blackie CA, Korb DR. *Blinking Exercises Can Be Used to Decrease Partial Blinking and Improve Gland Function and Symptoms in Patients with Evaporative Dry Eye.* Denver, CO, USA: American Academy of Optometry; 2014.

57. Wang MT, Craig JP. Investigating the effect of eye cosmetics on the tear film: current insights. *Clin Optom.* 2018;10:33–40.

58. Bitton E, Ngo W, Dupont P. Eyelid hygiene products: a scoping review. *Contact Lens Anterior Eye.* 2019;42(6): 591–597.

59. Gao YY, Di Pascuale MA, Elizondo A, Tseng SC. Clinical treatment of ocular demodecosis by lid scrub with tea tree oil. *Cornea.* 2007;26(2):136–143.

60. Koo H, Kim TH, Kim KW, Wee SW, Chun YS, Kim JC. Ocular surface discomfort and Demodex: effect of tea tree oil eyelid scrub in Demodex blepharitis. *J Kor Med Sci.* 2012;27(12):1574–1579.

61. Liu W, Gong L. Anti-demodectic effects of okra eyelid patch in Demodex blepharitis compared with tea tree oil. *Exp Ther Med.* 2021;21(4):338.

62. Chen D, Wang J, Sullivan DA, Kam WR, Liu Y. Effects of terpinen-4-ol on meibomian gland epithelial cells in vitro. *Cornea.* 2020;39(12):1541–1546.

63. Sung J, Wang MTM, Lee SH, et al. Randomized double-masked trial of eyelid cleansing treatments for blepharitis. *Ocul Surf.* 2018;16(1):77–83.

64. Siddireddy JS, Vijay AK, Tan J, Willcox M. Effect of eyelid treatments on bacterial load and lipase activity in relation to contact lens discomfort. *Eye Contact Lens.* 2020;46(4): 245–253.

65. Korb DR, Blackie CA. Debridement-scaling: a new procedure that increases Meibomian gland function and reduces dry eye symptoms. *Cornea.* 2013;32(12): 1554–1557.

66. Ngo W, Caffery B, Srinivasan S, Jones LW. Effect of lid debridement-scaling in sjogren syndrome dry eye. *Optom Vis Sci.* 2015;92(9):e316–320.

67. Albietz JM, Lenton LM. Effect of antibacterial honey on the ocular flora in tear deficiency and meibomian gland disease. *Cornea.* 2006;25(9):1012–1019.

68. Tan J, Jia T, Liao R, Stapleton F. Effect of a formulated eye drop with Leptospermum spp honey on tear film properties. *Br J Ophthalmol.* 2020;104(10):1373–1377.

69. Craig JP, Cruzat A, Cheung IMY, Watters GA, Wang MTM. Randomized masked trial of the clinical efficacy of MGO Manuka Honey microemulsion eye cream for the treatment of blepharitis. *Ocul Surf.* 2020;18(1):170–177.

70. Muntz A, Sandford E, Claassen M, et al. Randomized trial of topical periocular castor oil treatment for blepharitis. *Ocul Surf.* 2021;19(1):145–150.

71. Holzchuh FG, Hida RY, Moscovici BK, et al. Clinical treatment of ocular Demodex folliculorum by systemic ivermectin. *Am J Ophthalmol.* 2011;151(6):1030–1034 e1031.

72. Olson MC, Korb DR, Greiner JV. Increase in tear film lipid layer thickness following treatment with warm compresses in patients with meibomian gland dysfunction. *Eye Contact Lens.* 2003;29(2):96–99.

73. Turnbull PRK, Misra SL, Craig JP. Comparison of treatment effect across varying severities of meibomian gland dropout. *Contact Lens Anterior Eye.* 2018;41(1):88–92.

74. Bilkhu PS, Naroo SA, Wolffsohn JS. Randomised masked clinical trial of the MGDRx EyeBag for the treatment of meibomian gland dysfunction-related evaporative dry eye. *Br J Ophthalmol.* 2014;98(12):1707–1711.

75. Borchman D. The optimum temperature for the heat therapy for meibomian gland dysfunction. *Ocul Surf.* 2019;17(2):360–364.

76. Wang MT, Gokul A, Craig JP. Temperature profiles of patient-applied eyelid warming therapies. *Contact Lens Anterior Eye.* 2015;38(6):430–434.

77. Wang MT, Jaitley Z, Lord SM, Craig JP. Comparison of self-applied heat therapy for meibomian gland dysfunction. *Optom Vis Sci.* 2015;92(9):e321–326.

78. Lacroix Z, Leger S, Bitton E. Ex vivo heat retention of different eyelid warming masks. *Contact Lens Anterior Eye.* 2015;38(3):152–156.

79. Murakami DK, Blackie CA, Korb DR. All warm compresses are not equally efficacious. *Optom Vis Sci.* 2015; 92(9):e327–333.

80. Jones L, Downie LE, Korb D, et al. TFOS DEWS II management and therapy report. *Ocul Surf.* 2017;15(3):575–628.

81. Geerling G, Tauber J, Baudouin C, et al. The international workshop on meibomian gland dysfunction: report of the subcommittee on management and treatment of meibomian gland dysfunction. *Invest Ophthalmol Vis Sci.* 2011;52(4):2050–2064.

82. Korb DR, Blackie CA. Meibomian gland therapeutic expression: quantifying the applied pressure and the limitation of resulting pain. *Eye Contact Lens.* 2011;37(5): 298–301.

83. Wang MTM, Feng J, Wong J, Turnbull PR, Craig JP. Randomised trial of the clinical utility of an eyelid massage device for the management of meibomian gland dysfunction. *Contact Lens Anterior Eye.* 2019;42(6): 620–624.

84. Karpecki P, Wirta D, Osmanovic S, Dhamdhere K. A prospective, post-market, multicenter trial (CHEETAH) suggested TearCare((R)) system as a safe and effective blink-assisted eyelid device for the treatment of dry eye disease. *Clin Ophthalmol.* 2020;14:4551–4559.

85. Greiner JV. A single LipiFlow(R) thermal pulsation system treatment improves meibomian gland function and reduces dry eye symptoms for 9 months. *Curr Eye Res.* 2012;37(4):272–278.

86. Tauber J, Owen J, Bloomenstein M, Hovanesian J, Bullimore MA. Comparison of the iLUX and the LipiFlow for the treatment of meibomian gland dysfunction and symptoms: a randomized clinical trial. *Clin Ophthalmol.* 2020;14:405–418.

87. Greiner JV. Long-term (3 year) effects of a single thermal pulsation system treatment on meibomian gland function and dry eye symptoms. *Eye Contact Lens.* 2016; 42(2):99–107.

88. Craig JP, Blades K, Patel S. Tear lipid layer structure and stability following expression of the meibomian glands. *Ophthalmic Physiol Opt.* 1995;15(6):569–574.

89. Kaiserman I, Rabina G, Mimouni M, et al. The effect of therapeutic meibomian glands expression on evaporative dry eye: a prospective randomized controlled trial. *Curr Eye Res.* 2021;46(2):195–201.

90. Craig JP, Chen YH, Turnbull PR. Prospective trial of intense pulsed light for the treatment of meibomian gland dysfunction. *Invest Ophthalmol Vis Sci.* 2015; 56(3):1965–1970.

91. Xue AL, Wang MTM, Ormonde SE, Craig JP. Randomised double-masked placebo-controlled trial of the cumulative treatment efficacy profile of intense pulsed light therapy for meibomian gland dysfunction. *Ocul Surf.* 2020; 18(2):286–297.

92. Yan S, Wu Y. Efficacy and safety of Intense pulsed light therapy for dry eye caused by meibomian gland dysfunction: a randomised trial. *Ann Palliat Med.* 2021;10(7): 7857–7865.

93. Seo KY, Kang SM, Ha DY, Chin HS, Jung JW. Long-term effects of intense pulsed light treatment on the ocular surface in patients with rosacea-associated meibomian gland dysfunction. *Contact Lens Anterior Eye.* 2018; 41(5):430–435.

94. Shin KY, Lim DH, Moon CH, Kim BJ, Chung TY. Intense pulsed light plus meibomian gland expression versus intense pulsed light alone for meibomian gland dysfunction: a randomized crossover study. *PLoS One.* 2021; 16(3):e0246245.

95. Liu R, Rong B, Tu P, et al. Analysis of cytokine levels in tears and clinical correlations after intense pulsed light treating meibomian gland dysfunction. *Am J Ophthalmol.* 2017;183:81–90.

96. Cheng SN, Jiang FG, Chen H, Gao H, Huang YK. Intense pulsed light therapy for patients with meibomian gland dysfunction and ocular Demodex infestation. *Curr Med Sci.* 2019;39(5):800–809.

97. Fishman HA, Periman LM, Shah AA. Real-time video microscopy of in vitro Demodex death by intense pulsed light. *Photobiomodul Photomed Laser Surg.* 2020;38(8): 472–476.

98. Maskin SL. Intraductal meibomian gland probing relieves symptoms of obstructive meibomian gland dysfunction. *Cornea.* 2010;29(10):1145–1152.

99. Kheirkhah A, Kobashi H, Girgis J, Jamali A, Ciolino JB, Hamrah P. A randomized, sham-controlled trial of intraductal meibomian gland probing with or without topical antibiotic/steroid for obstructive meibomian gland dysfunction. *Ocul Surf.* 2020;18(4):852–856.

100. Magno M, Moschowits E, Arita R, Vehof J, Utheim TP. Intraductal meibomian gland probing and its efficacy in the treatment of meibomian gland dysfunction. *Surv Ophthalmol.* 2021;66(4):612–622.

101. Ferrari G, Colucci A, Barbariga M, Ruggeri A, Rama P. High frequency electrotherapy for the treatment of meibomian gland dysfunction. *Cornea.* 2019;38(11): 1424–1429.

102. ClinicalTrials.gov. *Clinical Evaluation of Safety and Efficacy of Radio Frequency (Forma Eye) Treatment for Dry Eye Disease Due to Meibomian Gland Dysfunction.* 2019. NCT04120584.

103. ClinicalTrials.gov. *Evaluation of AZR-MD-001 in Patients with Meibomian Gland Dysfunction (MGD).* 2020. NCT04391959.

104. Yoo SE, Lee DC, Chang MH. The effect of low-dose doxycycline therapy in chronic meibomian gland dysfunction. *Kor J Ophthalmol.* 2005;19(4):258–263.

105. Ta CN, Shine WE, McCulley JP, Pandya A, Trattler W, Norbury JW. Effects of minocycline on the ocular flora of patients with acne rosacea or seborrheic blepharitis. *Cornea.* 2003;22(6):545–548.

106. Onghanseng N, Ng SM, Halim MS, Nguyen QD. Oral antibiotics for chronic blepharitis. *Cochrane Database Syst Rev.* 2021;6:CD013697.

107. Alikhan A, Kurek L, Feldman SR. The role of tetracyclines in rosacea. *Am J Clin Dermatol.* 2010;11(2):79—87.

108. Foulks GN, Borchman D, Yappert M, Kakar S. Topical azithromycin and oral doxycycline therapy of meibomian gland dysfunction: a comparative clinical and spectroscopic pilot study. *Cornea.* 2013;32(1):44—53.

109. Foulks GN, Borchman D, Yappert M, Kim SH, McKay JW. Topical azithromycin therapy for meibomian gland dysfunction: clinical response and lipid alterations. *Cornea.* 2010;29(7):781—788.

110. De Benedetti G, Vaiano AS. Oral azithromycin and oral doxycycline for the treatment of Meibomian gland dysfunction: a 9-month comparative case series. *Indian J Ophthalmol.* 2019;67(4):464—471.

111. Kashkouli MB, Fazel AJ, Kiavash V, Nojomi M, Ghiasian L. Oral azithromycin versus doxycycline in meibomian gland dysfunction: a randomised double-masked open-label clinical trial. *Br J Ophthalmol.* 2015; 99(2):199—204.

112. Greene JB, Jeng BH, Fintelmann RE, Margolis TP. Oral azithromycin for the treatment of meibomitis. *JAMA Ophthalmol.* 2014;132(1):121—122.

113. Tao T, Tao L. Systematic review and meta-analysis of treating meibomian gland dysfunction with azithromycin. *Eye.* 2020;34(10):1797—1808.

114. Al-Namaeh M. A systematic review of the effect of omega-3 supplements on meibomian gland dysfunction. *Ther Adv Ophthalmol.* 2020;12, 2515841420952188.

115. Craig JP, Purslow C, Murphy PJ, Wolffsohn JS. Effect of a liposomal spray on the pre-ocular tear film. *Contact Lens Anterior Eye.* 2010;33(2):83—87.

116. Craig JP, Muntz A, Wang MTM, et al. Developing evidence-based guidance for the treatment of dry eye disease with artificial tear supplements: a six-month multicentre, double-masked randomised controlled trial. *Ocul Surf.* 2021;20:62—69.

117. Guthrie SE, Jones L, Blackie CA, Korb DR. A comparative study between an oil-in-water emulsion and nonlipid eye drops used for rewetting contact lenses. *Eye Contact Lens.* 2015;41(6):373—377.

118. Steven P, Scherer D, Krosser S, Beckert M, Cursiefen C, Kaercher T. Semifluorinated alkane eye drops for treatment of dry eye disease—a prospective, multicenter non-interventional study. *J Ocul Pharmacol Therapeut.* 2015; 31(8):498—503.

119. Muntz A, Marasini S, Wang MTM, Craig JP. Comparing the prophylactic action of lipid and non-lipid containing tear supplements in adverse environmental conditions: a randomised crossover trial. *Ocul Surf.* 2020;18(4): 920—925.

120. Gokul A, Wang MTM, Craig JP. Tear lipid supplement prophylaxis against dry eye in adverse environments. *Contact Lens Anterior Eye.* 2018;41(1):97—100.

CHAPTER 9

Systemic Pain Conditions and Dry Eye Disease

JELLE VEHOF, MD, PHD, FEBO • CHRISTOPHER JOHN HAMMOND, MD, FRCOPHTH

THE LINK BETWEEN SYSTEMIC PAIN CONDITIONS AND DRY EYE

Introduction

Chronic pain is a pain that persists or recurs for longer than 3 months. With an estimated 20% prevalence in the general population worldwide it is highly common. It comes with significant direct and indirect costs for society. In the United States, these costs are higher than the combined costs of cancer, diabetes, and heart disease, and are estimated to be over $500 billion per year.[1–4] In the new ICD-11 classification chronic pain is systematically classified as either primary pain, including disorders such as chronic widespread pain (CWP), chronic musculoskeletal pain, primary headache disorders, chronic pelvic pain, and irritable bowel syndrome (IBS), or as secondary pain including disorders such as cancer-related pain, postsurgical pain, neuropathic pain, secondary headache or orofacial pain, visceral pain, and secondary musculoskeletal pain.[5] There is increasing recognition that many chronic pain conditions often coexist, leading to the concept of chronic overlapping pain conditions (COPCs).[6]

Indeed, numerous systemic pain conditions have been associated with dry eye disease and dry eye (like) symptoms, suggesting dry eye might be a COPC as well. Fig. 9.1 illustrates this overlap. There are many similarities and shared pathophysiological mechanisms between dry eye and these disorders that may underlie this association.[7] Increased awareness and recognition of associated systemic pain conditions and their pathophysiological mechanisms might help an ophthalmic practitioner fully understand the clinical picture of dry eye and optimize patient's treatment. Similarly, physicians looking after patients with systemic pain should be aware of dry eye disease being a prevalent comorbidity with serious impact.

Shared Epidemiological Factors

Both dry eye and systemic pain conditions are much more prevalent in women. Other important risk factors are also largely similar, such as older age, mental health problems, sleep disturbance, reduced physical activity, a history of smoking, heritable factors, nutrition, surgical interventions, and a history of trauma.[8–10] A classical twin study in the United Kingdom investigated genetic and environment interrelations between fibromyalgia (FM), IBS, chronic pelvic pain, and DED. It revealed that these four disorders share a latent underlying factor that is highly heritable (66%), which accounts for clustering of these conditions in patients. This underlying

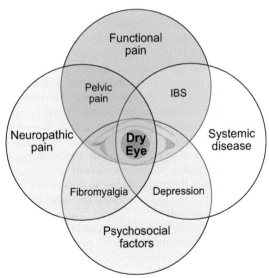

FIG. 9.1 An example of how dry eye overlaps with other chronic pain conditions. (*Created by Emily Moschowits.*)

Dry Eye Disease. https://doi.org/10.1016/B978-0-323-82753-9.00008-4

latent factor of *chronic pain predisposition* accounted for 15% of the variance of DED in the investigated population. This indicates that both shared genetic and shared environmental factors with other systemic pain conditions underlie dry eye, explaining the overlap of disorders in patients.[11]

Shared Clinical Characteristics

Both dry eye and systemic pain conditions are chronic diseases, and both show a lack of response to treatment.[7] Symptoms of both often include dysesthesias (meaning "abnormal sensations") such as a burning or throbbing feeling, or the feeling of pins and needles. One of the hallmarks of both is discordance between subjective symptoms and objective signs. Moreover, a study of 648 dry eye patients (83% women) in the Netherlands found systemic pain conditions to be the strongest predictor of discordance between symptoms and signs of dry eye.[12] IBS, FM, and chronic pelvic pain were all highly associated with greater symptoms compared to signs. In addition, depression and osteoarthritis were also associated with more symptoms than signs. A similar study in the United States, in men only, found similar results with greater symptoms than signs in persons with arthritis, chronic pain outside the eye, posttraumatic stress disorder (PTSD), anxiety, and depression.[13]

Neuropathic Pain

Neuropathic pain is pain caused by a lesion or disease of the somatosensory nervous system, and often plays a role in chronic pain. Somatosensory dysfunction may be the origin of dry eye symptoms, particularly in patients with limited or no abnormalities of the ocular surface with a standard eye exam. This dysfunction may be either at the periphery (e.g., corneal nerves) or central, within the central nervous system. At the periphery, corneal nerve abnormalities can lead to a spectrum of disease, ranging from hyposensitivity and neurotrophy with epitheliopathy to hypersensitivity with pain.[14] Inflammation at the ocular surface in dry eye can lower the threshold of neuron activation, and both intensity and duration of pulses can increase with time. When acute pain becomes chronic, it can undergo centralization: despite limited input from the peripheral nervous system, the central nervous system responds as if there are high levels of painful stimuli and patients become hypersensitive to pain. This process is often referred to as the wind-up or temporal summation. Patients can experience neuropathic pain from stimuli that are normally not painful (allodynia) or have an increased sensitivity to painful stimuli (hyperalgesia), but pain may also arise spontaneously.

Increased Pain Sensitivity and Nerve Abnormalities

Altered findings on quantitative sensory testing (QST) testing, such as lower pain tolerance and higher pain sensitivity, are very common with neuropathic pain and in systemic pain conditions.[15–18] Also dry eye has been associated with altered QST. In a UK cohort QST using a heat stimulus on the forearm was used to assess pain sensitivity and pain tolerance in 1635 females. Both pain sensitivity was higher and pain tolerance was lower in those with DED than in those without DED. Participants with a below median pain sensitivity were found to have almost twice as often dry eye pain symptoms such as light sensitivity, gritty feeling, and painful eyes than persons with an above median pain sensitivity.[19] Similar results were found in a predominantly male cohort in the United States, with severity of neuropathic-like dry eye pain (symptoms such as burning and evoked pain to wind and light) particularly correlating with QST. Moreover, increased pain sensitivity, as measured by QST metrics, was also associated with more symptoms compared to signs.[20] In addition, dry eye and neuropathic pain share similarities in altered nerve anatomy such as nerve density and length.[7]

Comorbid Mental Health Disorders

Systemic pain conditions, neuropathic pain, and dry eye are also highly comorbid with mental health disorders and influenced by psychological factors that can impact symptoms and an individual's experience of pain.[10,21,22] In a US cohort it was found that dry eye symptoms align more with nonocular pain and PTSD scores than with dry eye signs, explaining 35%–40% of the variability of symptoms.[23] A Korean study found that depression scores correlated with dry eye symptoms scores, but not with dry eye signs.[24] Another study in patients with symptoms of dry eye found that in those with high neuropathic ocular pain symptoms pain intensity ratings were higher, and mental health scores more abnormal compared to those with low or no neuropathic ocular symptoms.[25]

Inflammatory Factors

Finally, both neuropathic pain and dry eye may share similarities in inflammatory mechanisms. Among the studies that investigated inflammatory mediators in various systemic pain conditions, levels of PGE_2, IL-1, IL-6, TNF, are among the most consistently increased. These mediators have also been found to be increased in tears of DED patients, and may play a role in sensitization of peripheral corneal nociceptors.[26]

The findings above suggest that increased pain sensitivity, neuropathic pain, and other pain modifying mechanisms are responsible for a share of the symptom burden of dry eye, particularly in patients with comorbid systemic pain and mental health disorders. Fig. 9.2 schematically summarizes mechanisms underlying the link between systemic pain conditions and DED. Although pain management may fall outside the scope of practice of many eye practitioners, it is important to recognize neuropathic pain, particularly when symptoms are worse than clinical signs. When recognized, patients can be educated about the origin of their symptoms and their treatment can be optimized by a multidisciplinary approach including pain specialists. The TFOS DEWS II Definition and Classification Report added neuropathic pain and referral for pain management in its main clinical decision algorithm and classification scheme of DED. Box 9.1 presents an overview of systemic pain conditions that have been associated with an increased prevalence of DED and/or dry eye symptoms in clinical and population-based studies. The systemic pain disorders most studied in this context will be discussed in the next section.

SYSTEMIC PAIN CONDITIONS ASSOCIATED WITH DRY EYE

Fibromyalgia

FM is a chronic disorder and probably a subgroup of CWP, which is characterized by widespread musculoskeletal pain in all four quadrants of the body, and in the neck and back. FM is CWP of more than a 3-month duration, with mechanical hyperalgesia at least 11 tender-point sites. It is accompanied by symptoms such as fatigue and sleep and mood problems. Its etiology is largely unknown, but genetic factors, stressful life events, and peripheral and central mechanisms play a role. The prevalence in the general population is around 2%–5%, with women six times more affected than men. Over half of patients will have a diagnosis of depression in their life, and other chronic pain conditions such as head and jaw pain and IBS are also highly prevalent.[27,28] The revised 2010 diagnostic criteria of FM by the American College of Rheumatology included numerous somatic symptoms as additional minor criteria, including blurred vision and dry eye.[29]

Of all systemic pain disorders, FM is probably the most studied in relation to DED. Several studies have

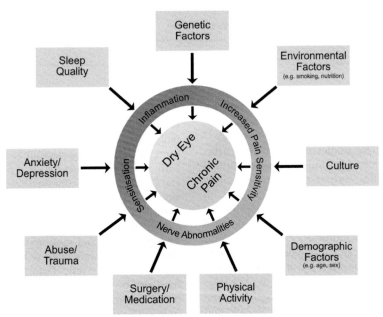

FIG. 9.2 Dry eye and chronic pain share many external and internal risk factors that contribute to the complex nature of both. (*Created by Emily Moschowits.*)

BOX 9.1
Overview of Pain (Modifying) Conditions That Have Been Associated With an Increased Prevalence of Dry Eye Disease and/or Dry Eye Symptoms

Functional Pain Disorders	Headache Disorders	Other
Fibromyalgia	Migraine	Small fiber neuropathy
Irritable bowel syndrome	Tension-type headache	Osteoarthritis
Chronic pelvic pain	Cluster headache	Trigeminal neuralgia
Chronic fatigue syndrome	Paroxysmal hemicrania	RSI
Temporomandibular joint disorders	Short-lasting unilateral neuralgiform headache attacks with conjunctival injection and tearing (SUNCT)	Carpal tunnel syndrome
Central pain syndrome		Disc herniation
Complex regional pain syndrome		Trigeminal neuralgia
Mental health disorders (modifying pain amplification)	**Ocular and (peri)orbital disorders mimicking dry eye symptoms**	
Depression	Sinusitis	
Anxiety disorder	Cavernous carotid fistula	
Posttraumatic stress disorder (PTSD)	Tolosa Hunt syndrome	
Insomnia	Refractive error	
Burn out	Digital eye strain	
Autism	Intermittent angle closure	
	Posterior scleritis	

shown dry eye prevalence to be much higher in FM patients than in controls and vice versa.[30–34] FM disease activity was found to correlate with dry eye severity.[35] In addition, half a dozen studies on corneal nerve structures in FM patients have uniformly reported abnormalities in nerve structures, such as a lower nerve density and nerve count compared to controls. Findings on corneal sensitivity, however, were less consistent among studies.[14] A recent study showed that one-third of FM patients with dry mouth and/or dry eye tested positive for Sjögren's syndrome autoantibodies. The majority of these only tested positive for the novel tissue-specific autoantibodies, that are observed in early stage Sjögren's syndrome, such as SP-1, CA6, and PSP, and not for the classic autoantibodies such as SS-A/Ro and SS-B/La. This indicates that autoimmunity and early-stage Sjögren's syndrome may be involved in at least some FM patients.[36]

Irritable Bowel Syndrome

IBS is a functional gastrointestinal disorder with recurrent symptoms of abdominal pain and a change in form or frequency of stool. It is a common disorder, with an estimated prevalence of 5%–10% in the general population. Its pathophysiology is not well understood, but it is widely accepted that there is dysfunctional communication between the brain and the gut that leads to visceral hypersensitivity, altered CNS processing and motility disturbances. Pain sensitivity, bacterial overgrowth of the small intestine, neurotransmitters, genetic factors, and food sensitivity have also been proposed to play a role.[37] Diagnosis is based on symptoms and exclusion of signs of other disorders. The most important risk factors of IBS include acute enteric infection, female sex, and psychological comorbidities.[37]

IBS has been associated with dry eye in clinical and population studies.[30,31,38,39] Not only dry eye symptoms but also signs such as Schirmer test and TBUT have been found to be significantly worse in IBS patients compared to controls, which may also suggest a common inflammatory pathogenesis. Like in dry eye, proinflammatory cytokines, such as IL-1, IL-6, and TNF-α, and T-cell activation have been shown to be increased in IBS patients.[39] Also, the transient receptor potential cation channel subfamily M member 8 (TRPM8) has been described in the pathophysiology of both IBS and dry eye. This channel is the primary thermoreceptor for responses to cold stimuli and can be found in multiple organs, including the gut where it plays a role in colonic spontaneous motility and the cornea where it plays a role in regulating basal tear flow.[40] Dysfunction may lead to inflammatory or neuropathic pain and cold allodynia and hyperalgesia.[41]

Chronic Pelvic Pain and Bladder Pain

Chronic pelvic pain is a disabling, persistent pain within the pelvis in women, lasting more than 6 months. Its prevalence lies between 4% and 16% in women. Centralized pain is widely considered as the main pathophysiology. It may or may not be associated with initial local pelvic pathology. It can, for example, originate from endometriosis, where acute pain associated with this condition becomes centralized after several months. IBS and bladder pain syndrome are also highly comorbid in women who suffer chronic pelvic pain. It has a strong association with previous physical and emotional trauma.[42] Although the link between DED and CPP has not been studied as much as other pain conditions, it was among the strongest risk factors of dry eye in population-based studies that included it in the set of investigated risk factors.[30–32] It was also one of the three pain disorders that were found to have shared genetic factors with DED (in addition to FM and IBS).[11]

An overactive bladder and bladder pain syndrome (interstitial cystitis) have been associated with systemic autoimmune disease, particularly Sjögren's syndrome, in several clinical samples.[43–45] Recurring cystitis was found as an independent risk factor of dry eye symptoms in a large population-based study.[31] Autoantibodies to the muscarinic M3 receptor, which plays a role in tear secretion and bladder contraction, may underlie these associations.[45]

Migraine and Other Headache Disorders

Migraine is considered a neurovascular condition that clinically manifests as recurrent headache attacks with a duration of 4–72 h. Typical features are a mostly unilateral, pulsating head pain, aggravation by physical activity, and accompanying symptoms such as nausea, vomiting, photo- and phonophobia, and visual and hemisensory disturbances. It has an estimated 1-year prevalence of around 15% in the general population, with females being more affected than males (3:1). Its pathogenesis is poorly understood, but the trigeminal nerve and its axonal projections to the trigeminovascular system are involved.[46] As such, in both migraine and dry eye pathways of the trigeminal system are involved, with photophobia being a shared common symptom. Numerous studies have found an increased risk of a dry eye diagnosis or dry eye symptoms in migraine patients.[30,31,47–51] Altered tear function or other objective signs of dry eye in migraine patients are however less apparent.[47,51–53]

Corneal nerves have been studied in the context of migraine, but results are not uniform and may vary between populations.[54] Corneal nerve lengths were found to be lower in individuals with migraine and concomitant photophobia than in controls or in individuals with migraine without photophobia.[55] One study found lower nerve density in migraine patients compared to controls,[52] while another study found higher corneal nerve density.[56] Only one study investigated corneal sensitivity and found borderline significant higher sensitivity in migraine patients compared to controls.[57] No shared genetic factors were found between migraine and other chronic pain syndromes including DED in a twin study, suggesting that other factors may play a role in the association between the two. For example, some authors suggest inflammatory processes could underlie the association between the two, such as T-lymphocyte—mediated inflammation and increased levels of inflammatory mediators such as calcitonin gene-related peptide and interleukines.[47,48] In migraine, inflammatory mediators may lead to hypersensitivity of trigeminal ganglion neurons via increased plasma extravasation. Also, increased sensitivity to pain, cold, and heat was found in individuals with migraine.[28,29] Migraine has also been associated with Sjögren's syndrome and other connective tissue diseases.

Other primary headache disorders may also give eye pain, tearing, or periocular pain that may mimic dry eye symptoms, such as tension-type headaches and the trigeminal autonomic cephalalgias (cluster headache, paroxysmal hemicrania, and short-lasting unilateral neuralgiform headache attacks with conjunctival injection and tearing).[58]

Osteoarthritis

Osteoarthritis is a complex progressive degenerative disease of multiple joint tissues. It can affect any joint and can lead to severe pain, stiffness, and disability. Older age and female sex are important risk factors. Similar to dry eye, it has a vicious circle of pathophysiology, that includes tissue inflammation, changes in synovial fluid, articular cartilage degeneration, and osteochondral alterations, leading to bone changes and damage.[59] A handful of studies have investigated the link between osteoarthritis and dry eye, and found a clearly increased risk of DED in patients with osteoarthritis.[30,32,60,61] Osteoarthritis may be comorbid with or misdiagnosed for arthritis in connective tissue disease, which may explain part of the associated risk found in studies. It was, however, also found to be a highly significant independent risk factor of dry eye, after correction for numerous autoimmune and connective tissue disorders in a large population-based study.[31] Similar to DED, osteoarthritis is associated with increased pain sensitivity on QST.[17,61] Another link between the two may be impaired function of the viscoelastic properties of both the tears and the synovial fluid, via, e.g., hyaluronic acid or lubricin. Hyaluronic acid plays an important role as a lubricant in the human body has the highest concentrations found in the joints and eyes, and promotes corneal epithelial wound healing.[62] One study found a diagnosis of tear film dysfunction twice as often in persons with osteoarthritis compared to controls, indicating that their link is not limited to just increased pain sensitivity.[32]

Temporomandibular Joint Disorders

Temporomandibular joint disorders (TMDs) are characterized by pain or dysfunction of the temporomandibular joint and the muscles of mastication. Their prevalence is around 5%−12% in the general population.[63] The disorders have associated symptoms such as headache, earache, restricted mandibular movement, and noises during jaw movement. The typical headache associated with TMD is pain that radiates to the jaw, temple, or forehead.[64] Chronic TMD is considered a biopsychosocial pain condition with many features similar to other chronic pain disorders, including lower pain tolerance than controls, a poor correlation between pain severity and tissue pathology, and a link with anxiety, depression, posttraumatic stress, and a history of abuse. FM and IBS are also highly comorbid.[64] In a large retrospective study investigating ICD-codes in the United States, TMD was associated with a 2.4 times higher risk of dry eye.[32] TMD is also more common in patients with Sjögren's syndrome, which may explain part of the associated risk of dry eye.[65,66]

Small Fiber Neuropathy

Small fiber neuropathy (SFN) is a subtype of neuropathy characterized by selective involvement of thinly myelinated and unmyelinated sensory fibers.[67] The neuropathy manifests clinically with isolated sensory disturbances, isolated autonomic disorders, or both. Persons can have severe pain attacks that typically start in the hands or feet, but can increase to a more generalized body pain. Its pathophysiology is complex, with immune-mediated, metabolic, toxic, and genetic factors likely playing a role. It has been associated with many autoimmune disorders, including Sjögren's syndrome, and also with hyperalgesia, allodynia, and several chronic pain syndromes.[68] The condition is further associated with urinary and bowel disorders, palpitations, orthostatic hypertension, and also dry eye and mouth.[69] An in vivo corneal confocal microscopy study found signs of trigeminal nerve injury in patients with SFN, with reduced corneal nerve fiber density and decreased total number of corneal nerves.[70]

Central Pain Syndrome

Central pain syndrome is a neurological condition consisting of constant pain due to sensitization of the pain system after damage to the CNS, e.g., by an accident, surgery, stroke, or autoimmune disease.[71] A diagnosis of central pain syndrome was associated with a two times higher risk of dry eye.[32]

Complex Regional Pain Syndrome

The complex regional pain syndrome (CRPS) is a neuropathic pain syndrome after injury, characterized by disabling pain, swelling, and impaired motor function. It is most prevalent in extremities but can also present in the orofacial region.[72] Pain and hyperalgesia can spread to uninjured sites of the ipsilateral side of the body, and even to the whole body. Visual discomfort and photophobia are common in patients with CRPS. A study investigating visual discomfort thresholds to a light source that increased in intensity found lower thresholds in patients than in controls. Thresholds were also found to be lower on the CRPS-affected than unaffected side.[73] Indeed, a diagnosis of CRPS was highly associated with a dry eye diagnosis in a US veteran population.[32] Visual discomfort in CRPS may be explained by abnormal processing of nociceptive input in the ipsilateral trigeminal−medullary region of the brainstem.[73]

Other Systemic Pain Conditions

There are several other pain conditions that have been associated with dry eye that point to a much more widespread association between chronic pain conditions and DED. A large population-based study in the Netherlands with over 78,000 participants found repetitive strain injury, disc herniation, carpal tunnel syndrome, and chronic back pain all to be independently associated with dry eye, even after correction for confounding disorders such as depression, FM, IBS, and osteoarthritis.[31] Multiple chemical sensitivity (sometimes called sick building syndrome) is another disorder highly associated with sensitization, that can also lead to burning or sore eyes. It is characterized by nonspecific symptoms in multiple organ systems due to exposure to low-level chemicals.[74]

Mental Health Disorders and Psychological Factors that can Influence Pain

The perception of pain can be highly influenced by psychological factors and mental health disorders such as depression, anxiety, and stress.[75] Underlying mechanisms include disinhibition of the central pain regulatory system and inhibition of the central pleasure system and of the psychomotor facilitatory system.[76,77] Comorbidity between chronic pain and depression was found to be higher in women.[78] Interestingly, in depressed people there is a particular increased pain sensitivity for exteroceptive stimuli, which are also important in the etiology of dry eye.[79-81] Depression and anxiety are also highly prevalent in dry eye.[82,83] A systematic review found an average prevalence of depression of 29% in dry eye patients, which was the highest rate among several common eye disorders investigated.[83] The association between depression and dry eye is likely to be bidirectional, with dry eye symptoms leading to depressive symptoms as well.

PTSD has also been associated with a highly increased risk of dry eye symptoms. PTSD not only shares similarities with depression but also leads to amplified emotional reactions including responses to painful stimuli.[84] Chronic fatigue syndrome (CFS), also known as myalgic encephalomyelitis, is a complex disease with a constellation of symptoms such as a disabling fatigue, postexertional malaise, muscle and joint pain, headaches, and cognitive impairment.[85] Several studies showed an increased prevalence of dry eye in persons with CFS.[31,32,86]

Poor sleep quality can also increase pain sensitivity.[87,88] Insomnia is a common comorbid disorder of both dry eye and neuropathic pain.[89,90] Every component of sleep quality was found to be highly affected in dry eye patients, particularly in those with frequent symptoms, even after correction for comorbid pain and psychiatric disorders.[91] As for depression, the relationship between sleep quality and dry eye is also likely to be bidirectional.

Referred Pain and Other Ocular and Orbital Disorders Mimicking Dry Eye Symptoms

An often-overlooked etiology of dry eye symptoms is the group of disorders that give referred pain or produce symptoms that mimic dry eye. Headache disorders are an important group, and have been discussed in section Migraine and Other Headache Disorders above. Trigeminal neuralgia is characterized by spontaneous and severe shock-like face pain lasting for seconds to minutes. It can also present with a less severe constant burning or throbbing pain between attacks.[92] The maxillary nerve (v2) is most often affected, but all branches including the ophthalmic nerve (v1) may be affected.[93] Sinusitis was found to be an independent risk factor of dry eye in a large population-based study. It may give a throbbing pain or pressure around the eyes that might be confused with dry eye.[31] Similarly, odontogenic pain and oral surgery may affect trigeminal function and give referred ocular pain.[94] Ocular motor cranial nerve palsies due to ischemia may produce a frontal headache pain, brow pain, and ocular pain.

Other ocular and orbital disorders that may produce similar (pain) symptoms as dry eye and that are often overlooked by standard ocular exams are trochleodynia, intermittent angle closure, posterior scleritis, Tolosa Hunt syndrome, and cavernous carotid fistula. Benign essential blepharospasm may not only be caused by dry eye but can also produce dry eye like symptoms.[72,93] It is also important to rule out any refractive error problem (e.g., latent hypermetropia) in patients who have both headache and dry eye like symptoms. Digital eye strain (also called trigeminal dysphoria) is another cause that can give both symptoms of headache and dry eye.

MEDICATIONS IN SYSTEMIC PAIN CONDITIONS THAT MAY AGGRAVATE DRY EYE

A number of medications that are used in the treatment of systemic pain conditions have been described to be associated with and/or cause DED.[95] Some of these medications may be secreted in tears and may lead to irritation or increased tear evaporation. Anticholinergic drugs, such as antispasmodics used in IBS, have been linked to decreased tear production and lower tear film quality by decreased mucus production.[95] Similarly, antidepressants may have anticholinergic actions, particularly the classical tricyclic antidepressants.[96] However, next to possible anticholinergic side effects, antidepressants may also have a positive effect on dry eye symptomatology by lowering depression scores and pain sensitivity.[31,97] Several analgesics, such as NSAIDs and cannabinoid and opioid analgesics, have also been proposed to affect tear function and production, although evidence is more limited.[95] Proton pump inhibitors, frequently used by patients with IBS, were found to be the most significantly associated medication group in a large population-based study investigating dry eye symptoms that corrected for over 50 comorbidities, suggesting PPIs could be causally related to dry eye.[97] It is important to identify medication use in every patient with dry eye, particularly in those with comorbid pain conditions. Where possible, a stop or a switch to a medication group with an alternative mechanism should be considered.[95]

CONCLUSIONS AND CLINICAL IMPLICATIONS

The pathophysiology of DED and symptomatic dry eye is highly multifactorial and extends beyond the ocular surface. Mechanisms such as peripheral and central sensitization and psychological factors may play important roles in patients' symptom experience. A holistic view when assessing a dry eye patient is required to understand the complete clinical picture and to optimize treatment. Systemic pain conditions, increased pain sensitivity, and mental health disorders that modulate symptom experience are highly prevalent in patients with DED and are among the most important risk factors in population-based studies. A detailed medical history and specifically designed pain questionnaires may provide important clues about a neuropathic origin of symptoms of dry eye, particularly in patients where clinical signs are limited or less apparent than symptoms. Application of in vivo corneal confocal microscopy of nerve status and corneal esthesiometry may be valuable tools in clinical practice, but further studies are needed to determine their exact value. Patients with associated systemic pain conditions could possibly benefit from nonocular treatment modalities, including medications aimed at neuropathic and chronic pain, and therapy aimed at coping strategies, such as cognitive behavioral therapy and mindfulness (see Chapter 15).

REFERENCES

1. Treede RD, Rief W, Barke A, et al. A classification of chronic pain for ICD-11. *Pain.* 2015;156(6):1003−1007.
2. Nahin RL. Estimates of pain prevalence and severity in adults: United States, 2012. *J Pain.* 2015;16(8):769−780.
3. Alford DP, Krebs EE, Chen IA, Nicolaidis C, Bair MJ, Liebschutz J. Update in pain medicine. *J Gen Intern Med.* 2010;25(11):1222−1226.
4. Pizzo PA, Clark NM. Alleviating suffering 101−pain relief in the United States. *N Engl J Med.* 2012;366(3): 197−199.
5. Treede RD, Rief W, Barke A, et al. Chronic pain as a symptom or a disease: the IASP classification of chronic pain for the international classification of diseases (ICD-11). *Pain.* 2019;160(1):19−27.
6. Maixner W, Fillingim RB, Williams DA, Smith SB, Slade GD. Overlapping chronic pain conditions: implications for diagnosis and classification. *J Pain.* 2016;17(9 Suppl):T93−T107.
7. Galor A, Moein HR, Lee C, et al. Neuropathic pain and dry eye. *Ocul Surf.* 2018;16(1):31−44.
8. van Hecke O, Torrance N, Smith BH. Chronic pain epidemiology - where do lifestyle factors fit in? *Br J Pain.* 2013; 7(4):209−217.
9. Mills SEE, Nicolson KP, Smith BH. Chronic pain: a review of its epidemiology and associated factors in population-based studies. *Br J Anaesth.* 2019;123(2):e273−e283.
10. Stapleton F, Alves M, Bunya VY, et al. TFOS DEWS II epidemiology report. *Ocul Surf.* 2017;15(3):334−365.
11. Vehof J, Zavos HM, Lachance G, Hammond CJ, Williams FM. Shared genetic factors underlie chronic pain syndromes. *Pain.* 2014;155(8):1562−1568.
12. Vehof J, Sillevis Smitt-Kamminga N, Nibourg SA, Hammond CJ. Predictors of discordance between symptoms and signs in dry eye disease. *Ophthalmology.* 2017; 124(3):280−286.
13. Ong ES, Felix ER, Levitt RC, Feuer WJ, Sarantopoulos CD, Galor A. Epidemiology of discordance between symptoms and signs of dry eye. *Br J Ophthalmol.* 2018;102(5): 674−679.
14. Patel S, Hwang J, Mehra D, Galor A. Corneal nerve abnormalities in ocular and systemic diseases. *Exp Eye Res.* 2021; 202:108284.
15. Pfau DB, Geber C, Birklein F, Treede RD. Quantitative sensory testing of neuropathic pain patients: potential mechanistic and therapeutic implications. *Curr Pain Headache Rep.* 2012;16(3):199−206.
16. Uddin Z, MacDermid JC. Quantitative sensory testing in chronic musculoskeletal pain. *Pain Med.* 2016;17(9): 1694−1703.
17. Frey-Law LA, Bohr NL, Sluka KA, et al. Pain sensitivity profiles in patients with advanced knee osteoarthritis. *Pain.* 2016;157(9):1988−1999.
18. Russo A, Coppola G, Pierelli F, et al. Pain perception and migraine. *Front Neurol.* 2018;9:576.

19. Vehof J, Kozareva D, Hysi PG, et al. Relationship between dry eye symptoms and pain sensitivity. *JAMA Ophthalmol.* 2013;131(10):1304–1308.

20. Galor A, Levitt RC, McManus KT, et al. Assessment of somatosensory function in patients with idiopathic dry eye symptoms. *JAMA Ophthalmol.* 2016;134(11):1290–1298.

21. IsHak WW, Wen RY, Naghdechi L, et al. Pain and depression: a systematic review. *Harv Rev Psychiatr.* 2018;26(6):352–363.

22. Hooten WM. Chronic pain and mental health disorders: shared neural mechanisms, epidemiology, and treatment. *Mayo Clin Proc.* 2016;91(7):955–970.

23. Galor A, Felix ER, Feuer W, et al. Dry eye symptoms align more closely to non-ocular conditions than to tear film parameters. *Br J Ophthalmol.* 2015;99(8):1126–1129.

24. Kim KW, Han SB, Han ER, et al. Association between depression and dry eye disease in an elderly population. *Invest Ophthalmol Vis Sci.* 2011;52(11):7954–7958.

25. Crane AM, Levitt RC, Felix ER, Sarantopoulos KD, McClellan AL, Galor A. Patients with more severe symptoms of neuropathic ocular pain report more frequent and severe chronic overlapping pain conditions and psychiatric disease. *Br J Ophthalmol.* 2017;101(2):227–231.

26. Belmonte C, Acosta MC, Gallar J. Neural basis of sensation in intact and injured corneas. *Exp Eye Res.* 2004;78(3):513–525.

27. Kleykamp BA, Ferguson MC, McNicol E, et al. The prevalence of psychiatric and chronic pain comorbidities in fibromyalgia: an ACTTION systematic review. *Semin Arthritis Rheum.* 2020;51(1):166–174.

28. Sarzi-Puttini P, Giorgi V, Marotto D, Atzeni F. Fibromyalgia: an update on clinical characteristics, aetiopathogenesis and treatment. *Nat Rev Rheumatol.* 2020;16(11):645–660.

29. Wolfe F, Clauw DJ, Fitzcharles MA, et al. The American College of Rheumatology preliminary diagnostic criteria for fibromyalgia and measurement of symptom severity. *Arthritis Care Res.* 2010;62(5):600–610.

30. Vehof J, Kozareva D, Hysi PG, Hammond CJ. Prevalence and risk factors of dry eye disease in a British female cohort. *Br J Ophthalmol.* 2014;98(12):1712–1717.

31. Vehof J, Snieder H, Jansonius N, Hammond CJ. Prevalence and risk factors of dry eye in 79,866 participants of the population-based Lifelines cohort study in The Netherlands. *Ocul Surf.* 2021;19:83–93.

32. Lee CJ, Levitt RC, Felix ER, Sarantopoulos CD, Galor A. Evidence that dry eye is a comorbid pain condition in a U.S. veteran population. *Pain Rep.* 2017;2(6):e629.

33. Chen CH, Yang TY, Lin CL, et al. Dry eye syndrome risks in patients with fibromyalgia: a National Retrospective Cohort Study. *Medicine.* 2016;95(4):e2607.

34. Schuster AK, Wettstein M, Gerhardt A, Eich W, Bieber C, Tesarz J. Eye pain and dry eye in patients with fibromyalgia. *Pain Med.* 2018;19(12):2528–2535.

35. Turkyilmaz K, Turkyilmaz AK, Kurt EE, Kurt A, Oner V. Dry eye in patients with fibromyalgia and its relevance to functional and emotional status. *Cornea.* 2013;32(6):862–866.

36. Applbaum E, Lichtbroun A. Novel Sjogren's autoantibodies found in fibromyalgia patients with sicca and/or xerostomia. *Autoimmun Rev.* 2019;18(2):199–202.

37. Ford AC, Sperber AD, Corsetti M, Camilleri M. Irritable bowel syndrome. *Lancet.* 2020;396(10263):1675–1688.

38. Barton A, Pal B, Whorwell PJ, Marshall D. Increased prevalence of sicca complex and fibromyalgia in patients with irritable bowel syndrome. *Am J Gastroenterol.* 1999;94(7):1898–1901.

39. Asproudis I, Tsoumani AT, Katsanos KH, et al. Irritable bowel syndrome might be associated with dry eye disease. *Ann Gastroenterol.* 2016;29(4):487–491.

40. Amato A, Terzo S, Lentini L, Marchesa P, Mule F. TRPM8 channel activation reduces the spontaneous contractions in human distal colon. *Int J Mol Sci.* 2020;21(15).

41. Liu Y, Mikrani R, He Y, et al. TRPM8 channels: a review of distribution and clinical role. *Eur J Pharmacol.* 2020;882:173312.

42. Fall M, Baranowski AP, Elneil S, et al. EAU guidelines on chronic pelvic pain. *Eur Urol.* 2010;57(1):35–48.

43. Lee CK, Tsai CP, Liao TL, et al. Overactive bladder and bladder pain syndrome/interstitial cystitis in primary Sjogren's syndrome patients: a nationwide population-based study. *PLoS One.* 2019;14(11):e0225455.

44. Pereira ESR, Romao VC, Neves M, et al. Overactive bladder symptom bother and health-related quality of life in patients with systemic lupus erythematosus and primary Sjogren syndrome. *Lupus.* 2019;28(1):27–33.

45. van de Merwe JP. Interstitial cystitis and systemic autoimmune diseases. *Nat Clin Pract Urol.* 2007;4(9):484–491.

46. Ashina M. Migraine. *N Engl J Med.* 2020;383(19):1866–1876.

47. Farhangi M, Diel RJ, Buse DC, et al. Individuals with migraine have a different dry eye symptom profile than individuals without migraine. *Br J Ophthalmol.* 2020;104(2):260–264.

48. Ismail OM, Poole ZB, Bierly SL, et al. Association between dry eye disease and migraine headaches in a large population-based study. *JAMA Ophthalmol.* 2019;137(5):532–536.

49. Yang S, Kim W, Kim HS, Na KS, Epidemiologic Survey Committee of the Korean Ophthalmologic Society. Association between migraine and dry eye disease: a nationwide population-based study. *Curr Eye Res.* 2017;42(6):837–841.

50. Wang TJ, Wang IJ, Hu CC, Lin HC. Comorbidities of dry eye disease: a nationwide population-based study. *Acta Ophthalmol.* 2012;90(7):663–668.

51. Koktekir BE, Celik G, Karalezli A, Kal A. Dry eyes and migraines: is there really a correlation? *Cornea.* 2012;31(12):1414–1416.

52. Kinard KI, Smith AG, Singleton JR, et al. Chronic migraine is associated with reduced corneal nerve fiber density and symptoms of dry eye. *Headache.* 2015;55(4):543–549.

53. Wong M, Dodd MM, Masiowski P, Sharma V. Tear osmolarity and subjective dry eye symptoms in migraine sufferers. *Can J Ophthalmol.* 2017;52(5):513–518.

54. Patel S, Felix ER, Levitt RC, Sarantopoulos CD, Galor A. Dysfunctional coping mechanisms contribute to dry eye symptoms. *J Clin Med.* 2019;8(6).

55. Erie JC, McLaren JW, Patel SV. Confocal microscopy in ophthalmology. *Am J Ophthalmol.* 2009;148(5):639–646.

56. Shen F, Dong X, Zhou X, Yan L, Wan Q. Corneal subbasal nerve plexus changes in patients with episodic migraine: an in vivo confocal microscopy study. *J Pain Res.* 2019;12:1489–1495.

57. Aykut V, Elbay A, Esen F, Kocaman G, Savran Elibol E, Oguz H. Patterns of altered corneal sensation in patients with chronic migraine. *Eye Contact Lens.* 2018;44(Suppl 2):S400–S403.

58. Friedman DI. The eye and headache. *Continuum.* 2015;21(4 Headache):1109–1117.

59. Di Nicola V. Degenerative osteoarthritis a reversible chronic disease. *Regen Ther.* 2020;15:149–160.

60. Roh HC, Lee JK, Kim M, et al. Systemic comorbidities of dry eye syndrome: the Korean National Health and Nutrition Examination Survey V, 2010 to 2012. *Cornea.* 2016;35(2):187–192.

61. Suokas AK, Walsh DA, McWilliams DF, et al. Quantitative sensory testing in painful osteoarthritis: a systematic review and meta-analysis. *Osteoarthritis Cartilage.* 2012;20(10):1075–1085.

62. Bayer IS. Hyaluronic acid and controlled release: a review. *Molecules.* 2020;25(11).

63. Valesan LF, Da-Cas CD, Reus JC, et al. Prevalence of temporomandibular joint disorders: a systematic review and meta-analysis. *Clin Oral Invest.* 2021;25(2):441–453.

64. Yin Y, He S, Xu J, et al. The neuro-pathophysiology of temporomandibular disorders-related pain: a systematic review of structural and functional MRI studies. *J Headache Pain.* 2020;21(1):78.

65. Crincoli V, Di Comite M, Guerrieri M, et al. Orofacial manifestations and temporomandibular disorders of Sjogren syndrome: an observational study. *Int J Med Sci.* 2018;15(5):475–483.

66. List T, Stenstrom B, Lundstrom I, Dworkin SF. TMD in patients with primary Sjogren syndrome: a comparison with temporomandibular clinic cases and controls. *J Orofac Pain.* 1999;13(1):21–28.

67. Basantsova NY, Starshinova AA, Dori A, Zinchenko YS, Yablonskiy PK, Shoenfeld Y. Small-fiber neuropathy definition, diagnosis, and treatment. *Neurol Sci.* 2019;40(7):1343–1350.

68. Shoenfeld Y, Ryabkova VA, Scheibenbogen C, et al. Complex syndromes of chronic pain, fatigue and cognitive impairment linked to autoimmune dysautonomia and small fiber neuropathy. *Clin Immunol.* 2020;214:108384.

69. Hovaguimian A, Gibbons CH. Diagnosis and treatment of pain in small-fiber neuropathy. *Curr Pain Headache Rep.* 2011;15(3):193–200.

70. Bucher F, Schneider C, Blau T, et al. Small-fiber neuropathy is associated with corneal nerve and dendritic cell alterations: an in vivo confocal microscopy study. *Cornea.* 2015;34(9):1114–1119.

71. Bowsher D. Central pain: clinical and physiological characteristics. *J Neurol Neurosurg Psychiatry.* 1996;61(1):62–69.

72. Ebrahimiadib N, Yousefshahi F, Abdi P, Ghahari M, Modjtahedi BS. Ocular neuropathic pain: an overview focusing on ocular surface pains. *Clin Ophthalmol.* 2020;14:2843–2854.

73. Drummond PD, Finch PM. Photophobia in complex regional pain syndrome: visual discomfort is greater on the affected than unaffected side. *Pain.* 2021;162(4):1233–1240.

74. Graveling RA, Pilkington A, George JP, Butler MP, Tannahill SN. A review of multiple chemical sensitivity. *Occup Environ Med.* 1999;56(2):73–85.

75. Conejero I, Olie E, Calati R, Ducasse D, Courtet P. Psychological pain, depression, and suicide: recent evidences and future directions. *Curr Psychiatr Rep.* 2018;20(5):33.

76. Carroll BJ. Brain mechanisms in manic depression. *Clin Chem.* 1994;40(2):303–308.

77. Klein DF. Endogenomorphic depression. A conceptual and terminological revision. *Arch Gen Psychiatr.* 1974;31(4):447–454.

78. Gambassi G. Pain and depression: the egg and the chicken story revisited. *Arch Gerontol Geriatr.* 2009;49(Suppl 1):103–112.

79. Adler G, Gattaz WF. Pain perception threshold in major depression. *Biol Psychiatr.* 1993;34(10):687–689.

80. Klauenberg S, Maier C, Assion HJ, et al. Depression and changed pain perception: hints for a central disinhibition mechanism. *Pain.* 2008;140(2):332–343.

81. Thompson T, Correll CU, Gallop K, Vancampfort D, Stubbs B. Is pain perception altered in people with depression? A systematic review and meta-analysis of experimental pain research. *J Pain.* 2016;17(12):1257–1272.

82. Wan KH, Chen LJ, Young AL. Depression and anxiety in dry eye disease: a systematic review and meta-analysis. *Eye.* 2016;30(12):1558–1567.

83. Zheng Y, Wu X, Lin X, Lin H. The prevalence of depression and depressive symptoms among eye disease patients: a systematic review and meta-analysis. *Sci Rep.* 2017;7:46453.

84. Fernandez CA, Galor A, Arheart KL, et al. Dry eye syndrome, posttraumatic stress disorder, and depression in an older male veteran population. *Invest Ophthalmol Vis Sci.* 2013;54(5):3666–3672.

85. Sharif K, Watad A, Bragazzi NL, et al. On chronic fatigue syndrome and nosological categories. *Clin Rheumatol.* 2018;37(5):1161–1170.

86. Chen CS, Cheng HM, Chen HJ, et al. Dry eye syndrome and the subsequent risk of chronic fatigue syndrome-a prospective population-based study in Taiwan. *Oncotarget.* 2018;9(55):30694–30703.

87. Sivertsen B, Lallukka T, Petrie KJ, Steingrimsdottir OA, Stubhaug A, Nielsen CS. Sleep and pain sensitivity in adults. *Pain.* 2015;156(8):1433–1439.

88. Staffe AT, Bech MW, Clemmensen SLK, Nielsen HT, Larsen DB, Petersen KK. Total sleep deprivation increases

pain sensitivity, impairs conditioned pain modulation and facilitates temporal summation of pain in healthy participants. *PLoS One.* 2019;14(12):e0225849.

89. Galor A, Seiden BE, Park JJ, et al. The association of dry eye symptom severity and comorbid Insomnia in US veterans. *Eye Contact Lens.* 2018;44(Suppl 1):S118–S124.

90. Husak AJ, Bair MJ. Chronic pain and sleep disturbances: a pragmatic review of their relationships, comorbidities, and treatments. *Pain Med.* 2020;21(6):1142–1152.

91. Magno MS, Utheim TP, Snieder H, Hammond CJ, Vehof J. The relationship between dry eye and sleep quality. *Ocul Surf.* 2021;20:13–19.

92. Cruccu G, Di Stefano G, Truini A. Trigeminal neuralgia. *N Engl J Med.* 2020;383(8):754–762.

93. Mehra D, Cohen NK, Galor A. Ocular surface pain: a narrative review. *Ophthalmol Ther.* 2020;9(3):1–21.

94. Rosenthal P, Borsook D, Moulton EA. Oculofacial pain: corneal nerve damage leading to pain beyond the eye. *Invest Ophthalmol Vis Sci.* 2016;57(13):5285–5287.

95. Gomes JAP, Azar DT, Baudouin C, et al. TFOS DEWS II iatrogenic report. *Ocul Surf.* 2017;15(3):511–538.

96. Isik-Ulusoy S, Ulusoy MO. Influence of different antidepressants on ocular surface in patients with major depressive disorder. *J Clin Psychopharmacol.* 2021;41(1):49–52.

97. Wolpert LE, Snieder H, Jansonius NM, Utheim TP, Hammond CJ, Vehof J. Medication use and dry eye symptoms: A large, hypothesis-free, population-based study in the Netherlands. *Ocul Surf.* 2021;22:1–12.

CHAPTER 10

Glaucoma and Dry Eye Syndrome: Double Trouble

SARAH R. WELLIK, MD

INTRODUCTION

Glaucoma is an optic neuropathy that most commonly presents clinically with loss of peripheral visual field.[1] 60 million people are estimated to have glaucoma worldwide making it the second most common cause of blindness.[2,3] The burden of this visually devastating disease is only expected to increase amid the rapid growth of the aging population, with an estimated 112 million people affected by the year 2040.[4] Glaucomatous visual loss is incurable but its progression can be mitigated with proper intraocular pressure (IOP) control which is the only modifiable risk factor proven to prevent the progression of glaucoma.[5] Current first-line therapy for treatment of this devastating disorder consists of daily drop regimens and/or laser trabeculoplasty. Surgical intervention is traditionally reserved for more advanced or poorly controlled disease although this has changed somewhat in the last several years with the increasing popularity of minimally invasive glaucoma surgery or MIGS as it has been coined.[6]

Although dry eye syndrome (DES) is not generally a blinding disorder, it is incredibly common and has significant morbidity, particularly in the elderly population. Ocular surface disease has an estimated prevalence of approximately 19% in those over the age of 75 and often presents with symptoms of discomfort and blurred vision.[7] Glaucoma and dry eye are two of the most prevalent issues facing ophthalmology patients and they often present together to form a "perfect storm" of trouble. Both glaucoma and dry eye increase with age so it is expected that many patients carry both diagnoses and patients on topical glaucoma medications are known to be at greater risk for ocular surface symptoms.[8] This is at least in part due to the use of preservative agents such as benzalkonium chloride (BAK) in glaucoma drugs which have a toxic effect on the corneal epithelium.[9] Dry eye is associated with both a decrease in quality of life and a concurrent decrease in compliance with glaucoma topical therapy.[10]

It is helpful to approach glaucoma patients from the perspective of identifying those at high risk for treatment failure because of ocular surface symptoms and target our regimen to optimizing the ocular surface. Likewise, we need to approach our patients presenting for dry eye evaluations that have concurrent glaucoma by optimizing the ocular surface without compromising treatment to optimal IOP to prevent vision loss. We have a significant knowledge gap still to overcome in terms of understanding the interaction of these two disorders. For example, when do the risks of undertaking more invasive glaucoma treatments outweigh the risks of glaucoma progression due to poor compliance? The current thinking on treatment of glaucoma is to increase compliance with therapy as much as possible by making treatment regimens tolerable. We can do this by decreasing the number of drops per day, decreasing the amount of preservative in glaucoma drops, and increasing our use of targeted laser and surgical treatments for glaucoma to decrease the number of drops needed. In addition, we can use our current understanding of dry eye to target treatments that improve the ocular surface so that our glaucoma treatments are better tolerated.

DRY EYE IN THE GLAUCOMA PATIENT

Dry eye is a multifactorial disease of the ocular surface characterized by a loss of homeostasis of the tear film. We see this clinically as tear film instability, ocular surface inflammation, and through our patients' complaints of ocular symptoms. Glaucoma drops find many "victims" in the tear film including goblet cells, epithelial cells, limbal stem cells, and even the corneal

Dry Eye Disease. https://doi.org/10.1016/B978-0-323-82753-9.00009-6

nerves and the eyelids and orbit can be affected.[11] Glaucoma specialists frequently overlook or accept that their treatments aimed at preventing glaucomatous vision loss can cause issues with the ocular surface. Rather than becoming singularly focused on control of IOP above all costs, patient care demands that we try to understand the tear film better. The most recent DEWS II report classifies dry eye into the categories of aqueous deficient, evaporative, and mixed.[11] In the aqueous deficient type, the lipid portion of the tear film is decreased or lacking. This includes Sjögren's syndrome and lacrimal deficiency or obstructions. The evaporative type can be further divided into intrinsic or extrinsic subtypes. Allergies to glaucoma drops and damage caused by topical drop preservatives fall under the category of extrinsic evaporative dry eye. Meibomian gland deficiency is also a very common sequelae of topical glaucoma medication use. This can be seen clinically as inspissated Meibomian glands with capping and increased telangiectasias at the lid margins.

Preservatives in our medications are understood to be one of the culprits in DES.[12,13] Allergic, toxic, and inflammatory mechanisms, as well as type IV allergy can all be involved. In addition to preservative-free glaucoma medications, alternatives to BAK have been used in some commercially available drugs and have shown some decrease in toxicity. In addition, there is some evidence that the active ingredients of both beta clockers and prostaglandins can contribute to DES.[14] Even glaucoma surgery can likewise influence the ocular surface by contributing to limbal stem cell deficiency through limbal-based surgery, cautery, application of antimetabolites, and by bleb formation which changes the contour of the ocular surface making it more difficult for smooth distribution of tears.[15,16]

To make the dry eye diagnosis we have several tools at our disposal. A thorough history is very important. We can quantify patient symptoms more precisely by using questionnaires such as the Ocular Surface Disease Index, Standardized Patient Evaluation of Eye Dryness questionnaire, or Dry Eye Questionnaire 5.[10,17] Objectively, tear production is commonly measured with Schirmer's test or by measuring tear meniscus height. We also quantify tear film stability and ocular surface integrity with fluorescein, rose bengal, or lissamine green dyes. Several commercial devices are available to quickly assess for tear osmolarity and matrix metalloprotein (MMP-0) which have been correlated to ocular surface disease. While these qualitative measures of dry eye can be useful, it is known that the objective severity and the degree of patient complaints do not always correlate. Glaucoma specialists should have a high

interest in dry eye as the prevalence of DES in glaucoma population is 40%−60% as compared to the prevalence in the general population of 10%−30%.[18] It has been shown that the number of glaucoma medication and dosing frequency are directly correlated to the prevalence of dry eye and that glaucoma-related dry eye is directly correlated to quality of life.[8] In addition, studies have shown that surgical outcomes for glaucoma procedures may be adversely affected by preexisting ocular inflammation due to glaucoma medications.[19] Many advocate for glaucoma medication holidays and/or pretreatment with topical corticosteroids prior to glaucoma surgery.[20]

There are many options when it comes to treating dry eye. Lubrication is the mainstay of ocular surface treatment, but we need to consider advocating for preservative-free artificial tears and using lubricants of increased viscosity when possible. This is particularly important for our glaucoma patients who are often already getting a dose of preservative in their glaucoma medications. In addition, use of pro-tear film agents such as cyclosporine and lifitegrast, serum tears, and limited use of topical corticosteroids is helpful.[20,21] Heat and massage of Meibomian glands can be particularly useful in those with a blepharitis component.[22] More specialized treatments such as in office thermal pulsation treatments and intense light therapy can be considered as well.[23] There has been increased use of scleral contact lenses and PROSE lenses; however, these may limit uptake of glaucoma topical medications and also can cause issues in the setting of previous trabeculectomy or glaucoma drainage device surgery.[24] With all these treatments available, we need to approach the treatment of dry eye in the glaucoma patient in a systematic way that incorporates both appropriate use of dry eye−specific therapies and also tailoring glaucoma therapy to limit ocular surface toxicities.

HOW TO TREAT GLAUCOMA IN THE DRY EYE PATIENT

Now that we have discussed how to diagnose and treat dry eye in the glaucoma patient, we will shift our focus toward how to treat glaucoma in our patients with dry eye issues. When both dry eye and glaucoma exist in the same patient, our attention is usually focused on the more vision threatening disease of glaucoma. Dry eye on the other hand tends to be more symptomatic so should not be ignored. Start by finding common ground with your patient. Make a conscious effort to look for dry eye signs and listen to patient symptoms. Studies have shown that most patients tend to tolerate one to two glaucoma medications without too much difficulty. Those patients who have issues tolerating even one topical medication should be offered laser trabeculoplasty early on.

Laser Treatment

Selective laser trabeculoplasty has several advantages. It has good efficacy, eliminates side effects related to topical treatment if used as a first-line approach, and has no adherence issues. Selective laser trabeculoplasty was first introduced in 1995 and received US FDA approval in 2001. It functions by reducing IOP by increasing aqueous outflow through the trabecular meshwork. Recently, a randomized controlled trial (LiGHT),[25] comparing topical medication to selective laser trabeculoplasty as initial treatment, has reaffirmed findings of previous trials showing that laser is an efficacious first-line treatment for primary open angle glaucoma.[25–28] In the LiGHT trial the majority of patients were drop free at 36 months in this treatment naïve group with no sight-threatening complications.[25] While these studies have not shown specific improvement in health-related quality of life indicators, a decrease in eyelid erythema and conjunctival hyperemia was present in the laser group as opposed to the topical medication group.[27] Laser trabeculoplasty is also not feasible in all types and stages of glaucoma. Finally, although rare, there are potential side effects to laser including inflammation, immediate postlaser elevated IOP, uveitis, and keratitis after laser that in rare cases could necessitate additional intervention.[25–28]

Medical Therapy

While one might expect the evidence for selective laser trabeculoplasty to promote its use as primary treatment, many patients are still hesitant to have laser as first-line therapy. Another approach would be to try to eliminate or reduce the BAK load on glaucoma patients. We can do this through use of preservative-free medications, BAK-free medications (those with an alternative preservative), and use of fixed combination drugs that reduces the total number of drops per day. Also, we can reduce frequency of medication administration such as use of beta-blocker once per day instead of twice per day, or CAI or alpha agonist twice per day instead of three times per day. Preservative-free medications that are currently available in the United States include tafluprost, timolol, and dorzolamide-timolol fixed combination. It is also possible to obtain glaucoma medications from compounding pharmacies which can prepare a variety of fixed combination and preservative-free compounded medications. All these medication

alternatives, while appealing, are often more expensive and/or more difficult to obtain. In addition to topical medications for glaucoma, recently approved in the United States is a sustained release medication therapy which can be administered intraocularly for continuous release over a period of months.[29] This form of delivery could eliminate the need for topical therapy in some patients. It is not clear how well accepted this treatment may be to patients. In addition, the treatment is currently only approved for one-time dosing which means patients may have to restart topical therapy once the effect of the treatment wears off.

Surgical Therapy

When surgical treatment is deemed necessary, we have several things to consider in our treatment paradigm. With the advent of MIGS, the choices for surgical glaucoma treatment have increased drastically and their use in the glaucoma treatment is increasing.[30] As stated previously, the true definition of MIGS is a matter of debate but it is generally agreed that these are glaucoma surgeries that have a more favorable risk profile than traditional trabeculectomy or glaucoma drainage device surgery. They have lower rates of hypotony, lower risk of both early and late infections, and lower risk of vision loss.[31,32] In addition, they are generally conjunctival sparing and so preserve the naïve conjunctiva for possible trabeculectomy surgery in the future.

Trabecular bypass MIGS are only approved in the United States for use in combination with cataract surgery and are best suited for controlled mild to moderate glaucoma. Studies comparing cataract surgery with or without a trabecular bypass stent utilize both pressure lowering and decreased need to topical glaucoma medications as endpoints. In the pivotal trial for one type of trabecular bypass system, glaucoma patients had a 7 mmHg average decrease in unmedicated IOP from baseline at 2 years follow-up and control patients with cataract surgery alone had a 5.4 mmHg decrease. In addition, a greater number of patients treated with trabecular bypass were medication free with and IOP ≤18 at 2 years when compared to patients who had cataract surgery alone.[33] Other MIGS include goniotomy which can be done from an ab interno approach via different techniques including Trabectome (MicroSurgical Technology, Redmond WA), Kahook Dual Blade (New World Medical, Rancho Cucamonga CA), Omni (Sight Sciences, Menlo Park CA), or threading a catheter or suture through Schlemm's canal internally often termed Gonioscopy-Assisted Transluminal Trabeculotomy. All these techniques have been shown to reduce IOP in glaucoma patients done either in conjunction with cataract surgery or as stand-alone procedures.[34–37]

Some would include cyclodestructive procedures in the MIGS category as they do not disrupt the conjunctiva. These can be performed via endocyclophotocoagulation (ECP), micropulse (mCPC), and transscleral routes (tsCPC).[38,39] Gel stents are another category of MIGS that shunt fluid from the anterior chamber to the subconjunctival space. These are like traditional trabeculectomy in that they shunt fluid to the subconjunctival space. However, they have a lower rate of hypotony because of the flow restriction of the stent.[40] These surgeries do utilize the conjunctiva and often use antimetabolites with its inherent risks but the bleb created is usually small and in the superonasal quadrant, still preserving the superotemporal conjunctival for potential more traditional glaucoma surgery if needed in the future. All three of the latter procedures discussed here, goniotomy, cyclodestruction, and gel stents, can be done with or without concurrent cataract surgery. There are also data to support use of these three procedures in more uncontrolled and/or advanced glaucomas as stand-alone procedures without cataract surgery.[34–40]

In the treatment spectrum of glaucoma surgery surrounding the MIGS space, there continues to be utility in cataract surgery alone as an IOP lowering technique. Cataract surgery alone as an IOP lowering procedure is supported by multiple studies showing a sustained decrease in IOP after cataract without any adjunct glaucoma procedure.[41–43] The amount and duration of IOP reduction varies greatly by type of glaucoma, preoperative IOP, and length of time after surgery. In the pivotal trial of ab interno trabecular microbypass system, the control group of cataract surgery alone had a >20% reduction in preoperative medication washout IOP in 62% of patients (compared to 76% of patients in the group receiving the trabecular bypass) sustained to 24 months.[33] There are multiple theories for why this may be the case. The cataract in many cases may have a phacomorphic component of angle closure. Secondly cataract surgery may partially clear the trabecular meshwork of microdebris and increase flow. It is important to remember that patients with uncontrolled, advanced, and/or medication resistant glaucoma are unlikely to get a significant pressure reduction from cataract surgery alone or cataract surgery with trabecular stent. These patients likely have a large degree of blockage or nonfunctionality of the trabecular meshwork and downstream drainage pathways.

When considering cataract surgery in severe dry patients, remember that those with dry eye may be more likely to have neuropathic pain with cataract surgery and may be more likely to have keratopathy specifically related to topical nonsteroidal antiinflammatory (NSAID) use.[44] We can preempt these issues by aggressively treating the dry eye prior to surgery with increased use of preservative-free lubricants. Starting treatment with steroidal antiinflammatories 1–2 weeks prior to surgery can be useful if we do not cause a steroid response in the IOP. To avoid keratopathy, it may be necessary to either use topical NSAIDs that are dosed fewer times per day and/or follow patients more frequently in the postoperative period to catch potential issues and intervene by either stopping the NSAID and/or using lubricant gel or ointments.

On the other end of the treatment spectrum, we have traditional glaucoma procedures including trabeculectomy and glaucoma drainage device surgery. These techniques have an excellent probability of success in terms of lowering IOP and decreasing dependence on topical glaucoma drops but can have significant postoperative complications such as hypotony, early- and late-onset infections, diplopia, erosions, and corneal decompensation.[45] As such, it should not be discounted, particularly in our glaucoma patients with severe dry eye. Trabeculectomy with use of antifibrotic agent remains one of the most effective procedures with a high chance of the patient needing few or no glaucoma drops postoperatively. Those dry eye patients who require two or more drops and have more advanced damage (and who may have already had more conservative laser trabeculoplasty) are likely to be on fewer glaucoma medications for the first 2 years of follow-up after trabeculectomy but do average one or more medications after 3 years. Glaucoma drainage device surgery patients consistently average of 1.3–1.4 glaucoma drops at all time points through 5 years after surgery.[46]

CONCLUSION

In summary, glaucoma and dry eye often coexist. Treatment of both is important as untreated dry eye can adversely impact adherence to glaucoma treatment. We must individualize treatment based on severity of both the glaucoma and severity of the dry eye understanding that the two disorders are intricately linked.

ACKNOWLEDGMENTS

I would like to thank Sunita Radhakrishnan, Robert Honkanen, and Sarah Weissbart for their valuable input on this topic. Thank you to Samuel Gurevich for helping in editing and being an endless source of support.

REFERENCES

1. Varma R, Lee PP, Goldberg I, Kotak S. An assessment of the health and economic burdens of glaucoma. *Am J Ophthalmol.* 2011;152:515–522.
2. Kingman S. Glaucoma is second leading cause of blindness globally. *Bull World Health Organ.* 2004;82(11):887–888.
3. Quigley HA, Broman AT. The number of people with glaucoma worldwide in 2010 and 2020. *Br J Ophthalmol.* 2006;90(3):262–267.
4. Tham YC, Li X, Wong TY, Quigley HA, Aung T, Cheng CY. Global prevalence of glaucoma and projections of glaucoma burden through 2040: a systematic review and meta-analysis. *Ophthalmology.* 2014;121:2081–2090.
5. Heijl A, Leske MC, Bengtsson B, et al. Reduction of intraocular pressure and glaucoma progression: results from the Early Manifest Glaucoma Trial. *Arch Ophthalmol.* 2002;120(10):1268–1279.
6. Manasses DT, Au L. The new era of glaucoma micro-stent surgery. *Ophthalmol Ther.* 2016;5(2):135–146.
7. Farrand KF, Fridman M, Stillman IÖ, Schaumberg DA. Prevalence of diagnosed dry eye disease in the United States among adults aged 18 years and older. *Am J Ophthalmol.* 2017;182:90–98.
8. Camp A, Wellik SR, Tzu JH, et al. Dry eye specific quality of life in veterans using glaucoma drops. *Contact Lens Anterior Eye.* 2015;38:220–225.
9. Anwar Z, Wellik SR, Galor A. Glaucoma therapy and ocular surface disease: current literature and recommendations. *Curr Opin Ophthalmol.* 2013;24(2):136–143.
10. Pouyeh B, Viteri E, Feuer W, et al. Impact of ocular surface symptoms on quality of life in a United States veterans affairs population. *Am J Ophthalmol.* 2012;153:1061–1066.
11. Willcox MDP, Argüeso P, Georgiev GA, et al. TFOS DEWS II tear film report. *Ocul Surf.* 2017;15(3):366–403.
12. Baudouin C, Labbé A, Liang H, Pauly A, Brignole-Baudouin F. Preservatives in eyedrops: the good, the bad and the ugly. *Prog Retin Eye Res.* 2010;29(4):312–334.
13. Tressler CS, Beatty R, Lemp MA. Preservative use in topical glaucoma medications. *Ocul Surf.* 2011;9(3):140–158.
14. Fechtner RD, Godfrey DG, Budenz D, Stewart JA, Stewart WC, Jasek MC. Prevalence of ocular surface complaints in patients with glaucoma using topical intraocular pressure-lowering medications. *Cornea.* 2010;29:618–621.
15. Flach AJ. Does medical treatment influence the success of trabeculectomy? *Trans Am Ophthalmol Soc.* 2004;102:219–223. discussion 223-4.
16. Li LX, Liu W, Ji J. The impact of trabeculectomy on ocular surface. *Zhonghua Yan Ke Za Zhi.* 2013;49(2):185–188.
17. Rossi GC, Tinelli C, Pasinetti GM, Milano G, Bianchi PE. Dry eye syndrome-related quality of life in glaucoma patients. *Eur J Ophthalmol.* 2009;19(4):572–579.
18. Garcia-Feijoo J, Sampaolesi JR. A multicenter evaluation of ocular surface disease prevalence in patients with glaucoma. *Clin Ophthalmol.* 2012;6:441–446.
19. Baudouin C. Mechanisms of failure in glaucoma filtering surgery: a consequence of antiglaucomatous drugs? *Int J Clin Pharmacol Res.* 1996;16(1):29–41.
20. Kallab M, Szegedi S, Hommer N, et al. Topical low dose preservative-free hydrocortisone reduces signs and symptoms in patients with chronic dry eye: a randomized clinical trial. *Adv Ther.* 2020;37(1):329–341.
21. Campos E, Versura P, Buzzi M, et al. Blood derived treatment from two allogeneic sources for severe dry eye associated to keratopathy: a multicentre randomised cross over clinical trial. *Br J Ophthalmol.* 2020;104(8):1142–1147.
22. Goto E, Monden Y, Takano Y, et al. Treatment of non-inflamed obstructive meibomian gland dysfunction by an infrared warm compression device. *Br J Ophthalmol.* 2002;86(12):1403–1407.
23. Cote S, Zhang AC, Ahmadzai V, et al. Intense pulsed light (IPL) therapy for the treatment of meibomian gland dysfunction. *Cochrane Database Syst Rev.* 2020;3(3).
24. Xu M, Randleman JB, Chiu GB. Long-Term descemetocele management with prosthetic replacement of the ocular surface ecosystem (PROSE) treatment. *Eye Contact Lens.* 2020;46(2):e7–e10.
25. Gazzard G, Konstantakopoulou E, Garway-Heath D, et al. Selective laser trabeculoplasty versus eye drops for first-line treatment of ocular hypertension and glaucoma (LiGHT): a multicentre randomised controlled trial. *Lancet.* 2019;393(10180):1505–1516.
26. Garg A, Vickerstaff V, Nathwani N, et al. Primary selective laser trabeculoplasty for open-angle glaucoma and ocular hypertension: clinical outcomes, predictors of success, and safety from the laser in glaucoma and ocular hypertension trial. *Ophthalmology.* 2019;126(9):1238–1248.
27. Ang GS, Fenwick EK, Constantinou M, et al. Selective laser trabeculoplasty versus topical medication as initial glaucoma treatment: the glaucoma initial treatment study randomised clinical trial. *Br J Ophthalmol.* 2020;104(6):813–821.
28. Katz LJ, Steinmann WC, Kabir A, et al. Selective laser trabeculoplasty versus medical therapy as initial treatment of glaucoma: a prospective, randomized trial. *J Glaucoma.* 2012;21(7):460–468.
29. Lee SS, Dibas M, Almazan A, Robinson MR. Dose-response of intracameral bimatoprost sustained-release implant and topical bimatoprost in lowering intraocular pressure. *J Ocul Pharmacol Therapeut.* 2019;35(3):138–144.
30. Olivier MMG, Smith O, Croteau-Chonka CC, et al. Demographic and clinical characteristics associated with minimally invasive glaucoma surgery use: an IRIS® registry retrospective cohort analysis. *Ophthalmology.* 2021;21:S0161–S6420, 00122–00126.
31. Shalaby WS, Bechay J, Myers JS, et al. Reoperation for complications within 90 Days of minimally invasive glaucoma surgery. *J Cataract Refract Surg.* 2021;47(7):886–891.
32. Yook E, Vinod K, Panarelli JF. Complications of micro-invasive glaucoma surgery. *Curr Opin Ophthalmol.* 2018;29(2):147–154.
33. Samuelson TW, Sarkisian Jr SR, Lubeck DM, et al. Prospective, randomized, controlled pivotal trial of an ab interno implanted trabecular micro-bypass in primary open-angle glaucoma and cataract: two-year results. *Ophthalmology.* 2019;126(6):811–821.

34. Francis BA, Akil H, Bert BB. Ab interno Schlemm's canal surgery. *Dev Ophthalmol.* 2017;59:127—146.

35. Ting JLM, Rudnisky CJ, Damji KF. Prospective randomized controlled trial of phaco-trabectome versus phaco-trabeculectomy in patients with open angle glaucoma. *Can J Ophthalmol.* 2018;53(6):588—594.

36. Wakil SM, Birnbaum F, Vu DM, McBurney-Lin S, ElMallah MK, Tseng H. Efficacy and safety of a single-use dual blade goniotomy: 18-month results. *J Cataract Refract Surg.* 2020;46(10):1408—1415.

37. Loayza-Gamboa W, Martel-Ramirez V, Inga-Condezo V, Valderrama-Albino V, Alvarado-Villacorta R, Valera-Cornejo D. Outcomes of combined prolene gonioscopy assisted transluminal trabeculotomy with phacoemulsification in open-angle glaucoma. *Clin Ophthalmol.* 2020;14:3009—3016.

38. Sheheitli H, Persad PJ, Feuer WJ, Sayed MS, Lee RK. Treatment outcomes of primary transscleral cyclophoto coagulation. *Ophthalmol Glaucoma.* 2021;21:S2589—S4196, 00002—8.

39. Michelessi M, Bicket AK, Lindsley K. Cyclodestructive procedures for non-refractory glaucoma. *Cochrane Database Syst Rev.* 2018;4(4):CD009313.

40. Do A, McGlumphy E, Shukla A, et al. Comparison of clinical outcomes with open versus closed conjunctiva implantation of the XEN45 gel stent. *Ophthalmol Glaucoma.* 2020;20:S2589—S4196, 30321—30325.

41. Young CEC, Seibold LK, Kahook MY. Cataract surgery and intraocular pressure in glaucoma. *Curr Opin Ophthalmol.* 2020;31(1):15—22.

42. Poley BJ, Lindstrom RL, Samuelson TW. Long-term effects of phacoemulsification with intraocular lens implantation in normotensive and ocular hypertensive eyes. *J Cataract Refract Surg.* 2008;34(5):735—742.

43. Poley BJ, Lindstrom RL, Samuelson TW, Schulze Jr R. Intraocular pressure reduction after phacoemulsification with intraocular lens implantation in glaucomatous and nonglaucomatous eyes: evaluation of a causal relationship between the natural lens and open-angle glaucoma. *J Cataract Refract Surg.* 2009;35(11):1946—1955.

44. Cabourne E, Lau N, Flanagan D, Nott J, Bloom J, Angunawela R. Severe corneal melting after cataract surgery in patients prescribed topical postoperative NSAIDs and dexamethasone/neomycin combination therapy. *J Cataract Refract Surg.* 2020;46(1):138—142.

45. Gedde SJ, Herndon LW, Brandt JD, et al. Postoperative complications in the Tube versus Trabeculectomy (TVT) study during five years of follow-up. *Am J Ophthalmol.* 2012;153(5):804—814.e1.

46. Gedde SJ, Schiffman JC, Feuer WJ, et al. Treatment outcomes in the Tube versus Trabeculectomy (TVT) study after five years of follow-up. *Am J Ophthalmol.* 2012;153(5):789—803.e2.

CHAPTER 11

Treatment of Dry Eye Disease in the United States

JENNIFER B. NADELMANN, MD • VATINEE Y. BUNYA, MD, MSCE • ILARIA MACCHI, MD • MINA MASSARO-GIORDANO, MD

INTRODUCTION

The treatment of patients with dry eye disease is based upon the severity of the patient's disease and symptoms. In addition, since there are several factors that can contribute to dry eye symptoms, it is critical to address the underlying cause.[1] Dry eye disease impacts patients' vision, quality of life, productivity, and activities of daily living and also has economic costs including the cost of medical appointments, treatments, and procedures.[2,3] The goals of treating dry eye disease are to improve patients' symptoms and quality of life, decrease inflammation, and prevent ocular surface damage. There have been several advances in treatment modalities in recent years that aim to decrease the effects of dry eye disease on patients' lives.

A stepwise approach is recommended to determine the most appropriate treatment for patients based upon the severity of their dry eye disease.[4] It is important for clinicians to consider each individual patient's symptoms to create a comprehensive treatment plan. Specifically, clinicians should evaluate meibomian gland physiology, tear film lipid quality, meibomian gland status, and tear production, loss, and runoff. It is also essential to ensure communication with other medical specialists to address multifactorial causes of dry eye disease. In 2017, the DEWS II Management and Therapy report put forth an algorithm for staged management recommendations for dry eye disease.[4] (Table 11.1).

NONPHARMACOLOGIC TREATMENTS

Patient Education

In patients with dry eye disease, removing exacerbating factors should be advised (e.g., antihistamine, diuretic use, cigarette smoking, air drafts, ceiling fans, and low humidity environments). Patients can employ environmental interventions including using indoor humidifiers, air filters, or cleaners to ameliorate dry eye symptoms by increasing air moisture and reducing particulates in the air.[5] Other conservative measures include but are not limited to the use of dry eye goggles, wrap-around sunglasses, and also limiting screen time.

Dietary Supplementation

Nutritional supplements that have antiinflammatory properties including essential fatty acids such as omega-3, linoleic acid (LA) and gamma-linoleic acids (GLAs) can be used in the management of ocular surface disease.[4] Omega 3 fatty acids from patients' diet or in the form of supplements have antiinflammatory properties that may aid in treating DED. Omega 3 fatty acids are present in fish and green leafy vegetables.[6] GLA and its precursor LA are used in chronic inflammatory disorders such as rheumatoid arthritis.[7]

Several studies have shown a potential benefit for the use of omega-3 fatty acids for the treatment of dry eye. Miljanović et al. studied the association between dietary intake of n − 3 and n − 6 fatty acids and dry eye syndrome in the Women's Health Study among 1546 subjects who reported a diagnosis of DES. Their study showed that patients who had higher dietary intake of n-3 fatty acids had a decreased incidence of dry eye syndrome.[8] In another study, a randomized trial of 28.5 mg LA plus 15 mg GLA twice daily in addition to substitute tears showed a significant decrease in DES symptoms, lissamine green staining, and ocular surface inflammation in patients with aqueous deficient

TABLE 11.1
Staged Management and Treatment Recommendations for Dry Eye Disease.[a–c]

Step 1:
- Education regarding the condition, its management, treatment, and prognosis
- Modification of local environment
- Education regarding potential dietary modifications (including oral essential fatty acid supplementation)
- Identification and potential modification/elimination of offending systemic and topical medications
- Ocular lubricants of various types (if MGD is present, then consider lipid-containing supplements)
- Lid hygiene and warm compresses of various types

Step 2:
If above options are inadequate consider
- Nonpreserved ocular lubricants to minimize preservative-induced toxicity
- Tea tree oil treatment for Demodex (if present)
- Tear conservation
  - Punctal occlusion
  - Moisture chamber spectacles/goggles
- Overnight treatments (such as ointment or moisture chamber devices)
- In-office, physical heating and expression of the meibomian glands (including device-assisted therapies, such as LipiFlow)
- In-office intense pulsed light therapy for MGD
- Prescription drugs to manage DED[d]
  - Topical antibiotic or antibiotic/steroid combination applied to the lid margins for anterior blepharitis (if present)
  - Topical corticosteroid (limited-duration)
  - Topical secretagogues
  - Topical nonglucocorticoid immunomodulatory drugs (such as cyclosporine)
  - Topical LFA-1 antagonist drugs (such as lifitegrast)
  - Oral macrolide or tetracycline antibiotics

Step 3:
If above options are inadequate consider
- Oral secretagogues
- Autologous/allogeneic serum eye drops
- Therapeutic contact lens options
  - Soft bandage lenses
  - Rigid scleral lenses

Step 4:
If above options are inadequate consider
- Topical corticosteroid for longer duration
- Amniotic membrane grafts
- Surgical punctal occlusion
- Other surgical approaches (e.g., tarsorrhaphy, salivary gland transplantation)

DED, dry eye disease; *MGD*, meibomian gland dysfunction.

[a] Potential variations within the disease spectrum are acknowledged to exist between patients and the management options listed above are not intended to be exclusive. The severity and etiology of the DED state will dictate the range and number of management options selected from one or more steps.

[b] One or more options concurrently within each category can be considered within that step of the dry eye disease state. Options within a category are not ranked according to importance and may be equally valid.

[c] It should be noted that the evidence available to support the various management options differs and will inevitably be lower for newer management options. Thus, each treatment option should be considered in accordance with the level of evidence available at the time management is instigated.

[d] The use of prescription drugs needs to be considered in the context of the individual patient presentation, and the relative level of evidence supporting their use for that specific indication, as this group of agents differs widely in mechanism of action.

Table and captions reproduced with permission from Jones L, Downie LE, Korb D, Benitez-del-Castillo JM, Dana R, Deng SX et al. TFOS DEWS II management and therapy report. *Ocular Surf*. 2017;15(3):575–628.

keratoconjunctivitis sicca.[7] A prospective, double-blind randomized trial of 264 eyes of patients with dry eye who received one capsule (500 mg) twice daily of 325 mg EPA and 175 mg DHA for 3 months compared to placebo showed significant improvement in the omega-3 group in symptoms compared to placebo. In addition, the omega-3 group also showed a significant change in Schirmer's test and TBUT values.[9] A multicenter, prospective, interventional, double-masked study randomized 105 subjects to receive a total of 1680 mg of eicosapentaenoic acid/560 mg of docosahexaenoic acid (omega-3 group) or a control of 3136 mg of LA daily for 12 weeks. The study showed that consumption of reesterified omega-3 fatty acids showed significant reduction in tear osmolarity, omega-3 index levels, TBUT, MMP-9, and OSDI symptom scores compared to controls.[10]

In contrast, other studies have not shown a benefit for omega-3 fatty acids in treating dry eye. The Dry Eye Assessment and Management trial, a large, multicenter, double-blind clinical trial sponsored by the National Eye Institute, compared the use of a daily oral dose of 3000 mg of fish-derived n-3 eicosapentaenoic and docosahexaenoic acids in 349 subjects to olive oil placebo in 186 subjects with moderate-to-severe dry eye disease. The study did not show significantly better outcomes after 12 months for the treatment group compared to placebo.[11]

There is also evidence that vitamin D deficiency may be a risk factor for dry eye disease as it is associated with worse subjective symptoms, tear film dysfunction, and decreased tear production. Future studies are indicated to determine if vitamin D has a protective effect on the development of dry eye diseases and if supplementation could be beneficial.[12–14]

Eyelid Hygiene
Warm compresses
The most common technique to relieve meibomian gland obstruction in evaporative dry eye is to apply heat to the eyelids and to physically manipulate the eyelids to express the contents of the meibomian glands. In patients with meibomian gland dysfunction (MGD), the lipid composition of the meibum, which is largely oil based, is altered causing an increased melting point with increased viscosity at lid temperature. Applying heat to the eyelids is thought to liquefy the lipids so they can be massaged out of the meibomian glands and secreted into the tear film with gentle pressure from a cotton swab or fingertip.[15,16] Warm compresses can be performed using a towel or cloth dipped in warm water or commercially available eyelid masks that are

microwaveable.[16] Studies have shown that the application of warm compresses increases the tear film lipid layer thickness within 5 min.[16,17]

Cleaning eyelids
Daily home treatments also include cleaning the eyelashes with tear-free baby shampoo such as Johnson's No More Tears (Johnson & Johnson, New Brunswick, NJ, USA) or using premedication scrubs or foams. Cleansers can be used to loosen oils and debris from the eyelids including premedicated wipes, such as OCuSOFT Lid Scrubs (OcuSOFT, Rosenberg, TX, USA) or Systane lid wipes (Alcon, Fort Worth, TX, USA). Foams can also be applied to the eyelid including TheraTears SteriLid (Akorn Pharmaceuticals, Lake Forest, IL, USA) or OCuSOFT foaming cleansers.[18]

In patients with chronic blepharitis, approximately 29%–74% of cases are thought to be attributed to *Demodex* mites infestation of the eyelashes.[18,19] Tea tree oil has been found to be efficacious against *Demodex*. The product Cliradex and Cliradex Complete (Biotissue, Doral, FL, USA) utilizes terpinen-4-ol, which is considered the most effective ingredient against *Demodex*, and is used one to two times daily for symptoms, for a treatment course of at least 2 months.[18,19]

Lubrication
Over-the-counter artificial tears are often the first line of pharmacotherapy for treating dry eye disease.[4,20] Artificial tears are used to replace and supplement patients' natural tears to improve ocular hydration.[4] As a result, treatment with artificial tears aims to reduce tear osmolarity and decrease evaporation to increase ocular lubrication.[5,21] Artificial tears alleviate symptoms of dry eye disease by improving lubrication between the eyelids and ocular surface, stabilizing the tear film, protecting corneal and conjunctival cells, decreasing evaporative loss, and improving wound healing.[6]

A systematic review of 43 randomized control trials showed that artificial tears are a safe measure to treat dry eye symptoms.[21] Treatment with artificial tears is considered to be effective in relieving symptoms and there has not been a significant difference in efficacy in comparing the different formulations.[21,22]

Dry eye products include various chemical formulations with a range of osmolarity, viscosity, and pH.[4] Artificial tears also vary in their electrolyte composition, the presence of preservatives and solutes.[6] The major component of artificial tears is an aqueous base.

While products with increased viscosity have a longer retention time, they can lead to blurred vision and increase debris.[23] Therefore, lower viscosity drops have better tolerability during the daytime, while higher viscosity formulations are often used at nighttime. Viscous enhancing agents help relieve symptoms in DED by enhancing tear retention, increasing goblet cell density, protecting the surface of the eye, increasing tear film thickness, and helping to restore corneal density.[4,24] Viscosity enhancing agents include carbomer 940 (polyacrylic acid), carboxymethyl cellulose (CMC), dextran, hyaluronic acid (HA), HP-guar, hydroxypropyl methylcellulose (HPMC), polyvinyl alcohol (PVA), polyvinylpyrrolidone (PVP), and polyethylene glycol.[4]

Some artificial tears products include preservatives including benzalkonium chloride (BAK), ethylenediaminetetraacetic acid (EDTA), and purite, which can be associated with toxicity and an allergic response. Preservatives are intended to prevent microbial growth. Artificial tears that contain preservatives should be used no more than 4–6 times daily.[23,25] Preservative-free drops are advised in patients that require frequent instillation of eye drops or who have preexisting corneal conditions.[4] However, preservative-free preparations, which come in unit dose containers, are often more expensive and may be difficult to use for some patients.[23] As such, the choice of an agent should be patient specific.

TheraTears and Bion Tears have an electrolyte profile similar to that of the natural tear film.[4]

Ointments and gels have the advantage of providing lubrication to the ocular surface for a longer duration of time, thereby, extending relief for the patient; however, they blur vision and are usually used before bedtime.[23]

Lacrisert (Bausch & Lomb, Rochester, NY, USA) is a water soluble, preservative-free, hydroxypropyl cellulose ophthalmic insert, used in patients with moderate-to-severe DED, that is placed in the inferior cul-de-sac beneath the base of the tarsus and dissolves over 12 h to improve lubrication of the eye (Fig. 11.1). A multicenter center study showed that the inserts significantly improved clinical signs (e.g., keratitis, conjunctival staining, and tear volume) and reduced symptoms in patients with dry eye syndrome.[26]

The lipid layer of the tear film controls the evaporation rate of tears. In patients with MGD, they have a deficiency of lipid in the tear film composition. Lipid-containing lubricants include eye drops, and lipid-containing sprays (formulations that contain liposomes).[27] Lipid-containing eye drops, which are formulated as emulsions, are being used at an increased frequency as they are thought to prevent tear evaporation.[4] Lee et al. conducted a systematic review of lipid-containing lubricants and concluded that most studies showed efficacy in improving signs of dry

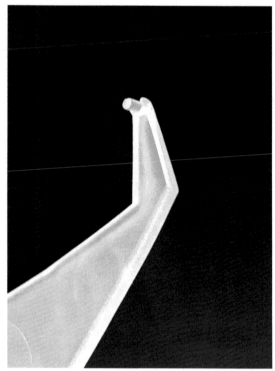

FIG. 11.1 Lacrisert (Bausch & Lomb, Rochester, NY, USA) ophthalmic insert and applicator.

eye.[27] Cationic oil-in-water (o/w) nanoemulsions are made of positively charged oil nanodroplets dispersed in water.[4] Armane et al. showed Cationorm was well tolerated in patients with mild to moderate dry eye.[28]

Punctal Plugs

The insertion of punctal plugs into the tear ducts (puncta) of the upper or lower eyelids aims to decrease the drainage of tears from the ocular surface to increase lubrication of the ocular surface.[29–31] Punctal plugs, which include absorbable and nonabsorbable devices, can be placed at the level of the punctual opening or deeper within the canaliculus (either the vertical or horizontal canaliculus).[4,32] There is a large collection of punctal and canalicular plugs available in the market that are made of a range of materials including collagen, silicone, hydrogel, polydioxanone, and acrylic.[32] Punctal occlusion can be utilized when combined with other dry eye treatments in patients refractory to topical lubricants alone.[4,33]

Collagen-based plugs absorb in 1 to 16 weeks. Atelocollagen solution can be injected through the punctum, where it turns into a white-colored gel at body temperature. Succinylated collagen plugs and hypromellose 2% can also be used.[4]

Punctal plugs have a range of designs but usually have a head on the top to enable removal of the plug and then a thin neck and cone-shaped base.[32] Nonabsorbable plugs are often silicone-based which include the Freeman style plug (dumb-bell shaped punctal plug). Silicone plugs, which are available in a range of sizes, are often prescribed after a patient has reported symptomatic benefit from a collagen-based plug.[30,33] Punctal plugs can also be made of Teflon, hydroxyethyl methacrylate (HEMA), and polymethylmethacrylate (PMMA).[32]

Canalicular plugs are temporary and usually rod shaped.[32] The cylindrical SmartPlug is an intracanalicular plug made from a thermolabile polymer that changes its shape when inserted into the punctum. The FORM FIT (Oasis Medical, Glendora, CA, USA) vertical intracanalicular plug is made from an injectable hydrogel that expands after contacting the tear film into the shape of the canaliculus. The plug is inserted using a preloaded inserter.[4,32] Cyanoacrylate adhesives can also be used for temporary punctal occlusion.[4] Thermosensitive acrylic canalicular plugs (Medennium Smart Plug) can also be used. Horizontal canalicular plugs exist in temporary or permanent forms. The Herrick canalicular plug is made of silicone and is described as having a "golf tee" shape.[32]

Complications of punctal plugs include plug extrusion, infection (e.g., canaliculitis and dacryocystitis), canalicular migration of the plug, pyogenic granuloma, punctal and canalicular stenosis, biofilm formation, allergic reaction, and punctual enlargements. Infections are more common with intracanalicular options.[4,32,33] Canalicular plugs have a higher risk of migration.[32,33]

A systematic review of randomized controlled trials of collagen and silicone punctal plugs in patients with dry eye syndrome or aqueous tear deficiency was inconclusive in determining whether punctal plugs improve dry eye symptoms.[30]

PRESCRIPTION DRUGS
Antiinflammatories
Cyclosporine
Cyclosporine (Restasis) helps to decrease inflammation in DED.[6] The US Food and Drug Administration (FDA) approved the 0.05% solution of cyclosporine A (CsA) to increase tear production in patients with dry eye disease.[29,34] Cyclosporine is an anti-inflammatory agent that acts by entering T cells and binding to cyclophilins, which inhibits calcineurin, a calcium-

dependent phosphatase, inhibiting nuclear factor of activated T cells, cytoplasmic 1 (NFATc1) dephosphorylation as shown in Fig. 11.2.[35] As a result, this reduces IL-2 levels and suppresses T-cell activation.[35,36] Cyclosporine has been shown to decrease IL-6 levels, reduce activated T lymphocytes, decrease the expression of inflammatory and apoptotic markers, and increase goblet cell numbers in the conjunctiva of patients with dry eye disease. Therefore, cyclosporine is thought to help to restore the homeostasis of the conjunctival epithelium.[37–40]

In the United States, CsA 0.05% (Restasis and Restasis multidose, Allergan, Irvine CA), a homogenous emulsion of glycerin (2.2%), castor oil (1.25%), polysorbate 80 (1.00%), carbomer copolymer type A (0.05%), and purified water (up to 100%), is approved to increase tear production in patients with ocular inflammation.[34,35] Results from clinical trials show that noticeable improvement usually takes 3 months.[34]

Chen et al. compared the efficacy and safety profile of topical cyclosporine 0.05% or vehicle twice daily for 8 weeks in a multicenter, randomized, double-blind, vehicle-controlled, parallel-group study of 223 dry eye patients. The study showed significant improvement in ocular dryness at week 8 foreign body sensation at weeks 4 and 8, corneal staining at weeks 4 and 8, and in the Schirmer test at week 4 compared to the vehicle. Overall, the study showed that cyclosporine 0.05% was effective and safe treatment for patients with moderate-to-severe dry eye.[41] Additional studies have shown cyclosporine's efficacy in patients with DED and Sjögren's syndrome (SS).[42]

Stevenson et al. reported on multicenter, double-masked, parallel-group, dose-response controlled trial of cyclosporine A (0.05%, 0.1%, 0.2%, and 0.04%) in 129 patients compared to the 33 patients who received the vehicle twice daily for 12 weeks. The study showed that CsA emulsions were all safe and well-tolerated and produced improvements in ocular signs and symptoms in patients with moderate-to-severe dry eye disease.[43]

Sall et al. compared the efficacy and safety of CsA 0.05% and 0.1% compared to vehicle in patients with moderate-to-severe dry eye disease for 6 months in two multicenter, randomized clinical trials with a total of 877 patients. The study reported that compared to vehicle, both CsA formulations produced significantly greater improvements in corneal staining and categorized Schirmer values while CsA 0.05% also had a significant improvement in three subjective measures.[44]

Baiza-Durán reported a multicenter, randomized, double-masked, vehicle controlled trial of CsA 0.1%, CsA 0.05%, or vehicle only including 183 patients

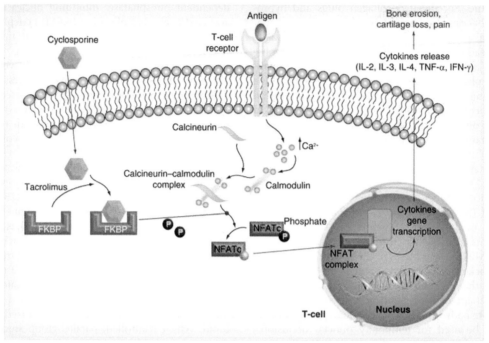

FIG. 11.2 **Cyclosporine acts by forming a complex with intracellular binding proteins after entering T cells**. This complex inhibits calcinuerin phosphatase, halting the activation of the transcription factor NFATc, thus preventing the production of cytokines including IL-2 and IFN-γ. (Figure and Caption courtesy of Ames P, Galor A. Cyclosporine ophthalmic emulsions for the treatment of dry eye: a review of the clinical evidence. *Clin Invest*. 2015;5(3):267–285.)

followed for 98 days and showed that both formulations of cyclosporine A decreased complaints and improved signs in patients with moderate-to-severe dry eye disease, with CsA 0.1% outperforming the other groups.[45]

Cequa (cyclosporine ophthalmic solution 0.09% (Sun Pharmaceuticals, Cranbury, NJ)) was approved by the US FDA to increase tear production in patients with dry eye disease. Cequa, also known as OTX-101, is a nanomicellar solution to enhance bioavailability of the drug to ocular tissues while decreasing systemic exposure.[46] Goldberg et al. reported the results of a randomized, multicenter, vehicle-controlled, double-masked, phase 3 clinical trial of OTX-101 0.09% including 744 patients that showed significant increase of 10 mm of more in Schirmer test score at day 84 and significant improvements in corneal and conjunctival staining compared to the vehicle.[47] Pooled analysis of randomized vehicle-controlled studies showed that OTX-101 twice daily led to significant improvements versus vehicle in corneal and conjunctival staining beginning at 4 weeks that were also seen up to 12 weeks and that the medication was well tolerated.[46,48,49]

Compounded cyclosporine-based formulations can be considered including Klarity-C (Imprimis Pharmaceuticals, San Diego, California), which is 0.1% CsA in a chondroitin sulfate emulsion. The possible advantages of using chondroitin sulfate as a lubricant include its antiinflammatory properties and it is thought to decrease corneal edema.[2]

Given that CsA may take 3 months for maximal effect, topical steroids have also been used before the initiation of long-term topical 0.05% cyclosporine as an induction agent and as an early maintenance agent to expedite relief of symptoms and improve ocular signs.[50,51] Side effects of topical cyclosporine include burning or stinging after instillation, conjunctival hyperemia, discharge, epiphora, eye pain, foreign body sensation, visual disturbance, or pruritus.[51]

Lifitegrast

Lifitegrast (Xiidra), approved in July 2016, is the second topical antiinflammatory agent approved by the US FDA for treatment of the signs and symptoms of dry eye.[34,36,52] Lifitegrast is a small lymphocyte function–associated antigen-1 (LFA-1) antagonist used to reduce

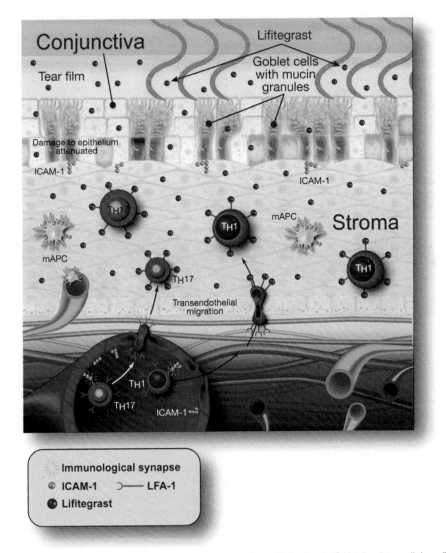

FIG. 11.3 **Mechanism of action (MOA) of lifitegrast at the cellular level.** ICAM-1 = intercellular adhesion molecule 1; LFA-1 = lymphocyte function-associated antigen 1; mAPC = mature antigen-presenting cell; T_H = T helper cell. Disclaimer: this figure illustrates the current understanding of the MOA of lifitegrast based on completed preclinical and clinical studies. Additional studies in the posterior ocular tissues and vascular system are required to further elucidate the MOA of lifitegrast. (Figure and caption courtesy of Perez VL, Pflugfelder SC, Zhang S, Shojaei A, Haque R. Lifitegrast, a novel integrin antagonist for treatment of dry eye disease. *Ocular Surf.* 2016;14(2):207–215.)

inflammation and manage dry eye symptoms.[53] The medication mimics the intercellular adhesion molecule-1 (ICAM-1) preventing the binding between ICAM-1 and lymphocyte functional–associated antigen-1 (LFA-1), inhibiting T-cell recruitment, activation, migration, and proinflammatory cytokine release.[2,4,54] The mechanism of action of Lifitegrast is demonstrated in Figs. 11.3 and 11.4.[36,55]

Studies have indicated that topical lifitegrast may have rapid effect, long-term safety as well as improvement in the signs and symptoms of dry eye disease.[2] Patients may experience mild instillation site irritation, pain and reaction, and dysgeusia.[34] Lifitegrast is preservative free and comes in single-unit dose ampule.[36]

The SONATA (Safety of a 5.0% concentration of lifitegrAst ophthalmic solution) study was a multicenter,

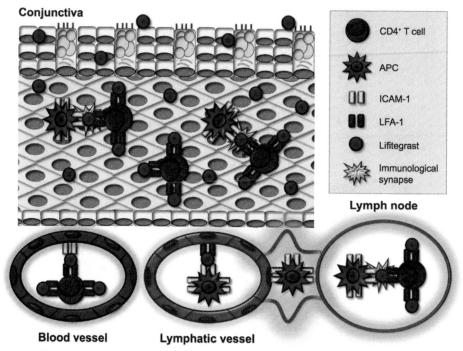

Conjunctiva

CD4+ T cell

APC

ICAM-1

LFA-1

Lifitegrast

Immunological synapse

Lymph node

Blood vessel   **Lymphatic vessel**

FIG. 11.4 **Mechanism of action of lifitegrast**. Notes: Lifitegrast blocks ICAM-1 and LFA-1 interaction, which is critical in migration of DCs to lymph nodes, naïve T-cell activation by DCs, and T-cell transmigration into the ocular surface. Abbreviations: *APCs*, antigen-presenting cells; *DC*, dendritic cell; *ICAM-1*, intercellular adhesion molecule; *LFA-1*, lymphocyte functional associated antigen-1. (Figure and caption courtesy of Lollett IV, Galor A. Dry eye syndrome: developments and lifitegrast in perspective. *Clin Ophthalmol*. 2018;12:125−139 originally published by Dove Medical Press.)

randomized, prospective, double-masked, placebo-controlled phase 3 study of 331 participants who evaluated the 1-year safety of twice-daily lifitegrast compared to placebo as measured by treatment-emergent adverse events. The study showed that lifitegrast was safe and well tolerated.[52]

Randomized control trials in the United States have evaluated the efficacy of lifitegrast: OPUS-1, OPUS-2, and OPUS-3.[54,56,57] Holland et al. reported on OPUS-3 a phase III, 12 week, double-masked, multicenter study of 711 participants that compared lifitegrast 5.0% ophthalmic solution to placebo. The study showed that lifitegrast significantly improved patient reported symptoms of eye dryness (measured by the EDS, eye dryness score) and was well tolerated.[54] Significant symptomatic improvement is reported to occur by 6 weeks and as early as 2 weeks (OPUS-2 and OPUS-3).[34]

Lifitegrast has high aqueous solubility, quick absorption into ocular tissues, and systemic elimination.[34]

Topical steroids

Topical corticosteroids target inflammatory pathways to improve symptoms in ocular surface disease.[29] Short-term therapy with corticosteroids such as loteprednol 0.5% (Lotemax) can be used to decrease inflammation at the ocular surface.[34] Topical corticosteroids bind to glucocorticoid receptors and modulate the expression of antiinflammatory and proinflammatory genes. NF-kB, which is a main transcription factor in inflammation, is suppressed by corticosteroids, which causes the suppression of proinflammatory mediators and induction of lymphocyte apoptosis.[36] Several studies have shown short-term benefit of topical corticosteroids in managing dry eye disease.

Loteprednol etabonate ophthalmic 0.5% suspension was approved by the US FDA in March 1998 for the treatment of corticosteroid-responsive conditions. A randomized, double-masked placebo-controlled trial of loteprednol etabonate ophthalmic 0.5% suspension four times daily in 64 patients with keratoconjunctivitis sicca and delayed tear clearance showed significant benefit after 2 weeks compared to the vehicle group in patients with at least moderate clinical inflammation.[58]

EYSUVIS (loteprednol etabonate ophthalmic suspension 0.25%) (Kala Pharmaceuticals Inc., Watertown, MA) was approved by the US FDA in 2020 for the short-term treatment of the signs and symptoms of dry eye disease. The medication is to be used four times daily for up to 2 weeks. EYSUVIS, also referred to as KPI-121, is an ophthalmic nanoparticle suspension of loteprednol etabonate that is formulated with a mucus-penetrating particle (MPP) technology to enhance ocular drug delivery. Specifically, MPP aims to prevent mucous binding and decrease mucous-driven clearance to improve ocular surface drug delivery. Korenfeld et al. reported on the results of four trials (one phase 2 and three phase 3 multicenter, randomized, double-masked, vehicle controlled trials) for a total of 2871 subjects. The results showed that the medication was safe and well tolerated when taken four times daily for 2−4 weeks with a low incidence of adverse events.[59]

A single-center, double-masked, randomized, vehicle-controlled clinical trial of 21 patients who received topical 0.1% fluorometholone (FML) compared to 19 patients who received topical polyvinyl alcohol group for 22 days in dry eye disease patients showed that the FML group had significant improvement in corneal and conjunctival staining, hyperemia, and TBUT compared to placebo. The study also showed that FML prevented ocular surface worsening in patients exposed to desiccating stress.[60]

Topical methylprednisolone and dexamethasone have been studied in dry eye disease.[61,62]

Risks of corticosteroid therapy include elevation of intraocular pressure and long-term use may lead to the development of cataracts.[58] Topical steroids can delay wound healing and cause corneal and scleral thinning. Topical steroids are contraindicated in patients with viral, mycobacterial, or fungal infections of the cornea and conjunctiva.

Antibiotics

Tetracyclines

Oral tetracyclines including doxycycline and minocycline, which block protein synthesis by inhibiting the binding of aminoacyl-tRNA to the mRNA-ribosome complex, have antibacterial and antiinflammatory properties.[4] Tetracyclines inhibit the production or bacterial lipases in order to improve the lipid profile of meibomian oils.[34] Tetracyclines reduce the activity of

collagenases, phospholipases, and matrix metalloproteinases. In addition, they block angiogenesis and suppress the production of IL-1 and TNF-α in the corneal epithelium, reducing meibomian lipid breakdown products.[5]

Tetracycline and its analogues are used to treat diseases associated with dry eye disease including blepharitis, MGD, and acne rosacea.[4] MGD is often associated with evaporative dry eye disease.[63]

Rosacea is an inflammatory disorder, which has been associated with MGD, blepharitis and Demodex. Ocular rosacea is characterized by meibomian gland inflammation and inspissation, conjunctival hyperemia, and lid margin telangiectasia, frequently leading to dry eyes.[4,64,65]

Several small studies have shown that tetracyclines may decrease symptoms and hyperemia in rosacea.[64] A comparative study of doxycycline 100 mg/day and tetracycline hydrochloride 1 g/day for the management of subjective symptoms of ocular rosacea in 24 patients showed that at 6 weeks all but one patient had symptomatic improvement.[66] A prospective study of 39 patients with cutaneous rosacea with ocular involvement who were given doxycycline 100 mg daily for 12 weeks showed improvement in ocular disease and increase in tear break-up time.[67] Määtä et al. showed that matrix metalloproteinase 8 (MMP-8) levels and activation were increased in tear fluid samples in 22 patients with ocular rosacea compared to 22 controls, which decreased after treatment with oral doxycycline at both 4 and 8 weeks.[65]

Blepharitis, a common ocular surface disorder, which involves inflammation of the eyelids can be managed with tetracyclines. A randomized, double-masked, placebo-controlled partial crossover trial studied topical fusidic acid gel and oxytetracycline in patients with symptomatic chronic blepharitis with and without rosacea. Fifty percent of patients with blepharitis and associated rosacea were symptomatically improved by oxytetracycline alone.[68]

MGD, a type of posterior blepharitis, is caused by structural changes or dysfunction of the meibomian glands.[69] A prospective open-label observational clinical trial demonstrated that topical therapy with azithromycin and oral therapy with doxycycline improved signs and symptoms of MGD and associated dry eyes and also reconstituted lipid properties of meibomian gland secretion.[63] A prospective randomized clinical trial of 60 patients with stage 3 or 4 MGD after 1 and 2 months of oral minocycline 50 mg and artificial tears compared to artificial tears alone showed statistically significant improvement in all clinical signs and symptoms measured. There were also significant reductions in IL-6, IL-1ß, IL-17α, TNF-α, and IL12p70 after 2 months of treatment.[69] Aronowicz also showed that tetracyclines may be efficacious in treating meibomianitis.[70]

Established side effects of tetracyclines include gastrointestinal effects and photosensitivity.[4]

Topical azithromycin

Azithromycin is a macrolide antibiotic, which has strong anti-inflammatory properties and good coverage against gram-negative microorganisms.[71] Topical azithromycin is considered a safe treatment for lid margin disease and MGD.[71] Azithromycin inhibits the production of TNF-alpha, IL-1beta, IL-8, RANTES (Regulated on Activation, Normal T Cell Expressed and Secreted), and MMP (MMP-1, MMP-3, and MMP-9) by inhibiting nuclear factor-kappaB activation in corneal epithelial cells.[72]

A study of 26 subjects with moderate-to-severe blepharitis who received azithromycin 1% ophthalmic solution for 4 weeks without warm compresses showed that topical azithromycin use was associated with significant improvement in several signs and symptoms of blepharitis.[73] Luchs et al. conducted an open-label study of 21 patients with posterior blepharitis that showed that topical azithromycin 1% combined with warm compresses showed significant improvement in ocular signs and symptoms compared to warm compresses alone.[74]

In patients with blepharoconjunctivitis, erythromycin ointment can also be considered.[75]

Oral azithromycin

Studies have shown that oral azithromycin may be beneficial in the treatment of MGD and can provide a treatment alternative in patients unable to take other oral antibiotics. In particular, azithromycin may be beneficial in patients with MGD who also have rosacea due to its antiinflammatory properties.[76–79] Side effects of systemic azithromycin include diarrhea, nausea, and vomiting.[4]

BLOOD PRODUCTS
Autologous and/or Allogenic Serum Drops

Autologous serum, which is devoid of blood's cellular components and clotting factors, has been shown to provide relief in symptoms and improvement of the ocular surface of DES in patients with severe ocular surface disease refractory to standard treatments.[80,81] Autologous serum eye drops are made from a patient's own blood by segregating the serum from cellular components.[82] An advantage of serum is that it has several biochemical similarities to natural tears.[4,29] In addition, it contains epitheliotropic and antimicrobial factors that are beneficial for corneal nutrition, growth, and development.[82] The topical use of serum was originally used to treat severe ocular surface diseases from SS, Stevens–Johnson syndrome, and chemical burns.[80,83–85] It is now also used to treat dry eyes after keratorefractive surgeries, recurrent erosions, persistent epithelial defects, neurotrophic keratopathy, chemical injuries, and superior limbic keratoconjunctivitis.[81]

Several clinical trials and case series investigating autologous serum conclude that it can be efficacious in the treatment of signs and symptoms of DED.[4] Mondy et al. showed that among 77 patients with dry eye and corneal epithelial defects, there were significant improvements in the symptoms frequency of dryness, ocular pain, and grittiness at 2 and 12 months.[82] A systematic Cochrane review reviewed five studies that compared autologous serum to artificial tears or saline showed that eye drops containing autologous serum may have short-term benefits at improving dry eye symptoms but that further studies are needed to evaluate long-term effects.[29]

Autologous serum eye drops are compounded from the patient's own serum. There is variability in the methods of preparation, storage, and administration. After blood is drawn and forms a clot, the supernatant is centrifuged to separate the serum from the solid components. The serum is then decanted and can be diluted to a specific concentration. Autologous serum is usually administered at a 20% concentration although higher concentrations (50%–100%) have been used.[29,80]

Serum tear preparation has rarely been associated with the risk of infection and microbial contamination (seen after extended use >30 days).[81] Autologous serum should be stored at 4°C for less than a month and then can be stored for up to 3 months at −20°C.[84] To prevent risk of viral transmission to others, it is advised that the donor be tested for blood-borne illnesses (e.g., human immunodeficiency virus (HIV), hepatitis B virus (HBV), hepatitis C virus (HVC), syphilis).[29,86]

Autologous serum may be cost prohibitive for patients. It also requires patients to provide blood samples at least every 3 months. In addition, the production of autologous serum is regulated by national laws that vary between countries.[4,81] In the United States, the Center for Biologics Evaluation and Research (CBER) of the FDA is responsible for the regulation of blood components and its derivatives.[29]

Allogenic serum may be used in patients with active inflammation, anemia, or other contraindications; however, allogenic serum may induce an immune response.[4]

Eye—Platelet-Rich Plasma and Plasma Rich in Growth Factors

Platelet preparations have been used to treat ocular surface disease, including platelet-rich plasma (PRP), plasma rich in growth factors (PRGFs), and platelet lysate.[4] The advantage of platelet preparations is that they contain an increased concentration of growth factor.

PRP is prepared from whole blood that is collected in the presence of a 3.2% sodium citrate anticoagulant solution, which is then centrifuged to isolate a platelet-enriched supernatant plasma. The PRP is divided into 3—4 mL aliquots and can be stored at 4°C for 1 week or a −20°C for an extended period.[53] The growth factors present in PRP are thought to activate macrophages, induce cell repair and angiogenesis.[87] In addition, these products, unlike serum drops, do not contain leukocytes that may increase levels of proinflammatory cytokines.[2] Alio et al. showed PRP was associated with improvement in dry eye symptoms and signs in 368 patients with moderate-to-severe dry eye at 6 week follow-up.[87]

PRGF is prepared by collecting whole blood in tubes containing 3.8% sodium citrate and then centrifuging the tubes using a soft spin at $460 \times g$ at room temperature for 8 min.[53] After the plasma supernatant is isolated, platelets are activated using 22.8 mM calcium chloride, which generates a fibrin clot and growth factors are released via platelet activation and degranulation. The growth factor—rich supernatant serum is filtered and is then diluted with 0.9% sodium chloride down to 20%.[53] The product can be stored at 4°C for up to 1 week and then at −20°C for longer periods. The drops are administered four times a day. PRGFs have also been shown to lead to symptom improvement in patients with moderate-to-severe dry eye.[88]

Platelet lysate has also been shown to be efficacious in the treatment of ocular graft-versus-host disease.[89]

EYELID PROCEDURES

Several in-office procedures can be utilized in patients with evaporative dry eye in the setting of MGD.

Intense Pulsed Light

Intense pulsed light (IPL) utilizes high-intensity light sources, which emit light extending from visible (515 nm) to the infrared spectrum (1200 nm), which is absorbed by the skin tissue and then converted to destructive heat.[2] Wavelengths can be customized for different targets. It is used in dermatology for the removal of hypertrichosis, benign cavernous hemangiomas, benign venous malformations, telangiectasia, pigmented lesions, acne rosacea, photo damaged skin, and port wine stain.[90,91]

A third-generation IPL device for periocular use is commercially available for treating severe MGD after being refractory to other therapies.[90] In 2021, the US FDA approved the Lumenis IPL device (Lumenis, Yokneam, Israel) for improving signs of DED from MGD. A randomized, double-masked, placebo-controlled trial evaluating IPL as a therapy for MGD showed a significant improvement in lipid layer grade, noninvasive tear break-up time, and in visual analogue symptoms scores from baseline with 86% of 28 subjects noting reduced symptoms in the treated eye by 45 days.[90] A 30-month retrospective study of IPL and gland expression for treatment of DED caused by MGD showed 93% of 91 patients reported posttreatment satisfaction in regard to dry eye symptoms.[92] A retrospective study of 35 patients with refractory dry eye treated with IPL and meibomian gland expression (MGX) showed significant reduction in Standard Patient Evaluation of Eye Dryness 2 (SPEED2) symptom survey scores and increase in meibomian gland evaluations (MGD) in the left eye after a minimum follow-up of 6 months.[91] A multicenter cohort study of 100 patients with MGD and dry eye who underwent IPL (with an average of four sessions) showed a significant decrease in lid margin edema, facial telangiectasia, lid margin vascularity, meibum viscosity, and OSDI score. There was also a significant increase in the measured oil flow score and TBUT.[93] A prospective study of IPL combined with MGX in 40 patients with moderate-to-severe MGD showed reduction in number and severity of symptoms and signs of dry eye after 15 weeks.[94]

It is important to note that IPL cannot be used in patients with a Fitzpatrick score greater than 4, the upper eyelid cannot be directly treated and the procedure can be cost prohibitive for some patients.[93]

Vectored thermal pulsation (LipiFlow)

Lipiflow Vectored thermal pulsation system (TearScience, Morrisville, NC, USA) clears blockages in the meibomian glands of patients with MGD by heating the glands to therapeutic levels of 42.5°C by applying localized heat to both inner eyelid surfaces (insulating the eye) while pulsating pressure is also applied to the outer eyelids through an inflatable air

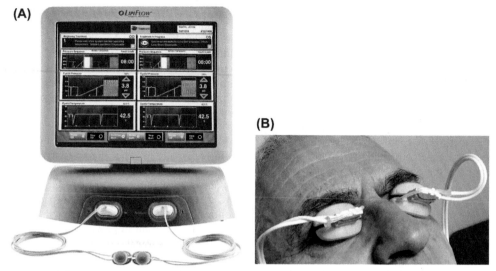

FIG. 11.5 **(A)** Lipflow vectored thermal pulsation system. **(B)** Clinical application of Lipiflow vectored thermal pulsation system. (Photograph for Fig. 11.5A Courtesy of Johnson & Johnson Vision Care, Inc.)

bladder. The procedure takes 12 min.[95] Studies have shown vectoral thermal pulsation can lead to sustained improvements in objective and subjective measures of dry eye disease.[15,95–99] Fig. 11.5 shows the Lipiflow device.

A prospective, multicenter, open-label clinical trial of 200 subjects that compared a single vectored thermal pulsation (VTP) treatment or twice daily, 3 month conventional warm compresses and eyelid hygiene therapy showed that the VTP group showed improved treatment outcomes. Specifically, at 3 months the treatment group had greater mean improvement in meibomian gland secretion and dry eye symptoms compared to the control group. In addition, at 12 months, the VTP group showed sustained improvement in both parameters.[95]

Finis et al. also describe a prospective, randomized, crossover observer masked trial of a single Lipiflow treatment compared to twice daily lid warming and massage for 3 months. At both 1 and 3 month follow-up, patients in the Lipiflow group had a significant decrease in OSDI score compared to the lid hygiene group while both groups had significant improvement in expressible meibomian glands compared to baseline. A total of 31 subjects were followed for 3 months.[99]

A retrospective study of 98 patients that underwent Lipflow showed that thermal pulsation treatment led to significant improvements in TBUT, OSDI score, and MMP-9 after a median follow-up of 64 days. In addition, in patients with baseline osmolarity >307 mOsm/L, there was significant improvement in mean tear osmolarity after treatment.[97]

iLux

The Systane iLux MGD Treatment System (Alcon, Fort Worth, TX) is an eyelid thermal pulsation system device that can be utilized in patients with MGD that applies localized heat and compression. The handheld battery-powered instrument is made of silicone with inner and outer pads that contact both the palpebral conjunctiva and external eyelid. Temperature sensors measure the temperature of the inner and outer eyelids and then remain at a temperature of 38–42°C to melt meibum. The procedure takes 8–12 min. The iLux device is demonstrated in Fig. 11.6.

Tauber et al. reported on a randomized, open-label, controlled, multicenter clinical trial of 142 patients that compared iLux to Lipiflow treatment. The study showed that both devices had significant improvement in meibomian gland scores (MGSs), TBUT and OSDI scores at 4 week follow-up, and there were no significant differences in effectiveness between the devices.[100]

MiBo Thermoflo

The MiBo Thermoflo (MiBo Medical Group, Dallas TX) is a therapeutic device that can be used in the office setting for the treatment of dry eye disease. MiBoFlo utilizes a handheld probe with a double eye pad attached with ultrasound gel to deliver thermoelectric heath through the eyelid to the meibomian glands. The protocol involves an initial 12 min treatment session per eyelid followed by a session 1 week later of 10 min per eyelid and then a third session 2 weeks following that is 8–10 min per lid. There are no published studies

(A)

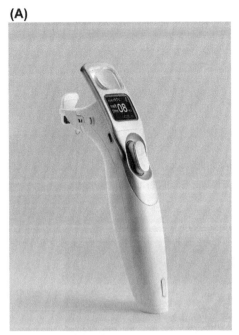

(B)

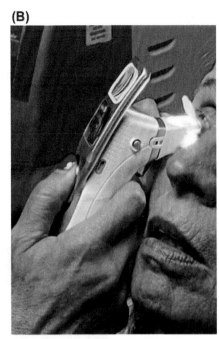

FIG. 11.6 **(A)** The Systane iLux MGD Treatment System. **(B)** Clinical application of the Systane iLux MGD Treatment System. (Photograph Courtesy of Alcon.)

available providing clinical data on this technology. Preliminary data from a 51-patient study showed statistically significant improvement from TBUT, osmolarity, OSDI, and SPEED scores at the 4-month visit.[2,101]

TearCare System

The TearCare System (Sight Sciences, Menlo Park, CA) is an in-office treatment that takes 12 min for patients with dry eye disease that utilizes four electrothermal iLid instruments that are affixed to the external surface of each eyelid through which regulated thermal energy is applied to the eyelids at a constant temperature (41−45°C) to melt meibum via a TearCare controller.[102] The SmartLids contain a silicon-based adhesive and are attached using a medical grade adhesive to the eyelids along the lid margins. The system also consists of a SmartHub controller and a charging adapter.[103] An advantage of the system is that the iLid devices conform the eyelid shape to enable patients to blink during the procedure, facilitating meibum expression through blinking. Following the thermal cycle, a manual MGX with expression forceps is performed to remove any residual obstructions.[102] The TearCare System is shown in Fig. 11.7.

A prospective, randomized, parallel group 6-month study of 24 subjects compared a single in-office

TearCare treatment with 4 weeks of daily warm compresses for 5 min. Subjects in the TearCare group showed significant improvement in TBUT from baseline at 1-month follow-up compared to patients with warm compress group who had average worsening in score. In addition, the TearCare group also had significantly greater improvement from baseline in MGSs, corneal and conjunctival staining, and dry eye symptoms.[102]

Badawi et al. also published an extension study during which at 6 months patients in the TearCare were reevaluated and then selected for a retreatment. Twelve subjects participated in the study and at 1 month after retreatment there was a significant improvement from baseline in mean TBUT at 1 month follow-up as well as significant reductions in MGSs, corneal and conjunctival staining cores, and dry eye symptoms following retreatment up until the conclusion of the study 6 months later.[104]

A multicenter, prospective, postmarket, interventional trial of 29 patients with MGD-related dry eye disease who received a single TearCare treatment showed statistically significant improvements in TBUT and mean baseline OSDI with a clinically meaningful improvement seen in 83% of subjects as per the Miller-Plugfeld definition and 66% improved by at least

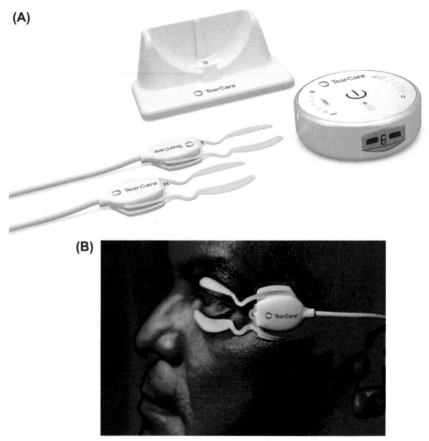

FIG. 11.7 **(A)** The TearCare System. **(B)** Clinical application of TearCare System. (Photographs Courtesy of Sight Sciences.)

one OSDI category. Significant improvements were also measured in total Meibomian Gland Secretion Score.[103]

Meibomian Gland Probing

Intraductal meibomian gland probing, described by Maskin in 2010, is performed at the slit lamp, during which a 2 mm probe is placed into each meibomian gland orifice to mechanically egress its contents.[18]

A retrospective review of 25 patients who underwent meibomian gland probing demonstrated that the procedure is safe and effective at causing relief of symptoms. Specifically, the study showed that all patients had relief of symptoms by 4 weeks, 80% only required one treatment and had an average of 11.5 month follow-up.[105]

Maskin et al. also published a retrospective study of 19 patients who showed that meibomian gland probing was associated with increased meibomian gland tissue area and growth of atrophied meibomian glands. Their study showed an overall incidence of 41.2% of eyelids showing individual meibomian gland growth between 4.5 and 12 months follow-up.[106]

Wladis et al. evaluated the role of intraductal meibomian gland probing in 40 eyelids of 10 patients with ocular rosacea. The study showed that all patients reported subjective improvement in symptoms with statistically significant improvement in OSDI scores at 1- and 6-months.[107]

Syed et al. described a modified technique of intraductal meibomian gland probing. The technique utilizes an operating microscope; after anesthesia is achieved, von Graefe fixation forceps are used to grasp the eyelid, traction is applied in a "milking manner," and then a 2 mm probe is used to dilate and then is passed into each orifice, followed by a 4 mm probe that is then used for deeper probing. In their retrospective review of 70 eyelids, 91.4% of cases had immediate symptomatic relief and there were no complications.[108]

Forced MGX can also be used to improve dry eye symptoms by expressing the eyelid margins to remove meibomian gland contents.[91]

BlephEx

BlephEx® (Scope Ophthalmics, London, UK) is a hand-held device used in the office setting for management of ocular surface disorders including blepharitis. The device contains a hand-held electromechanical unit and a disposable microsponge that is inserted and spins to cause debridement and exfoliation of the lash margin.[109] The BlephEx device is shown in Fig. 11.8.

Murphy et al. conducted a randomized controlled interventional treatment study of 86 patients who were treated with Tea Tree Face Wash, OcuSoft Lid Scrub Plus or lid scrub with the BlephEx device. All groups were also advised to clean their eyelids nightly for 4 weeks. The study showed that the quantity of *Demodex folliculorum* was significantly reduced after 4 weeks of treatment in all three groups with no difference in efficacy between the three treatments. In addition, symptoms significantly improved after 2 and 4 weeks of treatment.[109]

Epstein et al. reported on a randomized prospective double-masked trial of 46 patients with *Demodex*-positive blepharitis who underwent Microblepharoexfoliation with Blephex and randomized to masked lid scrubs (terpinen-4-ol or sham) twice daily for one month. The patients then returned for an additional BlephEx treatment with terpinen-4-ol scrubs twice daily for a month. The study showed that BlephEx treatments combined with either scrub caused statistically significant reduction in *D. folliculorum* infestations but that terpinen-4-ol scrubs showed no significant improvement over sham scrubs.[110]

DEVICES
Nasal Neurostimulation

Chemical or mechanical stimulation of the nasal mucosa leads to increased tear production by stimulating the nasolacrimal reflex. Therefore, neurostimulation can treat dry eye disease by inducing tear production.[4]

TrueTear Intranasal Tear Neurostimulator (INT, TrueTear Allergan, Dublin, Ireland), which was previously on the market, used neurostimulation in patients with aqueous tear deficiency to increase tear production.[34] The device was designed to utilize small electrical currents to stimulate mucosal nerves via the nasolacrimal reflex pathway of the lacrimal functional unit in order to augment natural tear production.[2,111] The device contained two small probes that were placed in each nostril. There were five levels of stimulation intensity.[2] Specifically, the device stimulated the nasociliary nerve to activate the nasolacrimal reflex and reach higher centers that act on the lacrimal functional unit through the efferent parasympathetic pathway as well as on goblet cells and meibomian glands. As such, it activated the nasolacrimal pathway that is involved in both basal and bolus tear secretion. The US FDA approved TrueTear™ that uses neurostimulation for the use of temporarily increasing tear production in adults.[111] Several studies showed intranasal neurostimulation to be effective at decreasing signs and symptoms of dry eye disease.[56,112–118] While the device was shown to be effective and safe, it was discontinued by Allergan.

The iTEAR 100 device (Olympic Ophthalmics Inc., Issaquah, WA) is an FDA-approved portable, sonic external neuromodulation device for the treatment of DED. The device uses a small unidirectional oscillating tip (frequency of 220–270 Hz and amplitude of

(A) 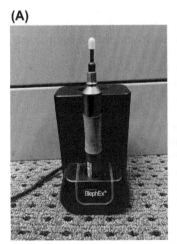 **(B)**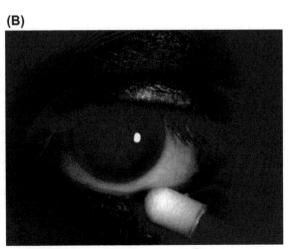

FIG. 11.8 **(A)** BlephEx®. **(B)** Clinical application of BlephEx®.

0.5–1 mm) to stimulate the external branch of the anterior ethmoidal nerve of the side of the nose, which activates the lacrimal functional unit to increase tear production. The device is placed on the lateral aspect of nasal skin between the nasal cartilage and nasal bone. A multicenter, open-label, single-arm clinical trial was conducted of 101 patients with DED treated by the device at least twice daily for 30 s bilaterally to the external nasal nerve and followed for 180 days. The study showed that the device was safe and efficacious for treating DED as demonstrated by the Schirmer index and change in OSDI score.[119]

OC-01 (Varenicline) Nasal Spray

The OC-01 nasal spray (Oyster Point Pharma, Inc., Princeton, NJ) uses varenicline, a highly selective nicotinic acetylcholine receptor agonist, which binds to the trigeminal nerve when administered in the nasal cavity to activate the parasympathetic nervous system to stimulate tear production. The United States FDA approved varenicline 0.03 mg solution (TYRVAYA Nasal Spray, Oyster Point Pharma, Inc.) in 2021 for the treatment of signs and symptoms DED. The ONSET-2 was a multicenter, double-masked, randomized, controlled Phase 3 study that compared OC-01 at two doses (0.6 mg/mL and 1.2 mg/mL) administered twice daily for 4 weeks compared to vehicle in 758 patients. The study showed a statistically significant improvement in increase in Schirmer's scores for both doses compared to vehicle. The MYSTIC and ONSET-1 were phase 2 studies of OC-01.[120,121]

Contact Lenses (Bandage Lenses and Rigid Gas Permeable Scleral Lenses)

Contact lens use for ocular surface disease often involves extended wear, which carries an increased risk of microbial keratitis as compared to daily wear.[4]

Bandage contact lenses aim to provide comfort and protect the ocular surface against adverse environmental factors. Bandage contact lenses should be used as an adjunct to other treatments and have been thought to work by stabilizing the tear film, restoring epithelial cell turnover, and insulating corneal nerves. They are also used in the management of recurrent corneal erosions, corneal abrasion, bullous keratopathy, lamellar lacerations, filamentous keratitis, Fuch's dystrophy, graft insufficiency, and following corneal surgery.[31,72,122–125] Advances in contact lens design have enabled higher oxygen diffusion capabilities that allows for a longer period of uninterrupted wear.[72] Extended wear soft bandage contact lenses can aid to resurface the corneal surface and protect sensitized

corneal receptors. However, once chronic pain develops, a bandage contact lens may be less effective in decreasing symptoms.[126]

A study of the Focus NIGHT & DAY (CIBA Vision, Duluth, GA) silicone hydrogel contact lens for seven patients with moderate-to-severe dry eye in the setting of graft-versus-host disease showed an improvement in subjective symptoms and visual acuity.[127]

A prospective randomized study of 37 patients with severe dry eye from SS showed that patients who received a bandage contact lens for 6 weeks had improvement in best-corrected visual acuity, Ocular Surface Disease Index score, quality of life measures, and corneal staining.[72]

Scleral lenses are situated on the sclera and create a constant fluid-filled reservoir over the cornea and can be used in severe ocular surface disorders to hydrate the corneal surface.[2] Fig. 11.9A shows improvement in conjunctival lissamine staining after scleral lens use. Fig. 11.9B shows a scleral lens and applicator.

The BostonSight PROSE (Prosthetic replacement of the ocular surface ecosystem, Boston Foundation for Sight, Needham, Massachusetts) is a fluid-filled rigid gas-permeable scleral lens that provides a precorneal nociceptive barrier that was approved by the FDA in 1994.[126] The lenses are custom designed using computer-assisted design and manufacture to ensure that they do not touch the apical or peripheral cornea. The lens is used to improve vision in individuals with severe keratoconus and is shown to be safe and efficacious when used in patients with refractory ocular surface disease, persistent epithelial defects, corneal ectasias, Steven–Johnson syndrome (SJS), chronic ocular graft-versus-host disease and those with decreased vision following penetrating keraoplasty, laser in situ keratomileusis, or other eye surgeries.[128–140]

A prospective study of 80 patients fitted with a Boston Ocular Surface Prosthesis showed a significant improvement in mean composite visual functioning scores.[129] A retrospective study of 121 patients who had used the PROSE lens showed that 89/121 had continued device wear at 5 years. At 5-year follow-up, those wearing the lens had a higher NEI VFQ-25 (National Eye Institute Vision Function Questionnaire) than those not wearing the lens.[132]

The EyePrintPro lens (Advanced Vision Technologies, Lakewood, Colorado) is another customizable highly oxygen transmissible scleral lens. It is created by using polyvinyl siloxane material to create an impression mold of the ocular surface, which is then scanned with a 3D scanner and then the posterior surface of the lens is created with lathe technology.

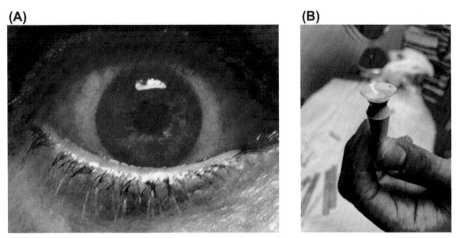

FIG. 11.9 **(A)** Lissamine green conjunctival staining after removal of scleral contact lens. **(B)** Scleral contact lens and applicator.

A retrospective study of 10 patients showed that most patients had improvement in BCVA and all patients reported improvement in dry eye symptoms.[141]

Amniotic Membrane

Cryopreserved amniotic membrane grafts may be used in moderate-to-severe ocular surface disease refractory to maximal medical treatments such as in patients with persistent epithelial defects, in cases of ocular cicatricial pemphigoid, neurotrophic ulcers, and in Stevens–Johnson syndrome.[4,142–144] They are also used in the treatment of filamentary keratitis, infectious keratitis, recurrent corneal erosion, corneal ulcers, chemical injury, pterygium excision, Salmann's nodular degeneration, post-DSEK for bullous keratopathy, and ocular surface reconstruction.[143] Amniotic membrane, which contains neuropeptides and neurotransmitters, has been shown to act as a therapeutic bandage to promote epithelialization and has antiinflammatory, antiscarring, and antiangiogenic effects.[143,145]

The commercially available forms of amniotic membrane include PROKERA (Bio-Tissue, Inc, Miami, FL), which is cryopreserved at −80°C AmbioDisk (Katena Products, Inc, Denville, NJ), which is sterilized, dehydrated, and stored at room temperature.

PROKERA, which has a ring that holds the amniotic membrane, can be placed on the ocular service as an in-office procedure. PROKERA products include PROKERA Slim, PROKERA, PROKERA Clear, and PROKERA Plus. PROKERA Slim is recommended for mild to moderate conditions, while the PROKERA Plus is recommended for more severe conditions. PROKERA Clear contains a 6 mm Clear-View aperture. Fig. 11.10 shows the PROKERA.

A retrospective review of 10 patients treated with PROKERA Slim for moderate-to-severe dry eye shows symptomatic relief (for a period of 4.2 ± 4.7 months), reduction in OSDI score, and decrease in use of topical medications, conjunctival hyperemia, corneal staining, and an improvement in visual acuity.[145] A retrospective study of 84 patients treated with amniotic membrane (PROKERA Slim) for dry eye disease who completed at least 3 month follow-up showed improvement in ocular surface as measured by reduction in the DEWS score.[146] A retrospective study of nine patients demonstrated amniotic membrane (PROKERA Slim/PROKERA Clear) showed improvement in neuropathic corneal pain with an average follow-up of 9.3 ± 0.8 months.[147]

SURGICAL PROCEDURES

Punctal Cautery

For patients who cannot tolerate punctal plugs, surgical punctal occlusion can be considered. Thermal methods that can be employed for punctal cauterization include cautery, diathermy, and use of an Argon laser, which can be used for both superficial and deep procedures. Surgical methods include canalicular ligation, extirpation of the canaliculus, punctal plug suturing, total or partial thermal cauterization, and punctal occlusion with a conjunctival flap or graft.[4] Complications of cauterization include epiphora and recanalization.[4]

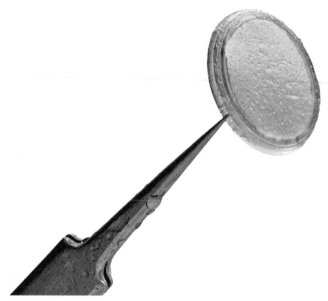

FIG. 11.10 PROKERA. (Photograph Courtesy of Bio-Tissue.)

Tarsorrhaphy

A tarsorrhaphy is a temporary or permanent surgical procedure to partially or completely close the eyelids. The advantage of tarsorrhaphy is that it can decrease exposure of the ocular surface in order to decrease evaporation. A tarsorrhaphy can be considered in patients who have severe dry eye disease that is refractory to medical treatments and is mainly in patients with persistent epithelial defects. A temporary tarsorrhaphy can be performed with sutures, adhesive tape, or levator paralysis via botulinum toxin injection.

Ectropion and Entropion Repair

Entropion and ectropion can both increase exposure of the ocular surface. Entropion is often associated with trichiasis, which can exacerbate symptoms of dry eye disease. Lower eyelid ectropion can be seen in the setting of facial nerve palsy, trauma, tumors, facial surgery, or age-related eyelid laxity. Repair of entropion or ectropion should be considered in patients with exposure keratopathy.[4]

Surgical Treatment for Conjunctivochalasis

Conjunctivochalasis refers to loose, excessive conjunctival tissue in the bulbar conjunctiva between the globe and the lower eyelid, which is age-related. The condition typically affects the inferior bulbar conjunctiva and is a common cause of ocular surface irritation. Conjunctivochalasis has a reported prevalence of 54% in patients with DED.[4] Conjunctivochalasis can cause tearing by mechanically interfering with the tear meniscus and the flow of tears along the lower eyelid into the punctum.[148] Patients with severe conjunctivochalasis that is symptomatic and refractory to medical management may benefit from resection of redundant conjunctival tissue.[149,150] Surgical techniques also include electrocoagulation or thermal cauterization, simple fixation to the sclera, and Argon green laser conjunctivoplasty.[4,150–153]

PIPELINE

The final section includes therapies that are currently being studied that may have therapeutic potential for treatment for dry eyes. The section includes several but not all investigational treatments for dry eye disease.

Recombinant Human Nerve Growth Factor

Nerve growth factor (NGF), which is naturally found in tears, plays a role in the regulation of growth, proliferation, and survival of neurons.[4] NGF, through activation of the receptor tyrosine kinase A (TrkA) and a common coreceptor p75 neurotrophin receptor (p75 NTR), has shown trophic effects on the ocular surface. NGF and TrkA are expressed by corneal epithelial cells and sensory neurons throughout the ocular surface.[154] Studies have shown the potential therapeutic role of topical

NGF in improving corneal sensitivity and increasing tear production in dry eye disease and that it may cause nerve regeneration.[155–157]

NGF (Oxervate) is currently authorized in United States for the treatment of neurotrophic keratitis, a rare corneal disease, caused by impaired trigeminal innervation, resulting in decreased corneal sensitivity, breakdown of the corneal epithelium, and progressive corneal damage.[156,158] A phase IIa, prospective, open label clinical trial of recombinant human nerve growth factor (rhNGF) in 39 patients with moderate-to-severe DED showed that rhNGF at 20 μg/mL or at 4 μg/mL was safe and improved signs of DED.[159]

Tavilermide (MIM-D3), a small molecule NGF peptidomimetic, which is a partial TrKA receptor agonist has been studied in a Phase 2 randomized clinical trial in which 150 patients with DED who were exposed to a Controlled Adverse Environment (CAE) chamber received MIM-D3 1%, 5%, or placebo twice daily for 28 days. Patients in the 1% MIM-D3 group did show significant improvement in fluorescein corneal staining at day 28 post-CAE compared to the pre-CAE. Patients in the 1% MIM-D3 group also had significant improvement versus placebo in both lissamine green staining and in inferior fluorescein staining after 14 and 28 days. Patients in the 5% MIM-D3 group had significant lower daily diary scores for ocular dryness compared to placebo. In a subgroup analysis of more symptomatic patients at baseline, both concentrations of MIM-D3 showed reduction in ocular staining and patient-reported symptoms. While the study did not meet its pre-specified primary endpoints, it showed the MIM-D3 had a favorable safety profile and was well-tolerated with twice daily dosing, leading to improvements in ocular surface staining and patient-reported symptoms.[154]

Lacritin

Lacritin is an endogenous tear glycoprotein that is mainly secreted by acinar cells of the lacrimal gland and promotes basal tearing. Lacritin has prosecretory and mitogenic properties and a cleavage-potentiated fragment has been appreciated for having bactericidal properties.[160]

A study by McNamara et al. showed that active tear lacritin was significantly reduced in patients with SS while inactive lacritin was increased. Nerve fiber density and length were also significantly decreased, where were highly correlated with reduced lacritin. Tear lacritin was also highly correlated with clinical signs of dry eye including Schirmers, ocular staining, and corneal sensitivity.[160]

Vijmasi et al. also determined that lacritin was significantly reduced in the tears of patients with SS. In a paired study, in autoimmune regulator (Aire) knockout

mice that were treated with lacritin, tear secretion significantly increased by 46% and lissamine green staining also significantly decreased.[161]

These studies show that topically administered lacritin may have therapeutic potential for treatment of dry eye disease.

Lubricin

Lubricin (proteoglycan-4) is a large mucin-like glycoprotein that is present in synovial fluid and also on the ocular surface and in meibomian glands.[4] Lubricin decreases friction between the cornea and the conjunctiva and eyelid.[2,162,163]

Lambiase et al. evaluated the efficacy and safety of recombinant human lubricin compared to 0.18% sodium hyaluronate eye drop twice daily for 7 days followed by instillation as needed for 7 days in 35 patients with moderate dry eye disease. The study showed that lubricin supplementation achieved a significant reduction in blurred vision and photophobia in at least one eye. They also observed a significant improvement in fluorescein staining, tear film breakup time, SANDE frequency, eyelid erythema, conjunctival erythema, and instillation compared to sodium hyaluronate. There were no adverse events observed.[162]

Thymosin β4

Thymosin β4, a naturally occurring G-actin–binding protein, which is found in most cells, is thought to enhance epithelial healing and reduce proinflammatory cytokines.[2,164] It is considered to have an important role in corneal repair. Thymosin β4 has been studied in the treatment of corneal neurotrophic defects.[165]

Sosne et al. reported the results of a small multicenter, randomized, double-masked, placebo-controlled study of nine patients with severe dry eye treated with Thymosin β4 eye drops (RGN-259) or a control six times daily for 28 days. They observed the RGN-259 treated group had significant reduction in ocular discomfort and total corneal fluorescein staining compared with control. The study suggested the RGN-259 drops were safe and showed improvement in dry eye.[164]

Kim et al. studied the effects of RGN-259 drops in a murine dry eye model compared to prescription drugs including cyclosporine A (CsA), diquafosol (DQS), and lifitegrast (LFA). In the study, RGN-259 led to recovery of mucins and reduction in antiinflammatory effects on the ocular surface. The study suggested that RGN-259 was comparable to other medications in improving signs of dry eye disease in a mouse model.[166]

Amniotic Membrane Extract Eye Drops

Amniotic membrane extract and amniotic membrane extract eye drops have been studied in cases of acute corneal injury, chemical burn ocular injury. Studies with animal models suggest that these drops may help promote reepithelialization in the treatment of corneal abrasion.[167] Amniotic membrane extract eye drops may provide a treatment alternative to amniotic membrane transplant in the future. These products are not commercially available for treatment of dry eye disease. Clinical trials are needed to evaluate its role in ocular surface disease.

Semifluorinated Alkane Eye Drops

Perfluorohexyloctane (F6H8, NovaTears) (Novaliq, Heidelberg, Germany), in the family of semifluorinated alkanes, is a novel nonaqueous liquid, nonblurring wetting agent commercialized in Europe (EvoTears by Ursapharm) and Australia and New Zealand (AFT Pharmaceuticals) for the treatment of evaporative dry eye disease. Perfluorohexyloctane demonstrates strong spreading properties due to low surface tension, facilitating small drop sizes and interacting with the lipophilic part of the tear film to form a layer at the film—air interface and prevent evaporation.[168] Steven et al. conducted an observational prospective, multicenter 6—8 week study of 61 patients with MGD and DED who received one drop of Perfluorohexyloctane four times daily. The study showed there was a significant reduction in corneal and conjunctival fluorescein staining, increase in number of expressible meibomian glands, increase in tear film break-up time, and improvement in severity of anterior and posterior blepharitis and improvement in OSDI score.[169]

NOVO3 (100% perfluorohexyloctane), an investigational drug in the United States, completed a Phase II study (SEECASE), a prospective, multicenter, randomized, double-masked, saline-controlled study of 336 DED patients. In the study, patients were randomized in a 2:2:1:1 manner to NOVO3 four times daily, NOVO3 twice daily, saline twice daily, and saline four times daily, respectively. The study met its primary endpoint of improvement in corneal fluorescein staining over control at 8 weeks and also showed significant improvement in symptoms.[170] Two Phase 3 studies are currently taking place in the United States for NOVO3.

Reproxalap Ophthalmic Solution

Reproxalap (Aldeyra Therapeutics, Inc., Lexington, MA) is a novel small-molecule immune-modulating covalent inhibitor of RASP (reactive aldehyde species) that is elevated in ocular and systemic inflammatory disease. RASP such as malondialdehyde (MDA) and 4-hydroxy-2-nonenal (HNE) covalently bind to amino and thiol groups on receptors and kinases, activating proinflammatory signaling cascades involving NF-kB, inflammasomes, scavenger receptor A, and other mediators. Elevated levels of RASP found in several inflammatory ocular diseases including Behcet's disease, SS, noninfectious uveitis, allergic conjunctivitis, and DED.[171]

Clark et al. report a randomized, double-masked parallel-group phase 2a trial of three ocular reproxalap formulations (0.1%, 0.5%, and 0.5% lipid ophthalmic solution) in 51 patients with DED treated four times daily for 28 days. Pooled data showed significant improvements in Symptoms Assessment in Dry Eye Disease Score, Ocular Discomfort Scale score, Ocular Discomfort Score, 4-Symptoms Questionnaire overall score, Schirmer's test, tear osmolarity, and lissamine green staining score.[171] A randomized double-masked, vehicle-controlled phase 2b trial of 300 patients with DED compared 0.1% topical reproxalap, 0.25% topical reproxalap, or vehicle treated four times daily for 12 weeks. The authors observed a dose-response with largest significant symptomatic improvement observed in ocular dryness and objective sign improvement in nasal fluorescein staining over 12 weeks. They also noted that improvements in symptoms were observed by the week 2 visit.[172]

Reproxalap is currently in phase 3 studies of the 0.25% ophthalmic solution for the treatment of dry eye and allergic conjunctivitis.

ALG-1007 (Risuteganib) Topical Ophthalmic Solution

ALG-1007 (Allegro Ophthalmics, San Juan Capistrano, CA, USA) is a topical application of risuteganib, a small peptide integrin regulator that modulates several integrin subunits such as integrin αM and β2, the subunits involved in complement 3 inflammatory pathways. Risuteganib is thought to decrease ocular surface inflammation by interfering with leukocyte adhesion and transendothelial migration. Based on preclinical studies, ALG-1007 is considered a potential candidate for treatment of dry eye disease. Lindstrom et al. report a Phase 1, prospective, open-label, 12 week study of 21 patients with DED who received 0.125%, 0.25%, 0.4%, or 0.6% ALG-1007 twice daily and were followed for 12 weeks. Improvement was seen in all groups in regards to TBUT, SICCA total ocular staining score, and Visual Analogue Scale. There was a significant improvement in the 0.6% group compared to the 0.125% in TBUT, conjunctiva staining SICCA, burning, discomfort, photophobia, and composite symptom score. The medication was well tolerated with no serious adverse effects.[173]

Peptide Melanocortin Receptor Agonist Ophthalmic Solution

PL9643 (Palatin Technologies Inc.), a peptide melanocortin receptor agonist at the melanocortin 1 and 5 receptors, is being investigated as a treatment for DED. Melanocortins are endogenous hormonal peptides cleaved from proopiomelanocortin (POMC), a precursor hormone. Melanocortin receptors are expressed by several cell types, have many physiologic roles, and are thought to have protective effects against infection and disease. Specifically, MC1r and MC3r have been shown to have antiinflammatory effects. Therefore, the antiinflammatory effects of melanocortin receptor agonists are currently being investigated in the treatment of chronic inflammatory and autoimmune conditions.[174]

A multicenter, randomized, double-masked, placebo-controlled Phase 2 study of 160 participants with dry eye disease treated with PL9643 or placebo three times daily took place over a 12-week period. The preliminary study results reported on the Palatin website showed that in patients with moderate-to-severe DED there was a significant improvement at week 2 and 12 in inferior, superior and total corneal staining, temporal, nasal and total conjunctival staining, tear film break-up time, and ocular discomfort.[175]

Ophthalmic Keratolytics

Ophthalmic keratolytics (Azura Ophthalmics) are being investigated for the treatment of MGD. Azura announced results from the ECLIPTIC study (not yet published), a Phase 2 clinical trial of twice weekly therapy of 1% AZR-MD-001 or vehicle in 26 patients with contact lens discomfort. AZR-MD-001 is a topical ointment applied to the lower eyelid to prevent abnormal keratinization to treat MGD. Azura reported statistically significant improvement in MGS after 2 week and at study completion. The AZR-MD-001 1% reached statistical superiority over the vehicle at 1.5 months in regards to MGS and meibomian glands yielding liquid secretion.[176]

CONCLUSION

In conclusion, there has been a large expansion in treatment modalities available to treat the different causes of dry eye disease. The treatment of dry eye should follow a stepwise approach based upon the patient's symptoms and the underlying physiology of their condition. Specifically, treatments should aim to address the underlying cause of dry eye disease including evaporative dry eye, aqueous deficiency, and inflammation. For patients with symptoms that are refractory to conservative measures and lubricants, there are several prescription medications that can be utilized. In addition, blood products are increasingly being used that have shown relief in symptoms and signs of dry eye disease. In office procedures can also play a helpful role in managing evaporative dry eye disease. For patients with advanced disease, contact lenses, amniotic membrane transplant, and neurostimulation can be considered. Furthermore, surgical procedures can help ameliorate symptoms for certain patients. Lastly, there is ongoing research on devices and novel therapeutics that are currently in clinical trials. While dry eye disease affects millions of patients, the advances that have been made in treating dry eye disease help decrease the burden of disease on patients' lives.

REFERENCES

1. Akpek EK, Amescua G, Farid M, et al. Dry eye syndrome preferred practice pattern®. *Ophthalmology.* 2019;126(1):286–334.
2. O'Neil EC, Henderson M, Massaro-Giordano M, Bunya VY. Advances in dry eye disease treatment. *Curr Opin Ophthalmol.* 2019;30(3):166–178.
3. Sarezky D, Massaro-Giordano M, Bunya VY. Novel diagnostics and therapeutics in dry eye disease. *Adv Ophthalmol Optometry.* 2016;1(1):1–20.
4. Jones L, Downie LE, Korb D, et al. TFOS DEWS II management and therapy report. *Ocul Surf.* 2017;15(3):575–628.
5. Dogru M, Tsubota K. Pharmacotherapy of dry eye. *Expet Opin Pharmacother.* 2011;12(3):325–334.
6. Lemp MA. Advances in understanding and managing dry eye disease. *Am J Ophthalmol.* 2008;146(3):350–356.e1.
7. Barabino S, Rolando M, Camicione P, et al. Systemic linoleic and γ-linolenic acid therapy in dry eye syndrome with an inflammatory component. *Cornea.* 2003;22(2):97–101.
8. Miljanović B, Trivedi KA, Dana MR, Gilbard JP, Buring JE, Schaumberg and DA. The relationship between dietary n-3 and n-6 fatty acids and clinically diagnosed dry eye syndrome in women. *Am J Clin Nutr.* 2005;82(4):887–893.
9. Bhargava R, Kumar P, Kumar M, Mehra N, Mishra A. A randomized controlled trial of omega-3 fatty acids in dry eye syndrome. *Int J Ophthalmol-Chi.* 2013;6(6):811–816.
10. Epitropoulos AT, Donnenfeld ED, Shah ZA, et al. Effect of oral Re-esterified omega-3 nutritional supplementation on dry eyes. *Cornea.* 2016;35(9):1185–1191.
11. Group DEA and MSR, Asbell PA, Maguire MG, et al. N–3 fatty acid supplementation for the treatment of dry eye disease. *N Engl J Med.* 2018;378(18):1681–1690.
12. Liu J, Dong Y, Wang Y. Vitamin D deficiency is associated with dry eye syndrome: a systematic review and meta-analysis. *Acta Ophthalmol.* 2020;98(8):749–754.

13. Demirci G, Erdur SK, Ozsutcu M, Eliacik M, Olmuscelik O, Aydin R, et al. Dry eye assessment in patients with vitamin D deficiency. *Eye Contact Lens.* 2018; 44(NA):S62–S65.

14. Yoon SY, Bae SH, Shin YJ, et al. Low serum 25-hydroxy-vitamin D levels are associated with dry eye syndrome. *PLoS One.* 2016;11(1):e0147847.

15. Finis D, König C, Hayajneh J, Borrelli M, Schrader S, Geerling G. Six-month effects of a thermodynamic treatment for MGD and implications of meibomian gland atrophy. *Cornea.* 2014;33(12):1265–1270.

16. Blackie CA, Solomon JD, Greiner JV, Holmes M, Korb DR. Inner eyelid surface temperature as a function of warm compress methodology. *Optom Vis Sci.* 2008; 85(8):675–683.

17. Olson MC, Korb DR, Greiner JV. Increase in tear film lipid layer thickness following treatment with warm compresses in patients with meibomian gland dysfunction. *Eye Contact Lens.* 2003;29(2):96–99.

18. Thode AR, Latkany RA. Current and emerging therapeutic strategies for the treatment of meibomian gland dysfunction (MGD). *Drugs.* 2015;75(11):1177–1185.

19. Tighe S, Gao Y-Y, Tseng SCG. Terpinen-4-ol is the most active ingredient of tea tree oil to kill Demodex mites. *Transl Vis Sci Technol.* 2013;2(7):2–8.

20. Bhojwani R, Cellesi F, Maino A, Jalil A, Haider D, Noble B. Treatment of dry eye: an analysis of the British Sjögren's Syndrome Association comparing substitute tear viscosity and subjective efficacy. *Contact Lens Anterior Eye.* 2011;34(6):269–273.

21. Pucker AD, Ng SM, Nichols JJ. Over the counter (OTC) artificial tear drops for dry eye syndrome. *Cochrane Db Syst Rev.* 2016;2(2).

22. Doughty MJ, Glavin S. Efficacy of different dry eye treatments with artificial tears or ocular lubricants: a systematic review. *Ophthalmic Physiol Opt.* 2009;29(6):573–583.

23. Caparas VL. Medical management of dry eye. In: Chan C, ed. *Dry Eye, A Practical Approach.* 2015.

24. Wegener AR, Meyer LM, Schönfeld C. Effect of viscous agents on corneal density in dry eye disease. *J Ocul Pharmacol Therapeut.* 2015;31(8):504–508.

25. Berdy GJ, Abelson MM, Smith LM, George MA. Preservative-free artificial tear preparations. *Arch Ophthalmol.* 1992;110:528–532.

26. McDonald M, D'Aversa G, Perry HD, Wittpenn JR, Nelinson DS. Correlating patient-reported response to hydroxypropyl cellulose ophthalmic insert (LACRI-SERT®) therapy with clinical outcomes: tools for predicting response. *Curr Eye Res.* 2010;35(10):880–887.

27. Lee S-Y, Tong L. Lipid-containing lubricants for dry eye. *Optom Vis Sci.* 2012;89(11):1654–1661.

28. Amrane M, Creuzot-Garcher C, Robert P-Y, et al. Ocular tolerability and efficacy of a cationic emulsion in patients with mild to moderate dry eye disease – a randomised comparative study. *J Français D'ophtalmologie.* 2014; 37(8):589–598.

29. Pan Q, Angelina A, Marrone M, Stark WJ, Akpek EK. Autologous serum eye drops for dry eye. *Cochrane Db Syst Rev.* 2017;2(2).

30. Ervin A, Law A, Pucker AD. Punctal occlusion for dry eye syndrome. *Cochrane Db Syst Rev.* 2017;6(6).

31. Foulks GN, Harvey T, Raj CVS. Therapeutic contact lenses: the role of high-Dk lenses. *Ophthlamol Clin North Am.* 2003;16(3):455–461. https://doi.org/10.1016/s0896-1549(03)00045-2.

32. Jehangir N, Bever G, Mahmood SMJ, Moshirfar M. Comprehensive review of the literature on existing punctal plugs for the management of dry eye disease. *J Ophthalmol.* 2016;2016:1–22.

33. Balaram M, Schaumberg DA, Dana MR. Efficacy and tolerability outcomes after punctal occlusion with silicone plugs in dry eye syndrome. *Am J Ophthalmol.* 2001;131(1):30–36.

34. Donnenfeld ED, Perry HD, Nattis AS, Rosenberg ED. Lifitegrast for the treatment of dry eye disease in adults. *Expet Opin Pharmacother.* 2017;18(14):1517–1524.

35. Ames P, Galor A. Cyclosporine ophthalmic emulsions for the treatment of dry eye: a review of the clinical evidence. *Clin Invest.* 2015;5(3):267–285.

36. Lollett IV, Galor A. Dry eye syndrome: developments and lifitegrast in perspective. *Clin Ophthalmol.* 2018;12: 125–139.

37. Turner K, Pflugfelder SC, Ji Z, Feuer WJ, Stern M, Reis and BL. Interleukin-6 levels in the conjunctival epithelium of patients with dry eye disease treated with cyclosporine ophthalmic emulsion. *Cornea.* 2000;19(4): 492–496.

38. Kunert K, Tisdale A, Stern M, Smith JA, Gipson E. *Analysis of Topical Cyclosporine Treatment of Patients with Dry Eye Syndrome.* Arch Ophthalmol. American Medical Assocation; 2000:118.

39. Kunert K, Tisdale A, Gipson I. Goblet cell numbers and epithelial proliferation in the conjunctiva of patients with dry eye syndrome treated with cyclosporine. *Arch Ophthalmol.* 2002;120:330–337.

40. Brignole F, Pisella P-J, De Saint Jean M, Goldschild M, Goguel A, Baudouin C. Flow cytometric analysis of inflammatory markers in KCS: 6-month treatment with topical cyclosporin A. *Invest Ophthalmol Vis Sci.* 2001; 42(1):90–95.

41. Chen M, Gong L, Sun X, Xie H, Zhang Y, Zou L, et al. A comparison of cyclosporine 0.05% ophthalmic emulsion versus vehicle in Chinese patients with moderate to severe dry eye disease: an eight-week, multicenter, randomized, double-blind, parallel-group trial. *J Ocul Pharmacol Therapeut.* 2010;26(4):361–366. https://doi.org/10.1089/jop.2009.0145.

42. Deveci H, Kobak S. The efficacy of topical 0.05 % cyclosporine A in patients with dry eye disease associated with Sjögren's syndrome. *Int Ophthalmol.* 2014;34(5): 1043–1048.

43. Stevenson D, Tauber J, Reis BL. Efficacy and safety of cyclosporin A ophthalmic emulsion in the treatment of moderate-to-severe dry eye disease: a dose-ranging, randomized trial. The Cyclosporin A Phase 2 Study Group. *Ophthalmology.* 2000;107(5):967–974.

44. Sall K, Stevenson OD, Mundorf TK, Reis BL, Two multicenter, randomized studies of the efficacy and safety of

cyclosporine ophthalmic emulsion in moderate to severe dry eye disease. CsA Phase 3 Study Group. *Ophthlamology.* 2000;107(4):631−639.

45. Baiza-Durán L, Medrano-Palafox J, Hernández-Quintela E, Lozano-Alcazar J, Alaniz J. A comparative clinical trial of the efficacy of two different aqueous solutions of cyclosporine for the treatment of moderate-to-severe dry eye syndrome. *Br J Ophthalmol.* 2010;94(10):1312.

46. Malhotra R, Devries DK, Luchs J, Kabat A, Schechter B, Lee BS, et al. Effect of OTX-101, a novel nanomicellar formulation of cyclosporine A, on corneal staining in patients with keratoconjunctivitis sicca: a pooled analysis of phase 2b/3 and phase 3 studies. *Cornea.* 2019;38(10):1259−1265.

47. Goldberg DF, Malhotra RP, Schechter BA, Justice A, Weiss SL, Sheppard JD. A phase 3, randomized, double-masked study of OTX-101 ophthalmic solution 0.09% in the treatment of dry eye disease. *Ophthalmology.* 2019;126(9):1230−1237.

48. Smyth-Medina R, Johnston J, Devries DK, et al. Effect of OTX-101, a novel nanomicellar formulation of cyclosporine A, on conjunctival staining in patients with keratoconjunctivitis sicca: a pooled analysis of phase 2b/3 and 3 clinical trials. *J Ocul Pharmacol Therapeut.* 2019;35(7):388−394.

49. Tauber J, Schechter BA, Bacharach J, et al. A Phase II/III, randomized, double-masked, vehicle-controlled, dose-ranging study of the safety and efficacy of OTX-101 in the treatment of dry eye disease. *Clin Ophthalmol.* 2018;12:1921−1929.

50. Byun Y, Kim T, Kwon SM, et al. Efficacy of combined 0.05% cyclosporine and 1% methylprednisolone treatment for chronic dry eye. *Cornea.* 2012;31(5):509−513.

51. Sheppard JD, Donnenfeld ED, Holland EJ, et al. Effect of loteprednol etabonate 0.5% on initiation of dry eye treatment with topical cyclosporine 0.05%. *Eye Contact Lens.* 2014;40(5):289−296.

52. Donnenfeld ED, Karpecki PM, Majmudar PA, et al. Safety of lifitegrast ophthalmic solution 5.0% in patients with dry eye disease: a 1-year, multicenter, randomized, placebo-controlled study. *Cornea.* 2016;35(6):741−748.

53. Drew VJ, Tseng C-L, Seghatchian J, Burnouf T. Reflections on dry eye syndrome treatment: therapeutic role of blood products. *Front Med.* 2018;5:33.

54. Holland EJ, Luchs J, Karpecki PM, et al. Lifitegrast for the treatment of dry eye disease results of a phase III, randomized, double-masked, placebo-controlled trial (OPUS-3). *Ophthalmology.* 2017;124(1):53−60.

55. Perez VL, Pflugfelder SC, Zhang S, Shojaei A, Haque R. Lifitegrast, a novel integrin antagonist for treatment of dry eye disease. *Ocul Surf.* 2016;14(2):207−215.

56. Sheppard JD, Torkildsen GL, Geffin JA, et al. Characterization of tear production in subjects with dry eye disease during intranasal tear neurostimulation: results from two pivotal clinical trials. *Ocul Surf.* 2019;17(1):142−150.

57. Tauber J, Karpecki P, Latkany R, et al. Lifitegrast ophthalmic solution 5.0% versus placebo for treatment

of dry eye disease results of the randomized phase III OPUS-2 study. *Ophthalmology.* 2015;122(12):2423−2431.

58. Pflugfelder SC, Maskin SL, Anderson B, et al. A randomized, double-masked, placebo-controlled, multicenter comparison of loteprednol etabonate ophthalmic suspension, 0.5%, and placebo for treatment of keratoconjunctivitis sicca in patients with delayed tear clearance. *Am J Ophthalmol.* 2004;138(3):444−457.

59. Korenfeld M, Nichols KK, Goldberg D, Evans D, Sall K, Foulks G, et al. Safety of KPI-121 ophthalmic suspension 0.25% in patients with dry eye disease: a pooled analysis of 4 multicenter, randomized, vehicle-controlled studies. *Cornea.* 2021;40(5).

60. Pinto-Fraga J, López-Miguel A, González-García MJ, Fernández I, López-de-la-Rosa A, Enríquez-de-Salamanca A, et al. Topical fluorometholone protects the ocular surface of dry eye patients from desiccating stress A randomized controlled clinical trial. *Ophthalmology.* 2016;123(1):141−153.

61. Jonisch J, Steiner A, Udell IJ. Preservative-free low-dose dexamethasone for the treatment of chronic ocular surface disease refractory to standard therapy. *Cornea.* 2010;29(7):723−726.

62. Marsh P, Pflugfelder SC. Topical nonpreserved methylprednisolone therapy for keratoconjunctivitis sicca in Sjogren syndrome. *Ophthlamology.* 1999;106(4):811−816.

63. Foulks GN, Borchman D, Yappert M, Kakar S. Topical azithromycin and oral doxycycline therapy of meibomian gland dysfunction. *Cornea.* 2013;32(1):44−53.

64. Pfeffer I, Borelli C, Zierhut M, Schaller M. Treatment of ocular rosacea with 40 mg doxycycline in a slow release form. *JDDG J der Deutschen Dermatol Gesellschaft.* 2011;9(11):904−907.

65. Määttä M, Kari O, Tervahartiala T, et al. Tear fluid levels of MMP-8 are elevated in ocular rosacea—treatment effect of oral doxycycline. *Graefe's Arch Clin Exp Ophthalmol.* 2006;244(8):957−962.

66. Frucht-Pery J, Sagi E, Hemo I, Ever-Hadani P. Efficacy of doxycycline and tetracycline in ocular rosacea. *Am J Ophthalmol.* 1993;116(1):88−92.

67. Quarterman MJ, Johnson MDW, Abele MDC, Lesher MJL, Hull MDS, Davis MLS. Ocular rosacea. *Arch Dermatol.* 1997;133:49−54.

68. Seal DV, Wright P, Ficker L, Hagan K, Troski M, Menday P. Placebo controlled trial of fusidic acid gel and oxytetracycline for recurrent blepharitis and rosacea. *Br J Ophthalmol.* 1995;79(1):42.

69. Lee H, Min K, Kim EK, Kim T-I. Minocycline controls clinical outcomes and inflammatory cytokines in moderate and severe meibomian gland dysfunction. *Am J Ophthalmol.* 2012;154(6):949−957.e1.

70. Aronowicz JD, Shine WE, Oral D, Vargas JM, McCulley JP. Short term oral minocycline treatment of meibomianitis. *Br J Ophthalmol.* 2006;90(7):856.

71. Foulks GN, Borchman D, Yappert M, Kim S-H, McKay JW. Topical azithromycin therapy for meibomian

gland dysfunction: clinical response and lipid alterations. *Cornea*. 2010;29(7):781–788.

72. Li J, Zhang X, Zheng Q, Zhu Y, Wang H, Ma H, et al. Comparative evaluation of silicone hydrogel contact lenses and autologous serum for management of sjögren syndrome-associated dry eye. *Cornea*. 2015;34(9), 1072–788.

73. Haque RM, Torkildsen GL, Brubaker K, et al. Multicenter open-label study evaluating the efficacy of azithromycin ophthalmic solution 1% on the signs and symptoms of subjects with blepharitis. *Cornea*. 2010;29(8):871–877.

74. Luchs J. Efficacy of topical azithromycin ophthalmic solution 1% in the treatment of posterior blepharitis. *Adv Ther*. 2008;25(9):858–870.

75. McCulley JP. Blepharoconjunctivitis. *Int Ophthalmol Clin*. 1984;24(2):65–77.

76. Igami TZ, Holzchuh R, Osaki TH, Santo RM, Kara-Jose N, Hida RY. Oral azithromycin for treatment of posterior blepharitis. *Cornea*. 2011;30(10):1145–1149.

77. Bakar Ö, Demircay Z, Toker E, Çakır S. Ocular signs, symptoms and tear function tests of papulopustular rosacea patients receiving azithromycin. *J Eur Acad Dermatol*. 2009;23(5):544–549.

78. Bakar Ö, Demirçay Z, Gürbüz and O. Therapeutic potential of azithromycin in rosacea. *Int J Dermatol*. 2004; 43(2):151–154.

79. Fernandez-Obregon A. Oral use of azithromycin for the treatment of acne rosacea. *Arch Dermatol*. 2004;140(4): 489–490.

80. Noble BA, Loh RSK, MacLennan S, et al. Comparison of autologous serum eye drops with conventional therapy in a randomised controlled crossover trial for ocular surface disease. *Br J Ophthalmol*. 2004;88(5):647.

81. Jeng BH. Use of autologous serum in the treatment of ocular surface disorders. *Arch Ophthalmol*. 2011; 129(12):1610–1612.

82. Mondy P, Brama T, Fisher J, et al. Sustained benefits of autologous serum eye drops on self-reported ocular symptoms and vision-related quality of life in Australian patients with dry eye and corneal epithelial defects. *Transfus Apher Sci*. 2015;53(3):404–411.

83. Semeraro F, Forbice E, Braga O, Bova A, Salvatore AD, Azzolini C. Evaluation of the efficacy of 50% autologous serum eye drops in different ocular surface pathologies. *BioMed Res Int*. 2014;2014:1–11.

84. Tsubota K, Goto E, Fujita H, Ono M, Inoue H, Saito I, et al. Treatment of dry eye by autologous serum application in Sjögren's syndrome. *Br J Ophthalmol*. 1999; 83(4):390.

85. Fox RI, Chan R, Michelson JB, Belmont JB, Michelson PE. Beneficial effect of artificial tears made with autologous serum in patients with keratoconjunctivitis sicca. *Arthritis Rheum*. 1984;27(4):459–461.

86. Kojima T, Higuchi A, Goto E, Matsumoto Y, Dogru M, Tsubota K. Autologous serum eye drops for the treatment of dry eye diseases. *Cornea*. 2008;27(Suppl 1):S25–S30.

87. Alio JL, Rodriguez AE, Ferreira-Oliveira R, Wróbel-Dudzińska D, Abdelghany AA. Treatment of dry eye disease with autologous platelet-rich plasma: A prospective, interventional, non-randomized study. *Ophthalmol Ther*. 2017;6(2):285–293.

88. López-Plandolit S, Morales M-C, Freire V, Grau AE, Durán JA. Efficacy of plasma rich in growth factors for the treatment of dry eye. *Cornea*. 2011;30(12): 1312–1317.

89. Pezzotta S, Fante CD, Scudeller L, Rossi GC, Perotti C, Bianchi PE, et al. Long-term safety and efficacy of autologous platelet lysate drops for treatment of ocular GvHD. *Bone Marrow Transplant*. 2017;52(1):101–106.

90. Craig JP, Chen Y-H, Turnbull PRK. *Prospective Trial of Intense Pulsed Light for the Treatment of Meibomian Gland Dysfunction*. The Association for Research in Vision and Ophthalmology, Inc.; 2015.

91. Vegunta S, Patel D, Shen JF. Combination therapy of intense pulsed light therapy and meibomian gland expression (IPL/MGX) can improve dry eye symptoms and meibomian gland function in patients with refractory dry eye: a retrospective analysis. *Cornea*. 2016; 35(3):318–322.

92. Toyos R, McGill W, Briscoe D. Intense pulsed light treatment for dry eye disease due to meibomian gland dysfunction; A 3-year retrospective study. *Photomed Laser Surg*. 2015;33(1):41–46.

93. Gupta PK, Vora GK, Matossian C, Kim M, Stinnett S. Outcomes of intense pulsed light therapy for treatment of evaporative dry eye disease. *Can J Ophthalmol J Can D'ophtalmologie*. 2016;51(4):249–253.

94. Dell SJ, Gaster RN, Barbarino SC, Cunningham DN. Prospective evaluation of intense pulsed light and meibomian gland expression efficacy on relieving signs and symptoms of dry eye disease due to meibomian gland dysfunction. *Clin Ophthalmol*. 2017;11:817–827.

95. Blackie C, Coleman C, Holland E. The sustained effect (12 months) of a single-dose vectored thermal pulsation procedure for meibomian gland dysfunction and evaporative dry eye. *Clin Ophthalmol*. 2016;10:1385–1396.

96. Lane SS, DuBiner HB, Epstein RJ, Ernest PH, Greiner JV, Hardten DR, et al. A new system, the LipiFlow, for the treatment of meibomian gland dysfunction. *Cornea*. 2012;31(4):396–404.

97. Kim MJ, Stinnett SS, Gupta PK. Effect of thermal pulsation treatment on tear film parameters in dry eye disease patients. *Clin Ophthalmol*. 2017;11:883–886.

98. Greiner JV. A single LipiFlow® thermal pulsation system treatment improves meibomian gland function and reduces dry eye symptoms for 9 months. *Curr Eye Res*. 2012;37(4):272–278.

99. Finis D, Hayajneh J, König C, Borrelli M, Schrader S, Geerling G. Evaluation of an automated thermodynamic treatment (LipiFlow®) system for meibomian gland dysfunction: a prospective, randomized, observer-masked trial. *Ocul Surf*. 2014;12(2):146–154.

100. Tauber J, Owen J, Bloomenstein M, Hovanesian J, Bullimore MA. Comparison of the iLUX and the LipiFlow for the treatment of meibomian gland dysfunction and symptoms: a randomized clinical trial. *Clin Ophthalmol.* 2020;14:405−418.

101. Kislan T. *New, Targeted Technology for Treating the Root Cause of Dry Eye Disease (DED) [Internet].* MiBo Medical; February 28, 2021. Available from: https://mibomedical group.com/articles/.

102. Badawi D. A novel system, TearCare®, for the treatment of the signs and symptoms of dry eye disease. *Clin Ophthalmol.* 2018;12:683−694.

103. Karpecki P, Wirta D, Osmanovic S, Dhamdhere K. A prospective, post-market, multicenter trial (CHEETAH) suggested TearCare® system as a safe and effective blink-assisted eyelid device for the treatment of dry eye disease. *Clin Ophthalmol.* 2020;14:4551−4559.

104. Badawi D. TearCare® system extension study: evaluation of the safety, effectiveness, and durability through 12 months of a second TearCare® treatment on subjects with dry eye disease. *Clin Ophthalmol.* 2019;13:189−198.

105. Maskin SL. Intraductal meibomian gland probing relieves symptoms of obstructive meibomian gland dysfunction. *Cornea.* 2010;29(10):1145−1152.

106. Maskin SL, Testa WR. Growth of meibomian gland tissue after intraductal meibomian gland probing in patients with obstructive meibomian gland dysfunction. *Br J Ophthalmol.* 2018;102(1):59.

107. Wladis EJ. Intraductal meibomian gland probing in the management of ocular rosacea. *Ophthalmic Plast Rec.* 2012;28(6):416−418.

108. Syed ZA, Sutula FC. Dynamic intraductal meibomian probing. *Ophthalmic Plast Rec.* 2017;33(4):307−309.

109. Murphy O, O'Dwyer V, Lloyd-McKernan A. The efficacy of tea tree face wash, 1, 2-Octanediol and microblepharoexfoliation in treating Demodex folliculorum blepharitis. *Contact Lens Anterior Eye.* 2018;41(1):77−82.

110. Epstein IJ, Rosenberg E, Stuber R, Choi MB, Donnenfeld ED, Perry HD. Double-masked and unmasked prospective study of terpinen-4-ol lid scrubs with microblepharoexfoliation for the treatment of Demodex blepharitis. *Cornea.* 2020;39(4):408−416.

111. Dieckmann G, Fregni F, Hamrah P. Neurostimulation in dry eye disease—past, present, and future. *Ocul Surf.* 2018;17(1):20−27.

112. Chayet A, Friedman N, Valdez KB, Silva NR, Loudin J, Baba S. A nonrandomized, open-label study to evaluate the effect of nasal stimulation on tear production in subjects with dry eye disease. *Clin Ophthalmol.* 2016;10: 795−804.

113. Gumus K, Schuetzle KL, Pflugfelder SC. Randomized, controlled, crossover trial comparing the impact of sham or intranasal neurostimulation on conjunctival goblet cell degranulation. *Am J Ophthalmol.* 2017;177: 159−168.

114. Cohn GS, Corbett D, Tenen A, Coroneo M, McAlister J, Craig JP, et al. Randomized, controlled, double-masked, multicenter, pilot study evaluating safety and efficacy of intranasal neurostimulation for dry eye disease. *Invest Ophthalmol Vis Sci.* 2019;60(1):147−153.

115. Pattar GR, Jerkins G, Evans DG, Torkildsen GL, Ousler GW, Hollander DA, et al. Symptom improvement in dry eye subjects following intranasal tear neurostimulation: results of two studies utilizing a controlled adverse environment. *Ocul Surf.* 2020;18(2):249−257.

116. Passi SF, Brooks CC, Thompson AC, Gupta PK. Optical quality and tear film analysis before and after intranasal stimulation in patients with dry eye syndrome. *Clin Ophthalmol.* 2020;14:1987−1992.

117. Farhangi M, Cheng AM, Baksh B, Sarantopoulos CD, Felix ER, Levitt RC, et al. Effect of non-invasive intranasal neurostimulation on tear volume, dryness and ocular pain. *Br J Ophthalmol.* 2020;104(9):1310−1316.

118. Pondelis N, Dieckmann GM, Jamali A, Kataguiri P, Senchyna M, Hamrah P. Infrared meibography allows detection of dimensional changes in meibomian glands following intranasal neurostimulation. *Ocul Surf.* 2020; 18(3):511−516.

119. Ji MH, Moshfeghi DM, Periman L, Kading D, Matossian C, Walman G, et al. Novel extranasal tear stimulation: pivotal study results. *Transl Vis Sci Technol.* 2020; 9(12), 23−23.

120. *Oyster Point Pharma Announces Positive Results in ONSET-2 Phase 3 Trial of OC-01 Nasal Spray for the Treatment of the Signs and Symptoms of Dry Eye Disease [Internet].* 2020; February 28, 2021. Available from: https://www. globenewswire.com/news-release/2020/05/11/2030882/ 0/en/Oyster-Point-Pharma-Announces-Positive-Results-in-ONSET-2-Phase-3-Trial-of-OC-01-Nasal-Spray-for-the-Treat ment-of-the-Signs-and-Symptoms-of-Dry-Eye-Disease.html? print=1.

121. Wirta D, Vollmer P, Paauw J, Chiu KH, Henry E, Striffler K, et al. ONSET-2 Study Group. Efficacy and safety of OC-01 (Varenicline) nasal spray on signs and symptoms of dry eye disease: the ONSET-2 phase 3, randomized trial. *Ophthalmology.* 2021. https://doi.org/ 10.1016/j.ophtha.2021.11.004.

122. Ahad MA, Anandan M, Tah V, Dhingra S, Leyland M. Randomized controlled study of ocular lubrication versus bandage contact lens in the primary treatment of recurrent corneal erosion syndrome. *Cornea.* 2013;32(10): 1311−1314.

123. Siu GDJ-Y, Young AL, Jhanji V. Alternatives to corneal transplantation for the management of bullous keratopathy. *Curr Opin Ophthalmol.* 2014;25(4): 347−352.

124. Grentzelos MA, Plainis S, Astyrakakis NI, Diakonis VF, Kymionis GD, Kallinikos P, et al. Efficacy of 2 types of silicone hydrogel bandage contact lenses after photorefractive keratectomy. *J Cataract Refract Surg.* 2009;35(12): 2103−2108.

125. Donnenfeld ED, Selkin BA, Perry HD, Moadel K, Selkin GT, Cohen AJ, et al. Controlled evaluation of a bandage contact lens and a topical nonsteroidal anti, inflammatory drug in treating traumatic corneal abrasions. *Ophthalmology.* 1995;102(6):979−984.

126. Goyal S, Hamrah P. Understanding neuropathic corneal pain—gaps and current therapeutic approaches. *Semin Ophthalmol.* 2016;31(1–2):59–70.

127. Russo PA, Bouchard CS, Galasso JM. Extended-wear silicone hydrogel soft contact lenses in the management of moderate to severe dry eye signs and symptoms secondary to graft-versus-host disease. *Eye Contact Lens.* 2007;33(3):144–147.

128. Heur M, Bach D, Theophanous C, Chiu GB. Prosthetic replacement of the ocular surface ecosystem scleral lens therapy for patients with ocular symptoms of chronic Stevens-Johnson syndrome. *Am J Ophthalmol.* 2014;158(1):49–54.

129. Stason WB, Razavi M, Jacobs DS, Shepard DS, Suaya JA, Johns L, et al. Clinical benefits of the Boston ocular surface prosthesis. *Am J Ophthalmol.* 2010;149(1):54–61.

130. Jacobs DS, Rosenthal P. Boston scleral lens prosthetic device for treatment of severe dry eye in chronic graft-versus-host disease. *Cornea.* 2007;26(10):1195–1199.

131. Romero-Rangel T, Stavrou P, Cotter J, Rosenthal P, Baltatzis S, Foster CS. Gas-permeable scleral contact lens therapy in ocular surface disease. *Am J Ophthalmol.* 2000;130(1):25–32.

132. Agranat JS, Kitos NR, Jacobs DS. Prosthetic replacement of the ocular surface ecosystem: impact at 5 years. *Br J Ophthalmol.* 2016;100(9):1171.

133. Dimit R, Gire A, Pflugfelder SC, Bergmanson JPG. Patient ocular conditions and clinical outcomes using a PROSE scleral device. *Contact Lens Anterior Eye.* 2013;36(4):159–163.

134. Theophanous C, Irvine JA, Parker P, Chiu GB. Use of prosthetic replacement of the ocular surface ecosystem scleral lenses in patients with ocular chronic graft-versus-host disease. *Biol Blood Marrow Transplant.* 2015;21(12):2180–2184.

135. DeLoss KS, Le H-G, Gire A, Chiu GB, Jacobs DS, Carrasquillo KG. PROSE treatment for ocular chronic graft-versus-host disease as a clinical network expands. *Eye Contact Lens.* 2016;42(4):262–266.

136. Papakostas TD, Le H-G, Chodosh J, Jacobs DS. Prosthetic replacement of the ocular surface ecosystem as treatment for ocular surface disease in patients with a history of Stevens–Johnson syndrome/toxic epidermal necrolysis. *Ophthalmology.* 2015;122(2):248–253.

137. Lim P, Ridges R, Jacobs DS, Rosenthal P. Treatment of persistent corneal epithelial defect with overnight wear of a prosthetic device for the ocular surface. *Am J Ophthalmol.* 2013;156(6):1095–1101.

138. Cressey A, Jacobs DS, Remington C, Carrasquillo KG. Improvement of chronic corneal opacity in ocular surface disease with prosthetic replacement of the ocular surface ecosystem (PROSE) treatment. *Am J Ophthalmol Case Rep.* 2018;10:108–113.

139. Takahide K, Parker PM, Wu M, Hwang WY, Carpenter PA, Moravec C, et al. Use of fluid-ventilated, gas-permeable scleral lens for management of severe keratoconjunctivitis sicca secondary to chronic graft-versus-host disease. *Biol Blood Marrow Transplant.* 2007;13(9):1016–1021.

140. Kloek CE, Jeng-Miller KW, Jacobs DS, Dunn IF. Prosthetic replacement of the ocular surface ecosystem treatment of ocular surface disease after skull base tumor resection. *World Neurosurg.* 2018;110:e124–e128.

141. Nguyen MTB, Thakrar V, Chan CC. EyePrintPRO therapeutic scleral contact lens: indications and outcomes. *Can J Ophthalmol.* 2018;53(1):66–70.

142. Shay E, Kheirkhah A, Liang L, Sheha H, Gregory DG, Tseng SCG. Amniotic membrane transplantation as a new therapy for the acute ocular manifestations of Stevens-Johnson syndrome and toxic epidermal necrolysis. *Surv Ophthalmol.* 2009;54(6):686–696.

143. Arya S, Bhala S, Malik A, Sood S. Role of amniotic membrane transplantation in ocular surface disorders. *Nepal J Ophthalmol.* 2010;2(2):145–153.

144. Shanbhag SS, Hall L, Chodosh J, Saeed HN. Long-term outcomes of amniotic membrane treatment in acute Stevens-Johnson syndrome/toxic epidermal necrolysis. *Ocul Surf.* 2020;18(3):517–522.

145. Cheng AMS, Zhao D, Chen R, Yin HY, Tighe S, Sheha H, et al. Accelerated restoration of ocular surface Health in dry eye disease by self-retained cryopreserved amniotic membrane. *Ocul Surf.* 2016;14(1):56–63.

146. McDonald MB, Sheha H, Tighe S, Janik SB, Bowden FW, Chokshi AR, et al. Treatment outcomes in the DRy eye amniotic membrane (DREAM) study. *Clin Ophthalmol.* 2018;12:677–681.

147. Morkin MI, Hamrah P. Efficacy of self-retained cryopreserved amniotic membrane for treatment of neuropathic corneal pain. *Ocul Surf.* 2018;16(1):132–138.

148. Liu D. Conjunctivochalasis. *Ophthalmic Plast Reconstr Surg.* 1986;2(1):25–28.

149. Petris CK, Holds JB. Medial conjunctival resection for tearing associated with conjunctivochalasis. *Ophthalmic Plast Rec.* 2013;29(4):304–307.

150. Nakasato S, Uemoto R, Mizuki N. Thermocautery for inferior conjunctivochalasis. *Cornea.* 2012;31(5):514–519.

151. Zhang X-R, Zhang Z-Y, Hoffman MR. Electrocoagulative surgical procedure for treatment of conjunctivochalasis. *Int Surg.* 2012;97(1):90–93.

152. Otaka I, Kyu N. A new surgical technique for management of conjunctivochalasis. *Am J Ophthalmol.* 2000;129(3):385–387.

153. Yang HS, Choi S. New approach for conjunctivochalasis using an argon green laser. *Cornea.* 2013;32(5):574–578.

154. Meerovitch K, Torkildsen G, Lonsdale J, Goldfarb H, Lama T, Cumberlidge G, et al. Safety and efficacy of MIM D3 ophthalmic solutions in a randomized placebo controlled phase 2 clinical trial in patients with dry eye. *Clin Ophthalmol.* 2013;7:1275–1285.

155. Coassin M, Lambiase A, Costa N, De Gregorio A, Sgrulletta R, Sacchetti M, et al. Efficacy of topical nerve growth factor treatment in dogs affected by dry eye. *Graefe's Arch Clin Exp Ophthalmol.* 2005;243(2):151–155.

156. Bonini S, Rama P, Olzi D, Lambiase A. Neurotrophic keratitis. *Eye.* 2003;17(8):989–995.

157. Ma K, Yan N, Huang Y, Cao G, Deng J, Deng Y. Effects of nerve growth factor on nerve regeneration after corneal nerve damage. *Int J Clin Exp Med*. 2014;7(11): 4584−4589.

158. Mastropasqua L, Massaro-Giordano G, Nubile M, Sacchetti M. Understanding the pathogenesis of neurotrophic keratitis: the role of corneal nerves. *J Cell Physiol*. 2017;232(4):717−724.

159. Sacchetti M, Lambiase A, Schmidl D, Schmetterer L, Ferrari M, Mantelli F, et al. Effect of recombinant human nerve growth factor eye drops in patients with dry eye: a phase IIa, open label, multiple-dose study. *Br J Ophthalmol*. 2020;104(1):127−135.

160. McNamara NA, Ge S, Lee SM, Enghauser AM, Kuehl L, Chen FY, et al. Reduced levels of tear lacritin are associated with corneal neuropathy in patients with the ocular component of Sjögren's syndrome dry eye alters tear lacritin and corneal nerves. *Invest Ophthalmol Vis Sci*. 2016; 57(13):5237−5243.

161. Vijmasi T, Chen FY, Balasubbu S, Gallup M, McKown RL, Laurie GW, et al. Topical administration of lacritin is a novel therapy for aqueous-deficient dry eye disease novel therapy for aqueous-deficient DED. *Invest Ophthalmol Vis Sci*. 2014;55(8):5401−5409.

162. Lambiase A, Sullivan BD, Schmidt TA, Sullivan DA, Jay GD, Truitt ER, et al. A two-week, randomized, double-masked study to evaluate safety and efficacy of lubricin (150 μg/mL) eye drops versus sodium hyaluronate (HA) 0.18% eye drops (Vismed®) in patients with moderate dry eye disease. *Ocul Surf*. 2017;15(1):77−87.

163. Schmidt TA, Sullivan DA, Knop E, Richards SM, Knop N, Liu S, et al. Transcription, translation, and function of lubricin, a boundary lubricant, at the ocular surface. *JAMA Ophthalmol*. 2013;131(6):766−776.

164. Sosne G, Dunn SP, Kim C. Thymosin b4 significantly improves signs and symptoms of severe dry eye in a phase 2 randomized trial. *Cornea*. 2015;34(5):491−496.

165. Dunn SP, Heidemann DG, Chow CY, Crockford D, Turjman N, Angel J, et al. Treatment of chronic nonhealing neurotrophic corneal epithelial defects with thymosin beta 4. *Arch Ophthalmol*. 2010;128(5): 636−638.

166. Kim CE, Kleinman HK, Sosne G, Ousler GW, Kim K, Yang J. RGN-259 (thymosin β4) improves clinically important dry eye efficacies in comparison with prescription drugs in a dry eye model. *Sci Rep-UK*. 2018;8(1): 10500.

167. Murri MS, Moshirfar M, Birdsong OC, Ronquillo YC, Ding Y, Hoopes PC. Amniotic membrane extract and eye drops: a review of literature and clinical application. *Clin Ophthalmol*. 2018;12:1105−1112.

168. Steven P, Scherer D, Krösser S, Beckert M, Cursiefen C, Kaercher T. Semifluorinated alkane eye drops for treatment of dry eye disease—a prospective, multicenter non-interventional study. *J Ocul Pharmacol Therapeut*. 2015; 31(8):498−503.

169. Steven P, Augustin AJ, Geerling G, Kaercher T, Kretz F, Kunert K, et al. Semifluorinated alkane eye drops for treatment of dry eye disease due to meibomian gland disease. *J Ocul Pharmacol Therapeut*. 2017;33(9): 678−685.

170. Tauber J, Wirta DL, Sall K, Majmudar PA, Willen D, Krösser S. A randomized clinical study (SEECASE) to assess efficacy, safety, and tolerability of NOV03 for treatment of dry eye disease. *Cornea*. 2020;40(9):1132−1140.

171. Clark D, Sheppard J, Brady TC. A randomized double-masked phase 2a trial to evaluate activity and safety of topical ocular reproxalap, a novel RASP inhibitor, in dry eye disease. *J Ocul Pharmacol Therapeut*. 2021;37(4): 193−199.

172. Clark D, Tauber J, Sheppard J, Brady TC. Early onset and broad activity of reproxalap in a randomized, double-masked, vehicle-controlled phase 2b trial in dry eye disease. *Am J Ophthalmol*. 2021;226(22−31).

173. Lindstrom R, Donnenfeld E, Holland E, Karageozian V, Park J, Sarayba M, et al. Safety and efficacy of ALG-1007 topical ophthalmic solution − a synthetic peptide that regulates inflammation, in patients with dry eye disease: an exploratory Phase I, open-label, single-center clinical study. *Am J Ophthalmic Clin Trials*. 2020;3(10): 1−9.

174. Spana C, Taylor AW, Yee DG, Makhlina M, Yang W, Dodd J. Probing the role of melanocortin type 1 receptor agonists in diverse immunological diseases. *Front Pharmacol*. 2019;9:1535.

175. *PL9643 for dry eye disease [Internet]*. 2020; February 28, 2021. Available from: https://www.palatin.com//assets/PL9643-DED-Phase-2-Clinical-Data-Presentation.pdf.

176. *Azura Ophthalmics Announces Primary Endpoints Met in Phase 2 Trial of Investigational Treatment for Contact Lens Discomfort [Internet]*. 2020; February 28, 2021. Available from: https://eyewire.news/articles/azura-ophthalmics-announces-primary-endpoints-met-in-phase-2-trial-of-investigational-treatment-for-contact-lens-discomfort/.

CHAPTER 12

Treatment of Dry Eye Disease in Asia

TAKASHI KOJIMA, MD, PHD • ZUGUO LIU, MD, PHD • MURAT DOGRU, MD, PHD •
NORIHIKO YOKOI, MD, PHD • KYUNG CHUL YOON, MD, PHD •
LOUIS TONG, MBBS, FRCS, MD, PHD • CHI CHIN SUN, MD, PHD •
VILAVUN PUANGSRICHARERN, MD • CHI HOANG VIET VU, MD, PHD •
KAZUO TSUBOTA, MD, PHD

INTRODUCTION

Dry eye disease (DED) is a significant public health problem in many parts of the world, not only because it causes restriction of social and daily activities but it causes undeniable economical burden due to health-related costs and loss of working hours.[1] DE has been reported to be more prevalent in Asia compared to the rest of the world, which might be related to genetics or lifestyles of Asians, and some ophthalmic diseases are more prevalent in Asia, such as myopia.[2] Recently, DE has been considered to be due to lifestyle changes such as increased use of visual display terminals (VDTs), using smartphones for longer hours, diet, lack of omega 3 fatty acid diet, lack of exercise, or sleep disorders.[3–7] Likewise, myopia is recently considered to be a lifestyle disorder and related to sleep, omega 3 fatty acid intake, exercise, outdoor activities, in addition to VDT use.[8,9] The overall prevalence of symptomatic DED in Asia ranged between 14.4% and 24.4%.[10–14] Symptomatic DE is also prevalent in high school students in China and Japan, where the prevalence ranged between 21% and 24%[11,14] which was considerably higher than rates in adults, of 9.8%–11.5% in men and 18.7%–19.4% in women.[11,13,14] South East Asian Studies using DE definition showed the highest prevalence rates of symptomatic DED, ranging from 20.0% to 52.4%.[15–18] In Singapore, two studies showed a prevalence of only 6.5% and 12.3%.[19,20] In Korea, using a strategy based on definition, the prevalence of symptomatic DED was reported to be around 20%.[21]

In the 1990s, tear deficiency was still the central concept in DE. Large-scale epidemiological studies performed in China, Singapore, Korea and Japan on the role of longer hours of VDT work and smart phone use suggesting a higher incidence of resultant short tear film break-up time (TBUT) type of DEs started to cause a paradigm shift in diagnosis and treatment of DED favoring the tear instability as a core factor in diagnosis and treatment. Japan, China, and Korea established the Asia Dry Eye Society (ADES) in 2012. As a result of successive meetings held in 2013 and 2014, the society published the definition in a separate report as "Dry eye is a multifactorial disease characterized by unstable tear film causing a variety of symptoms and/or visual impairment, potentially accompanied by ocular surface damage."[22] According to the new definition, presence of symptoms of either discomfort or visual disturbance is essential.[22] The ADES report concluded that DE questionnaires outlined in the DEWS report including Ocular Surface Disease Index (OSDI), McMonnies questionnaire, Women's Health Study Questionnaire or the recently reported DE-related quality of life (QOL) score (DEQS), appear as useful tools, but questionnaires assessing the visual impairment in daily life may provide additional and helpful information in the context of this new definition.[22]

Since tear film instability is pivotal in the definition of DE, the measurement of TBUT is a mandatory step.[22] The major problems in dealing with DED are a lack of consensus on the appropriate diagnostic criteria, classification of disease states, the aim of specific diagnostic tests, the role of symptoms in disease and treatment response assessment, and interpretation of results. Despite attempts to attain a consensus in diagnosis, classification, and treatment protocols of DED in Asia, there appears to be a significant regional variation in such protocols resulting from availability of different eye drops and cultural influences.

This chapter aims to provide an insight to DE diagnostic and treatment preferences in different parts of Asia.

Dry Eye Disease. https://doi.org/10.1016/B978-0-323-82753-9.00014-X

CURRENT DRY EYE THERAPIES IN CHINA

DE is the most common disease in eye clinics, with an incidence of 6.1%–59.1% in China.[23,24] The incidence of DE is higher compared to western countries. With the arrival of the era of "screen reading," the incidence of DE is fast increasing in China. Therapies for DE are diverse and complex in China. Individualized and comprehensive treatment is recommended to all patients.[25,26] A healthy lifestyle such as sufficient sleep, adequate exercise, and a healthy diet is emphasized in the treatment.

Pharmacotherapy

More than 20 commercial artificial tears are available in China, which include water and viscosity-enhancing agents such as sodium hyaluronate, carboxymethocel, hydroxypropyl methyl cellulose, poly-vinyl, povidone, polyethylene glycol, and capom 940 (polyacrylic Acid). Three percent diquafosol tetrasodium, a purinergic P2Y2 receptor agonist that stimulates water and mucin secretion, was approved as an ophthalmic solution for the mucin deficiency DE 3 years ago.[27] Eye drops that promote corneal epithelial healing are used for DE patients with corneal defects. Two such kinds of eye drops are fibroblast growth factor and epidermal growth factor eye drops.[28,29] They also show the effect of increasing the goblet cells and mucin secretion. An eyedrop from the deproteinized calf blood extract which was proved to promote corneal epithelial repair and improve microenvironment of ocular surface is also commercially available for moderate and severe DE patients. The autologous serum could be a treatment option for severe patients who do not react to routine treatment. A consensus on how to prepare the autologous serum was published recently.[30]

Glucocorticoids, nonsteroidal antiinflammatory drugs (NSAIDs), and immunosuppressants are commonly used antiinflammatory drugs for DE patients. Several glucocorticoids with different concentrations are available for clinician selection. The 0.05%, 1% cyclosporine A and 0.1% tacrolimus are prescribed for moderate to severe DE patients depending on their severity. NSAIDs are a common choice for mild and moderate DE patients who do not respond to artificial tears but have no related immune disorders. It is also used as an alternative choice for DE patients who cannot bear the side effects of glucocorticoids. Several antibiotics that have both antibacterial and antiinflammatory effects, such as tetracycline and azithromycin, are used for meibomian gland dysfunction (MGD) patients with abnormal eyelid and blepharitis.[31]

Physical Therapy

Physical therapies are very popular in China, which include a wide range of strategies, from lid hygiene, hot compress and fumigation, massage of meibomian gland, intense pulsed light, LipiFlow (LipiFlow Tear Science, Morrisville, NC, USA) to traditional Chinese medicine (TCM) therapies. Appropriate eyelid hygiene is important in managing lid conditions that cause DE (particularly blepharitis) and can reduce lipid by-products and lipolytic bacteria associated with lid diseases. Lid scrubs are gentle cleansers for helping lid hygiene, including a mild dilution of baby shampoo or professional eye wipes and cleaning fluids containing hypochlorous acid, tea tree oil,[32] and its derivatives 4-turpentine alcohol or okra. Heat from a warm compress can soften or liquefy the increased viscosity meibum and thus help patients with DE to improve or restore the meibomian gland function. Patients could receive domestic hot compress items such as hot towel, hot compress eye mask, heated steam mask, etc. Fumigation treatment performed by professional caregivers can promote meibum flow and remove obstruction. Under the guidance of TCM, special TCM ingredients can be prescribed to patients with DE, including wild chrysanthemum, mulberry leaf, or honeysuckle for fumigation. Meibomian gland massage is commonly used in treating DE patients, which includes finger massage for home use and professional massage in hospital using rigid objects such as glass rod, meibomian pad forceps, and squeezing. The purpose of meibomian gland massage is to improve and/or restore the function of the glands by ameliorating or removing ductal obstruction, thus allowing the glands to be functional. Intense pulsed light delivers intense pulses of noncoherent light from 500 to 1200 nm in wavelength and LipiFlow is also a common selection for the treatment of MGD and DE.[33]

Punctal occlusion, moisture chamber spectacles, and contact lenses are also available in China. Punctal occlusion is used for patients with aqueous-deficient DE, especially for moderate to severe DE patients whose symptoms cannot be relieved by artificial tears. Moisture chamber spectacles are able to reduce evaporation of the tears by providing a humid environment and minimizing airflow over the ocular surface.[34] Therapeutic soft contact lens with high oxygen permeability is preferable among patients with corneal epithelium injuries or noninfectious eyelid diseases.

Traditional Chinese Medicine

TCM is currently the best-preserved and most influential traditional medical system with the largest number of users worldwide. In recent years, the trend of adopting TCM in DE has increased greatly in China. The application of TCM in DEs includes herbal, natural products, and Chinese medicine and acupuncture.

Herbal or natural products and chinese medicine

Topical and oral herbal or natural products have been widely used in China for thousands of years. However, relatively few randomized clinical trials have compared herbal medicine with conventional therapies due to the inherent challenges of the way of prescribing herbal medicine. Many of these therapies are based on the traditional "yin" and "yang" theory of Chinese medicine, and practitioners usually treat DE patients with a combination of different Chinese herbs. Chinese medicine can be prepared and used in eye drops, eye patches, and steam inhalations. Chinese medicine eye drops have been applied in patients with DE for many years in China,[35] such as *houttuynia* eye drops and ZhenZhu-MingMuDiYanYe (HaiBao). Recently, a randomized, double-blinded, placebo-controlled clinical trial of our group showed *houttuynia* atomized liquid had good curative effects on MGD-related DE. Furthermore, Chinese medicine eye patch showed a significant improvement in symptoms of DE.[36]

Acupuncture

Acupuncture is a long-standing intervention in China to treat a wide variety of conditions. Studies have shown that stimulation of the peripheral nervous system with a concomitant central effect by acupuncture could be the mechanism of pain relief, which might then affect pain perception, alter inflammation or peripheral sensations, or "retrain" peripheral nerves in pain sensation.[37] Acupuncture has been reported to improve TBUT, Schirmer scores, and corneal staining to a greater degree than artificial tears.

Therapeutic Strategies for Different Types of Dry Eye in China

Strategies for managing DE are based on classification and grading of DE. DEs are classified into five types in China. Table 12.1 below shows the therapeutic choices.[25]

DRY EYE THERAPY IN JAPAN BASED ON TFOD AND TFOT

Introduction and Epidemiology

Since 1995, the DE diagnostic criteria in Japan focused on objective measures of tear stability, tear quantity assessment, and presence of positive vital stainings. Participation of Japan to the International DE workshop during 2004–07 resulted in recognition of the importance of symptom assessment which led to the incorporation of symptoms into Japanese diagnostic criteria and a surge of questionnaire-based epidemiological studies which revealed a prevalence of between 8.7% and 30.1%.[38] These studies also revealed that the short BUT type of DED especially among office workers and due to extensive use of smart phones was much more prevalent in Japan. Such findings of those epidemiological studies and introduction of mucin secretagogue eye drops in Japan resulted in a revision of Japanese DE diagnostic criteria which supports the conduct of TBUT tests and symptom assessment to diagnose the majority of DEs. The diagnostic recommendations include checking the vital stainings and tear quantity to diagnose the subtypes. Recently, classifying DEs from break up patterns is a hot topic of investigation in Japan. The section of DE management in Japan covers the logical reasons for the changes of diagnostic guidelines in Japan in alignment with ADES.

Through the accumulated report for the tears, tear film, and DE,[39] the primary mechanisms that are associated with subjective eye symptoms in DE are the instability of tear film and increased friction,[40] because a stable tear film can cover the ocular surface epithelium within the interpalpebral zone via the stability of tear film when the eye is kept open and tears function as a lubricant during blinking. Those primary mechanisms, when they are activated via the respective dysfunction of tear film or tears, may result in a variety of ocular surface epithelial damage, inflammation, and neurosensory response, each of which may explain a variety of symptoms in DE.[39–41] In this comprehensive understanding for DE, only unstable tear film and resultant epithelial damage can be visualized simply by fluorescein-assisted slit-lamp biomicroscopy. Thus, one of the objective signs, tear film break-up, can become a clue to understand not only the mechanism but also symptoms for DE.[42] Accordingly, unstable tear film, one of the visible characteristics in DE, from the clinical aspect, is emphasized in the definition and diagnostic criteria for DE not only in Asia but also in Western countries.[22,41,43–45]

Tear Film–Oriented Diagnosis and Tear Film–Oriented Therapy

In Japan, a paradigm shift has come in the diagnosis and therapy for DE, after new eye drops have become available from December 2010 to January 2012 as prescribed eye drops to treat DE, first in the world. Those

TABLE 12.1
Therapeutic Choices for Dry Eye in China.

Treatments/Classification	Pharmacotherapy	Physical Therapy and Others
Aqueous deficient type	1. Artificial tears 2. Topical secretagogues 3. Topical glucocorticoids or immunosuppressants 4. Autologous serum(severe corneal epithelium lesions)	1. Punctal occlusion 2. Moisture chamber spectacles 3. Treatments of systemic diseases 4. Surgical treatments
Abnormal lipid type	1. Artificial tears 2. Topical secretagogues 3. Topical sterilization of mites 4. Topical antibiotics and/or glucocorticoids or immunosuppressants 5. Oral administration of doxycycline or azithromycin	1. Moisture chamber spectacles 2. Nondrug and physical therapy of eyelid
Abnormal mucin type	1. Artificial tears containing no or less toxic preservatives 2. Topical secretagogues 3. Topical glucocorticoids or immunosuppressants	1. Punctal occlusion 2. Contact lenses 3. Moisture chamber spectacles
Abnormal tear dynamics type	1. Artificial tears containing no or less toxic preservatives 2. Topical glucocorticoids or immunosuppressants	1. Contact lenses 2. Treatments of systemic diseases 3. Surgical treatments
Mixed type	Comprehensive considerations	

new eye drops include diquafosol sodium and rebamipide which enable to, respectively, supplement aqueous fluid and mucins (both secretory and membrane associated), either of which contribute to the stabilization of tear film leading to the elongation of break-up time of tear film.[46] The availability of those eye drops facilitated the born of a new concept that are layer-by-layer diagnosis and therapy for DE that had not been appeared in the world.[40,47,48] Those new idea for the diagnosis and therapy for DE first born in Japan were coined, respectively, as Tear Film–Oriented Diagnosis (TFOD) and Tear Film–Oriented Therapy (TFOT) (Fig. 12.1)[40,47–49] which are currently expanding to the other Asian countries.

TFOD is a diagnostic method which suggests two points: (1) insufficient component of the ocular surface (aqueous tears, secretory mucins, membrane-associated mucins, and meibomian lipids) and (2) DE subtype of aqueous-deficient DE [ADDE], decreased wettability DE [DWDE], and/or increased evaporation DE [IEDE],

latter of those two constitute short TBUT DE,[50] based on the observation of the upward movement of fluorescein-stained aqueous tear film and the fluorescein break-up patterns (BUPs).[40,47,49,51] In addition, TFOD enables the clinician to propose the most effective treatment for DE, which is coined as TFOT, via the stabilization of tear film through the supplementation of insufficient components to the ocular surface in DE. It is reported that fluorescein BUPs are classified into essentially five categories comprising Area, Line, Spot, Dimple, and Random breaks and are caused by a different pathophysiology depending on the insufficient components of the ocular surface, including aqueous tears, secretory mucins in the aqueous tear film, membrane-associated mucins, and component of ocular surface epithelium.[49] Area and line breaks suggest that the insufficient component of the ocular surface is aqueous tears which are specific to ADDE as DE subtype and DE presenting area or line break can be treated, respectively, by punctal plugs or diquafosol

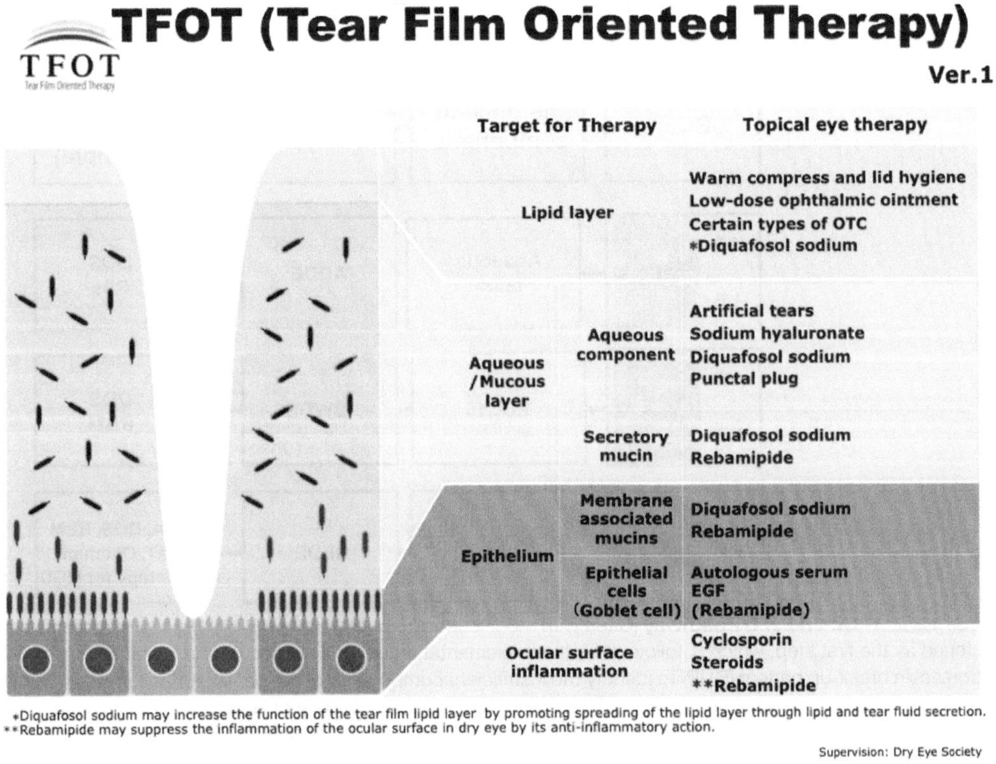

FIG. 12.1 **Concept of TFOT (Tear Film–Oriented Therapy)**. TFOT is a layer-by-layer therapy of the ocular surface for dry eye to treat unstable tear film resulting in dry eye symptoms via the supplementation of the insufficient components of the ocular surface. The topical treatment currently available in each country that can supplement the insufficient components can be selected. This scheme can be cited from the homepage (http://www.dryeye.ne.jp/tfot/index.html). (Figure courtesy of Dry Eye Society of Japan.)

sodium eye drops as TFOT. Spot and dimple breaks suggest the insufficiency of membrane-associated mucins, especially the longest mucin MUC16, corresponding to DWDE, can be treated via the supplementation of diquafosol sodium and/or rebamipide as TFOT. Random break suggests the insufficiency of MUC5AC and/or meibomian lipids, corresponding to IEDE, can be treated by either by hyaluronic acid having water-retentive property, diquafosol, or rebamipide via the increase of goblet cells, or treatment for MGD in DE cases with MGD. Therefore, through TFOD, insufficient components of ocular surface are looked through and DE subtypes are determined and either of which can propose the optimal treatment as TFOT for DE (Fig. 12.2).

In addition, in our recent progress, understanding for blink-related friction has been advancing and blink-related friction has become effectively treated using rebamipide, in which goblet cells at the lid wiper can be increased[52] to attenuate blink-related friction between the lid wiper and eye ball surface during blinking which lead to the attenuation of the symptoms associated with increased friction via the resolution of lid-wiper epitheliopathy,[53] filamentary keratitis,[54] superior limbic keratoconjunctivitis,[55] and conjunctival epithelial damage which are likely to be seen especially in ADDE.[56] Together with the progress in TFOD/TFOT concept, more optimal diagnosis and treatment has been advancing in Japan.

TREATMENT OF DRY EYE IN KOREA
Introduction
According to the Korea National Health and Nutrition Examination Survey 2010–11, the overall prevalence of patients with DE was reported to be 16% among 11,666 participants 19 years of age and older.[12] However, the prevalence of DE has a tendency to increase due to aging and environmental factors.

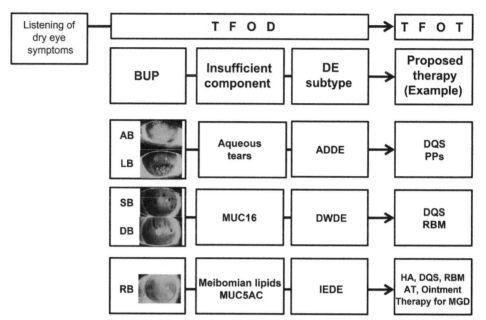

FIG. 12.2 **TFOD and TFOT pathway** (Cited with modification from references 40,49). Dry eye symptoms are listened as the first step, which is followed by the implementation of TFOD based on the classification of fluorescein break-up pattern (BUP) to identify the insufficient components of the ocular surface and to classify the dry eye subtype and as the final step, the most appropriate therapy to supplement the insufficient components with reference to the TFOT options. *AB*, Area break; *AT*, artificial tears; *BUP*, break-up pattern; *DB*, Dimple break; *DQS*, Diquafosol sodium; *HA*, hyaluronic acid; *LB*, Line break; *MGD*, meibomian gland dysfunction; *PPs*, Punctal plugs; *RB*, Random break; *RBM*, rebamipide; *SB*, Spot break.

In 2014, the Korean guideline for the diagnosis and management of DE, mainly based on the DEWS classification, was published by the Korean Corneal Disease Study Group (KCDSG).[57] According to the guideline, DED was defined as "a disease of the ocular surface that is associated with tear film abnormalities." It has been accepted that inflammation in the lacrimal functional unit composed of the ocular surface and lacrimal glands plays a key role in the pathogenesis of DED. According to the guidelines for diagnosis, patients should have at least one DE symptom including ocular and visual symptoms and one objective sign; the ocular surface staining score by the Oxford system was the most important sign, followed by TBUT and Schirmer-1 test score (Table 12.2).[58] DE treatment options were recommended for each particular level (I ~ IV), and the main treatment agents included preserved or nonpreserved artificial tears and antiinflammatory agents (topical corticosteroids and cyclosporine A). After the launching of topical secretagogues and the release of new perspectives on DE definition by the ADES in 2017,[44] the importance of unstable tear film and decreased TBUT

in the pathogenesis of DE was emphasized, and mucin secretagogue (diquafosol sodium) has been used as another main treatment agent. A new definition of DE reported by the TFOS DEWS II in 2017,[43] in which tear film instability and hyperosmolarity, ocular surface inflammation and damage, and neurosensory abnormalities play etiological roles, is now popularly accepted by Korean ophthalmologists. The resolution of theses etiological factors has become basic principles of DE treatment.

The treatment pattern of DE in Korea is interesting as preservative-free artificial tears (hyaluronic acid), antiinflammatory agents (cyclosporine A 0.05% and 0.1% emulsions), and secretagogues (diquafosol sodium) are the mainstay of treatment; these agents are frequently prescribed with insurance coverage, and treatment of MGD is popularly performed at the same time. In 2021, the Korean Dry Eye Society is establishing a revised guideline of DE diagnosis and treatment for DE subtypes including the aqueous deficiency dominant type, evaporation dominant type, and altered tear distribution type.

TABLE 12.2
The Guideline for Diagnosis and Grading of Dry Eye Disease by the Korean Corneal Disease Study Group in 2014.

		Level I	Level II	Level III	Level IV
Symptoms	Ocular symptoms	Sometimes	Often	Always	Daily life limited
	Visual symptoms	Sometimes	Often	Always	Daily life limited
Signs[b]	Staining score[a]	< Grade I	Grade II	Grade III	> Grade IV
	Tear film break-up time	Variable	6–10 s	1–5 s	Immediate
	Schirmer-1	Variable	5< ~ ≤10 mm	2< ~ ≤5 mm	<2 mm

[a] Oxford system.
[b] Positive ocular signs may include conjunctival injection, lid abnormalities (blepharitis, trichiasis, keratinization, and symblepharon), and tear film abnormalities (debris, decreased tear meniscus, and mucus clumping). However, these findings are not to be considered in the grading of disease severity.

Specific Dry Eye Treatment Agents
Artificial tears
The growth rate of the artificial tears market is approximately 15% annually, which is the highest in the ophthalmic market in Korea. Hyaluronic acid (90%) is the most commonly used formulation of artificial tears, followed by carboxymethylcellulose (8%). Hyaluronic acid lubricants have several advantages including 1) increased tear stability facilitated by high viscosity between blinks, 2) uninterrupted blinking due to reduced viscosity under shear stress, 3) resistance to dehydration by binding to water, and 4) promotion of epithelial wound healing which improves ocular surface damages. Many formulations of hyaluronic acid artificial tears are commercially available and can be selected according to the presence of preservatives (preservative-containing and preservative-free), concentration (0.1%, 0.15%, 0.18%, and 0.3%), and tonicity (isotonic and hypotonic).

Preservative-free hyaluronic acid occupies more than 90% of the hyaluronic acid market. The KCDSG recommended the use of preservative-free artificial tears when instillation frequency exceeds 4 times a day. The toxic effects of preservatives such as benzalkonium chloride on the ocular surface have been well accepted by Korean ophthalmologists since 2010. Factors affecting toxicity include concentration, frequency of dosing, amount of tear secretion, and severity of ocular surface diseases. Benzalkonium chloride can induce cellular necrosis and apoptosis and inflammation of the corneal and conjunctival epithelium at concentrations of 0.01% −0.1%. Therefore, it may lead to ocular discomfort on instillation, stinging sensation, foreign body sensation, tearing, and itchy eyelids, and it has been associated with superficial punctate keratitis, conjunctival hyperemia, blepharitis, as well as reduced tear production and TBUT. Compared to preserved formulations, preservative-free formulations have been reported to be more effective in improving symptoms and signs, decreasing ocular inflammation, and increasing tear antioxidant contents in patients with DE.[59,60]

Among the various concentrations of hyaluronic acid, 0.1% and 0.15% concentrations are the most frequently used, followed by 0.18% and 0.1% concentrations. In a clinical study comparing 0.1%, 0.15%, and 0.3% hyaluronic acid with 0.05% cyclosporine in Korean patients with DE, all three hyaluronic acids were effective in improving subjective symptoms and objective signs similar to 0.05% cyclosporine, and the 0.15% hyaluronic acid group showed a better improvement in Schirmer test scores at week 12 than the other groups.[61] In an animal study comparing 0.1%, 0.18%, and 0.3% hyaluronic acid eye drops in the treatment of experimental DE, 0.3% hyaluronic acid was more effective than 0.1% and 0.18% hyaluronic acid in improving tear film instability and ocular surface staining and irregularity, increasing conjunctival goblet cell density, and decreasing corneal epithelial apoptosis.[62] In clinical situations, higher concentrations of hyaluronic acid are preferred for aqueous deficient DE with moderate to severe corneal epithelial staining and evaporative DE with MGD.

Since 2015, the use of hypotonic hyaluronic acid drops has been gradually increasing in patients with inflammatory DE with ocular surface damage, especially those with Sjögren's syndrome. Comparative studies have shown that hypotonic 0.18% hyaluronic acid drops (Kynex II, Alcon Korea, Seoul, Korea) were more effective in improving tear film stability and ocular surface staining and decreasing inflammatory cytokines, chemokines, and cells on the ocular surface of experimental and clinical DE compared to isotonic 0.1% hyaluronic acid (Kynex, Alcon Korea) or 0.5% carboxymethylcellulose (Refresh plus, Allergan, Irvine, CA, USA).[63,64] Similarly, 0.3% hypotonic hyaluronic acid was superior to 0.3% isotonic hyaluronic acid in improving corneal staining scores, decreasing inflammatory molecules, and increasing goblet cell counts in experimental DE.[65] These data from Korean studies indicate that hypotonic artificial tears can be useful as an adjunctive treatment for inflammatory DE.

Ointments can be applied in moderate DE and are best used before bedtime since they cause blurring. Lipid-containing eye drops and ointments have grown in availability and can help restore the lipid layer in evaporative DE with MGD or lipid deficiency. Various lipid agents, such as mineral oil, lanolin, and carbomer with triglyceride, are commercially available in Korea.

Antiinflammatory agents

Based on the role of inflammation in DE, antiinflammatory agents, including corticosteroids and cyclosporine A, have been widely prescribed in Korea. Among topical corticosteroids, 0.1% fluorometholone is the most commonly used for treating acute DE, followed by 0.5% loteprednol. Recently, preservative-free 0.1% fluorometholone has been launched to reduce ocular damage and inflammation by benzalkonium chloride.[59] Since long-term use of topical corticosteroids is a risk for glaucoma or cataract, it is not recommended. Short-term treatment (4 times a day for 2 weeks) with topical 1% methylprednisolone is recommended for cases with moderate to severe DE associated with Sjögren's syndrome.

Topical cyclosporine A 0.05% anionic emulsion (Restasis, Allergan, Irvine, CA, USA), which can inhibit the activation of CD4+ T cells and consequently decrease HLA-DR, apoptosis markers, and inflammatory molecules in the ocular surface and lacrimal gland, was firstly launched in Korea in 2006. A prospective multicenter Korean study demonstrated that 3-month use of cyclosporine A 0.05% emulsion was tolerable and effective for the treatment of DE, as evidenced by improved ocular symptom scores, increased Schirmer scores, and decreased conjunctival staining and use of artificial tears.[66] The KCDSG recommended the use of topical 0.05% cyclosporine A for inflammatory DE patients with mild to moderate corneal epithelial staining that corresponds to severity levels II and III. Cyclosporine A 0.05% emulsion was also proven to be effective in improving symptoms and signs of DE associated

with graft-versus-host diseases and thyroid-associated ophthalmopathy as well as Sjögren's syndrome. Other ocular formulations of 0.05% cyclosporine A including micelle-based solution (TJ cyporin, Taejoon, Seoul, Korea) and nanoemulsion (Clacier, Huons, Seoul, Korea) have also been developed and are available in the Korean market.

Cyclosporine A 0.1% cationic emulsion (Ikervis, Santen, Evry, France) was launched in Korea in 2017. It has been generally accepted that cyclosporine A 0.1% cationic emulsion is effective in reducing epithelial staining and inflammatory markers in the ocular surface as well as symptom scores, especially in patients with moderate to severe DE with severe keratitis, due to its higher concentration, longer residence time, and higher ocular bioavailability in the tear film.

A common pattern of antiinflammatory treatment by Korean ophthalmologists is that the initial combination of topical corticosteroids and cyclosporine A, followed by tapering of the steroid and eventual discontinuation after 2–4 weeks, while cyclosporine A is continued for as long as necessary.

Mucin secretagogues

Diquafosol tetrasodium 3% (Diquas, Santen) which stimulates water and mucin secretion from conjunctival epithelial cells and goblet cells and consequently improves tear film stability in DE was introduced in Korea in 2013. Diquafosol has become a major therapeutic agent along with artificial tears and cyclosporine A. The main etiological target of diquafosol is unstable tear film, and the optimal indication of diquafosol use is short TBUT DE and evaporative DE with MGD.[67] In addition, diquafosol is used popularly for patients with DE after cataract and refractive surgery.[68] Preservative-free 3% diquafosol (Diquas-S, Santen), which was also developed for the management of patients with preexisting DE after cataract surgery, is commercially available in Korea.[69]

In comparison with 0.05% cyclosporine A, 3% diquafosol was more effective in improving TBUT; however, cyclosporine A was more effective in decreasing conjunctival staining.[70] Another clinical study demonstrated that diquafosol was more effective in increasing tear secretion, whereas cyclosporine A was more effective in improving optical aberrations in DE patients following cataract surgery.[71]

Serum

Serum contains essential tear components, growth factors, neurotrophic factors, vitamin A, fibronectin, prealbumin, and oil; it provides the corneal and conjunctival epithelium with basic elements for epithelial regeneration. Autologous serum eye drops (20%) have been recommended for the treatment of moderate to severe DE (level III or higher) in Korea since 2010. Yoon et al. found that umbilical cord serum contains a higher concentration of essential tear components, growth factors, and neurotrophic factors than autologous serum, and umbilical cord serum eye drops (20%) can be safely and effectively applied in severe DE with or without Sjögren's syndrome, graft-versus-host disease, persistent epithelial defects, neurotrophic keratopathy, recurrent corneal erosions, ocular chemical burn, and surface problems after corneal refractive surgery.[72–75]

Antioxidants

The role of oxidative stress in addition to inflammation in the lacrimal functional unit in the pathogenesis of DE has been well elucidated in Korea since 2000. Oxidative stress generates reactive oxygen species that can cause deleterious alterations in DNA, protein, and lipid of corneal and conjunctival epithelial cells and induce cellular damages and apoptosis, and, as a result, promote ocular surface inflammation that results in DE. In 2008, a prospective multicenter study demonstrated the clinical effectiveness of oral antioxidant dietary supplements in DE patients.[76]

Topical application of antioxidant medicinal plant extracts improved clinical signs, decreased inflammatory molecules and cells, and ameliorated oxidative stress markers and reactive oxygen species production on the ocular surface in a mouse model of experimental DE.[77] Antioxidant glasses (Eye Plus Alpha II, BM Korea, Gwangju, Korea) containing extracts of medicinal plants could effectively improve subjective symptoms and objective signs including TBUT in DE, and they were approved by the Korean Food and Drug Administration in 2013.[78]

Others

Punctal plugs (temporary and permanent) and therapeutic contact lenses are used in DE with higher severity levels. Periocular application of a TRMP8 agonist (Blephacool, Samil, Seoul, Korea) can increase tear secretion by activating efferent nerve signals and reduce ocular discomfort by inducing the perception of coolness.[79] The commercially available TRPM8 agonist may be a promising therapeutic agent in DE patients with Sjögren's syndrome and ocular neuropathic pain.

Proposed Treatment Guidelines

In 2014, the KCDSG developed the Korean guideline for DE management for the various levels (I ~ IV) of the disease severity (Table 12.3). The detailed treatment

TABLE 12.3
Treatment Recommendations According to the Severity Level of Dry Eye Disease by the Korean Corneal Disease Study Group in 2014.

Severity Level	Treatment recommendation[a]

Level I	Patient education, environmental control
	  Check systemic medications
	  (e.g., antihistamines, antidepressants,
	  or beta-blockers)
	  Fluid intake, psychological support
	Artificial tears (preserved or nonpreserved)
	  4 times a day, or incremental according
	  to patients' symptoms
	Allergy treatment, when necessary

Level II	Nonpreserved artificial tears Antiinflammatory therapy (e.g., topical cyclosporine A or topical corticosteroids) Oral supplements; essential fatty acid (e.g., omega-3-fatty acid or gamma linoleic acid) Gels/ointment (may be used in level I patients, when necessary)
Level III	Autologous serum Oral tetracycline (may be used in level II patients) Punctual plug/occlusion Contact lenses, goggles
Level IV	Surgery Systemic antiinflammatory medication

[a] Accompanying ocular surface disease such as blepharitis or ocular allergies should be treated for any level.

options for each severity level were recommended. This guideline was based on the DEWS guidelines and modified to simplify the grading scheme so that they could be used more easily in clinical practice. However, this guideline had several limitations, including the use of fewer topical therapeutic agents and their application for only aqueous deficient DE. The Korean Dry Eye Society is establishing a new guideline for DE diagnosis, classification, and management. DE can be diagnosed when ocular symptoms, TBUT <7 s, and/or low tear volume (Schirmer test value < 10 mm), and/or corneal or conjunctival staining exist. According to the proposed guideline, DE can be classified into three types: 1) aqueous deficiency dominant type including Sjögren's syndrome, 2) evaporation dominant type including MGD and blepharitis, and 3) altered tear distribution type such as lipid wiper epitheliopathy (Fig. 12.3). Regarding management of DE, a stepwise approach using therapeutic agents (steps I and II)

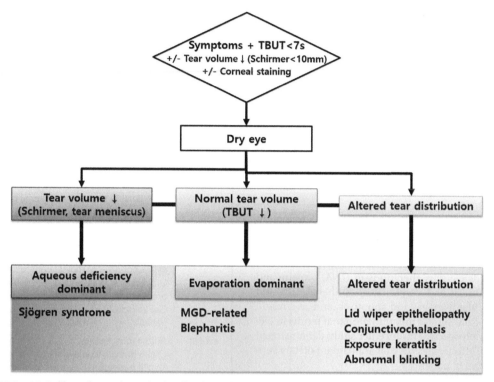

FIG. 12.3 New diagnosis and classification of dry eye proposed by the Korean Dry Eye Society. Abbreviations: *MGD*, Meibomian gland dysfunction; *TBUT*, tear film break-up time.

combined with procedures is recommended according to each type (Fig. 12.4). The key therapeutic agents are artificial tears, secretagogues, antiinflammatory agents (corticosteroids and cyclosporine A), and dietary modification (omega-3 and antioxidants).

Conclusions

Both ocular surface inflammation and tear film instability are considered as major pathophysiological factors to be corrected in the treatment of DE. Treatment of DE in Korea is unique, as cyclosporine A and diquafosol are major topical agents along with preservative-free hyaluronic acid (various concentrations and tonicity). Antioxidants are popularly used as adjunctive treatments, and management of combined MGD has been emphasized. The selection of these therapeutic agents can be modified depending on the types (aqueous deficiency dominant type, evaporation dominant type with MGD, and mixed type) and severity of DE.

DRY EYE THERAPY IN SINGAPORE

The treatment of DE is evolving in Singapore. Mild DE is generally treated in the community, either by patients

from retail pharmacy or directed by general practitioners from private primary care clinics or family physicians from the government polyclinics. The tertiary care DE cases are seen by specialists in public hospitals and private ophthalmologists. In Singapore National Eye Center (SNEC), which sees 60% of the tertiary eye care in Singapore, DE is managed by all ophthalmologists and more severe DE by cornea specialists. From mid-2006, a dedicated DE service in SNEC has been setup, providing care for referred, more severe DE. A prospective DE database began, which is useful to audit for risk factors of symptomatic DE.[80,81]

Prevalence of DE by symptoms in the latest study is 12.3% and 6-year incidence is 5.1%.[20,82] From the early 2000 (Fig. 12.5), newer artificial tears such as Systane eyedrops or transient gels have become available in Singapore.[83] Moisture occlusion chambers have also been advocated for evaporative DE.[84] Although cyclosporine at 0.5% (preserved eyedrops) have been available, an important milestone is the availability of 0.05% cyclosporine eyedrops in a commercial emulsion form (Restasis, Allergan). Some patients were prescribed oral doxycycline or azithromycin, but unfortunately the lowest strength doxycycline in Singapore is

	Aqueous deficiency dominant	Evaporation dominant	Altered tear distribution

Step I	• Education & Environmental modifications
	• Elimination of offending medications
	• Artificial tears & ointments (Preserved or non-preserved)
		• Education & Environmental modifications
		• Lid hygiene and warm compress
		• Artificial tears
		• Lipid containing agents
		• Topical secretagogues (Diquafosol)
			• Lid wiper epitheliopathy
			  - Ocular lubricants
			  - Lipid containing agents
			
			• Conjunctivochalasis
			  - Ocular lubricants

Step II	• Topical secretagogues (Diquafosol)
	• Topical steroids
	• Topical immunomodulatory drugs (Cyclosporine A etc)
	• Serum eye drops
	• Dietary modifications (Omega-3, antioxidants)
	• Oral secretagogues
		• Topical steroids
		• Topical immunomodulatory drugs (Cyclosporine A etc)
		• Dietary modifications (Omega-3, antioxidants)
		• Oral tetracycline antibiotics
			• Exposure keratitis
			  - Artificial ointment
			
			• Abnormal blinking
			  - Blinking education
			  - Blinking exercise

Procedures	• Punctal occlusion
	• Therapeutic contact lens
	• Goggles
		• Intense pulsed light
		• LipiFlow
		• Meibomian gland probing
			• Conjunctivochalasis
			  - Conjunctival excision
			  - Cautery / Argon laser
			
			• Exposure keratitis
			  - Tarsorrhaphy

FIG. 12.4 New dry eye treatment recommendations according to the classification proposed by the Korean Dry Eye Society.

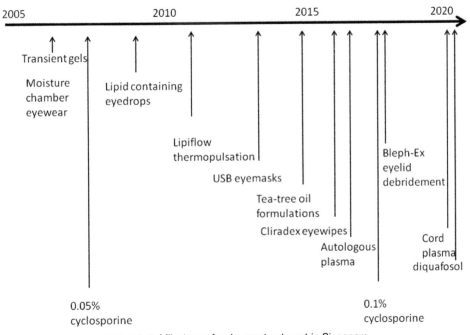

FIG. 12.5 Milestones for dry eye treatment in Singapore.

100 mg, which induces gastric intolerance. Patients with aqueous deficiency were also offered punctal plugs,[85,86] and some with corticosteroid eyedrops. In this clinic, the use of multiple modalities can eventually improve the central corneal staining of the severe DE patients.[87]

In around 2010, the use of autologous plasma tears using a closed system of preparation has been made available.[88] However, this turns out to be expensive because service providers include not only the hematology center in the general hospital but also the laboratory at the national blood bank. Recently this service converted to the use of more affordable cord plasma processed from cord blood, provided by the Singapore Cord Blood Bank.

Use of special contact lens solutions, such as those containing alginic acid, has been made available for tear film protection. However, wearing of contact lenses with such solutions over 1 week did not produce significant advantage over control.[89]

Another important milestone in the care of DE from 2010 is the provision of lipid-containing eyedrops like Endura (castor oil based), Catiornom (positive charged), and Artelac (negative charged).[90] These eyedrops, at least transiently, augment the tear lipid layer thickness, if the baseline level is low.[91] In the last 5 years, lipid-containing transient gels (Systane balance, Alcon) have been made available.[92] This is followed by the first regulatory-approved 0.1% cyclosporine for DE (Ikeryvis, Santen).[93]

From the year 2009 and later, advances have been made in the care of MGD in Singapore. To facilitate eyelid warming,[94] USB-powered eyemasks have been made more easily available, such as through vending machines. Lipiflo thermopulsation[95] was available from 2010, and at that time, diagnostic modalities such as TearLab osmometer, Lipiview interferometer,[96] and meibography[97] have been made available for research uses. Use of thermography for tear evaporation is able to predict response to eyelid warming.[88,98] These efforts were followed by the use of the Oculus Keratograph 5 for noninvasive tear break-up and other imaging.[99–101]

From 2019, eyelid microabrasion (Bleph-Ex) is provided in SNEC and by private ophthalmologists. This is performed for blepharitis, MGD, and demodex infestations. Cliradex eyewipes (containing the terpenoid-active ingredient of tea tree oil) are available for demodex infestations.[102] Late last year, SNEC physicians began to use the secretagogue diaquafosol eyedrops under a named patient basis, SNEC having participated in the previous randomized study by Santen on the same medication.[103]

Future directions of DE care will include technologies for community care of DE (imaging[104] or strip meniscometry[105]), telemedicine or telemonitoring for more stable cases,[106] and community care such as with TCM.[107] DE care will also incorporate strategies to improve sleep[108] and anxiety/depression,[109] and other holistic factors uncovered through focus groups.[110] Reasons for eyedrop intolerance such as acidity of eyedrops[111] have been disseminated and, hopefully, will help patients to select artificial tears.

In specialized centers, effort is made toward more patient advocacy. More focus will be directed toward cases of DE with conjunctivochalasis,[112] glaucoma,[113,114] ocular allergies,[115] and prevention of DE in ocular graft-versus-host disease. A noninvasive way to phenotype conjunctival T cells in DE patients has been developed.[116] In terms of medical education of practitioners, the recent Asia Dry Eye Disease framework will be adapted for use in Singapore and disseminated to all eye specialists. To ensure uniformity of protocols nationally, similar efforts which has already gained broad acceptance will be undertaken with professional bodies associated with optometrists and pharmacists. Digital medicine is employed in several areas, such as empowerment of general practitioners in a community network, and preoperative assessment of refractive cataract surgeries.

EPIDEMIOLOGY, DIAGNOSIS, AND TREATMENT OF DRY EYE DISEASE IN TAIWAN

Epidemiology

The increasing prevalence of DED has become a global public health issue.[117] DED imposes a significant economic burden on the patient and the society. The prevalence of DED range from 5% to 50%, which vary with different definitions and the characteristics of the study population.[117] The prevalence seems higher in individuals of Asian ethnicity,[117] and there is now an increased awareness of DED among young population.[118,119] In Taiwan, the prevalence rate of DED in patients older than 65 years is 33.7%.[120] In a population-based study excluding younger than 20 years, the overall prevalence rate was about 4.6%.[121] We recently analyzed the Taiwan National Health Insurance Database by selecting outpatients who had at least two ophthalmology clinic visits with the diagnoses of DED and had been prescribed eye lubricants (patients with a Schirmer test score of less than 5 mm) with follow-up period more than 1 year. We found that the overall prevalence of DED was 7.85%, higher among women (10.49%)

than men (4.92%), increased with age (0.53%, 3.94%, 10.08%, and 20.72% for ages of <18, 18−39, 40−64, and >65 years, respectively).[122] We also found that DED increases the risk of corneal surface damage, including recurrent corneal erosion, corneal ulcers, and corneal scars. The risk factors for corneal surface damage in DED are younger age (<18 years), female sex, DM, and autoimmune diseases.[122]

Diagnosis

A battery of diagnostic tools have been developed to evaluate the DED because of lacking a consistent and accurate diagnostic test.[22,123,124] Recently, an online questionnaire from 70 DE specialists in Taiwan was conducted to investigate the preferred diagnostic test in evaluating different subtypes of DED. The results showed that ocular surface fluorescein staining, Schirmer I test with anesthesia, and fluorescein TBUT were the most common diagnostic tests for DED in both medical center ophthalmologists and nonmedical center ophthalmologists in Taiwan. In previous researches that evaluated the presence of DED or monitor the progression of DED, these three diagnostic tests were also frequently used for such task, similar to our results.[43,125,126] Interestingly, Schirmer I test with anesthesia was thought as the most sensitive diagnostic test for aqueous deficiency DED, possibly because of the reimbursement guideline (Schirmer I test with anesthesia less than 5 mm in 5 min) set by the National Health Insurance Administration in Taiwan. For the evaporative DED, the most sensitive diagnostic test was fluorescein TBUT according to medical center ophthalmologists, but the nonmedical center ophthalmologists thought the noninvasive TBUT was the most sensitive diagnostic test in such condition, which may due to the fast-screening ability and the noninvasive nature.[127,128] About the most sensitive diagnostic test for mucin deficiency DED, fluorescein TBUT got the highest agreement in medical center ophthalmologists, while the ocular surface fluorescein staining had the highest votes in nonmedical center ophthalmologists. The secondary sensitive diagnostic test for mucin deficiency DED was impression cytology in both the medical center and nonmedical center ophthalmologists.

Treatment

About the management of DED, medical treatment is usually prescribed first and the surgical intervention is preserved for those with refractory or cicatricial DED that show minimal responsiveness to medications.[129] Lubrication agents such as artificial tears account for the majority of first-line DED therapy,[46,129] and the

topical immunomodulating agents as well as antiinflammatory medications like cyclosporin (CsA) and steroid have been prescribed for those with moderate to severe DED patients.[129,130] Other therapies such as autologous serum eye drops, punctal occlusion, and amniotic membrane transplantation would be applied in severe cases.[131] In Taiwan, the secondary popular treatment agent is the topical nonglucocorticoid immunomodulatory drugs like cyclosporine in both the medical center and the nonmedical center ophthalmologists. Recently, we retrospectively identified patients with moderate to severe DED who had shown inadequate response to twice-daily use of topical 0.05% CsA but showed significant improvement after switching to 0.1% CsA daily. In this study, after a 2-month course of treatment with topical 0.1% CsA, significant improvements were noted for corneal fluorescein staining ($P < 0.001$), corneal sensitivity ($P = 0.008$), and TBUT ($P = 0.01$) (manuscript submitted). Besides, steroid had been used in DED as concurrent treatment with CsA due to the antiinflammation effect.[132,133] Also, topical steroid with long duration use was recommended for patient with DED that CsA treatment is inadequate according to the report from Dry Eye Workshop.[129] However, researches concerning the effect of combined therapy with CsA and adjuvant steroid on severe DED are absent. We also demonstrated that the combined therapy of 0.05% CsA and steroid decreased the sign score in severe DED, while the concurrent 0.05% CsA and high-potency steroid can further decrease the symptom score in such subjects (manuscript submitted). However, further large-scale prospective study to evaluate the effect of other steroid and 0.05% CsA with different concentration and duration on the management of recalcitrant DED is mandatory. In Taiwan, most DE specialists regard that the complexity of DED pathophysiology is the most problematic issue during management, indicating that we still have a long way to go before satisfying our patients with DED.

DRY EYE THERAPY IN THAILAND

Epidemiology

DE is a common disease in Thailand. Thirty-four percent of out-patients, aged more than 40 years who came for an eye check-up at a tertiary care hospital in Bangkok, reported symptoms of DE.[134] This prevalence is high, compared to other Asian countries, ranging from 12% to 34%.[20,120,135] This difference may be due to several factors, such as age group, study-population, and diagnostic criteria.

Dry Eye Diagnosis

Diagnosis of DE can be made by a careful history taking of frequency and severity of DE symptoms. Several risk factors, such as previous ocular surgery, especially refractive surgery, contact lens wearing, preexisting systemic and ocular diseases, should be asked. In Thailand, due to air pollution problems in the big city, ocular allergy is common. Allergy itself, combined with antihistamine use, can worsen DE conditions, especially in a younger age group. Also, the increased screen time is a significant risk factor for DE in children and young adults.[136] The Cornea and Refractive Surgery Society of Thailand has developed a self-check DE test, available on Appstore (Fig. 12.6).[137] Within 5 minutes, the user can perform a self-check of DE through four items, blink rate, the longest time to keep the eyes open, vision test, and DE questionnaire. The individual score and demographic data will then be reported to the user immediately and to the central data reposition center for future evaluation and analysis.

A thorough ocular surface evaluation, using slit-lamp biomicroscopy, is essential for the diagnosis of DE. Eyelids and lashes evaluation, blinking function, including completeness of blink and blink rate, decrease tear meniscus height, and abnormal discharge in tear film are essential. The conjunctival redness findings and increased punctate stainings on conjunctival and corneal surfaces indicate the inflammatory component of DE. Dye staining using a fluorescein strip is a time-efficient test and offer useful information. Firstly, TBUT and patterns (TBUP) can be assessed. According to the diagnosis proposed by the ADES,[45] we agree with the cut-off value of TBUT <5 s to diagnose tear film instability. Secondly, ocular surface staining can then be graded. Fluorescein dye is a single dye that stains both the corneal and the conjunctival surface.

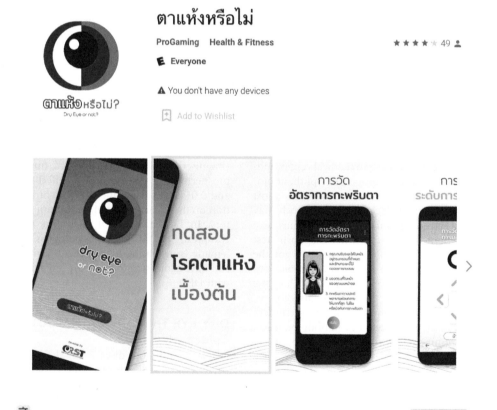

FIG. 12.6 The Cornea and Refractive Surgery Society of Thailand (CRST) mobile application "Dry Eye or Not?" This picture displays the "Dry Eye or Not?" application, which is available on App Store, both for Android and Apple.

The conventional cobalt blue illumination will show fluorescein-stainings (green) on a blue background, in which the image is less contrast and indistinguishable. Modern technology integrated into a digital slit-lamp microscope will make the stainings more pronounced. By combining a "blue-free" filter (optional) into the observation system, the blue background will be suppressed, giving a clearer image of green stainings on a black background.[138]

Together with enhanced system software, this superior contrast image will enable the observer to detect both the corneal and conjunctival stainings with confidence. The corneal and conjunctival staining and tear break-up patterns of different types of DE can easily be observed (Fig. 12.7A and B), thus avoiding the conventional use of rose-Bengal dye, which has intrinsic toxicity to the ocular surface. The same technique is also helpful in other diseases, such as detecting surface irregularities in limbal stem cell deficiency (Fig. 12.8A and B) and superior limbic keratoconjunctivitis (Fig. 12.9).

Dry Eye Treatment

Most doctors in Thailand approach treatment in a stepwise way, guiding by DE grading and severity. The mainstay therapy is artificial tears, with or without preservatives. Secretagogues, antiinflammatory agents, both concentration of 0.05% and 0.1% cyclosporine A are also available. Topical self-made nonpreserved steroids, such as 1% methylprednisolone and 0.1% dexamethasone, are prepared and used locally in several tertiary care centers. In severe cases, treatment with autologous serum, punctual plugs, and cauterization will be offered. Coexisting MGD can be treated with

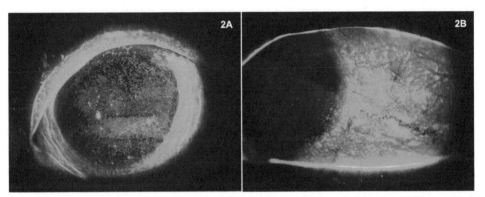

FIG. 12.7 **Fluorescein stainings in dry eye. (A)** Demonstrates diffuse fluorescein staining on the total corneal surface of a dry eye patient. **(B)** Shows moderate fluorescein staining on the temporal bulbar conjunctiva of a dry eye patient. The blue light from the background is filtered out using the "Blue-free" filter, mounted in the observation systems, making the green fluorescein staining spots on the conjunctiva prominent.

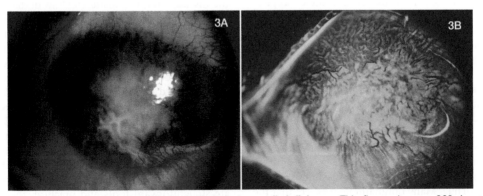

FIG. 12.8 **Ocular surface irregularity in limbal stem cell deficiency**. This figure shows a 360-degree corneal vascularization and superficial corneal scar found in a patient, which sustained a chemical injury **(A)**. When using a "Blue-free" technique, the corneal surface irregularity can be easily observed **(B)**.

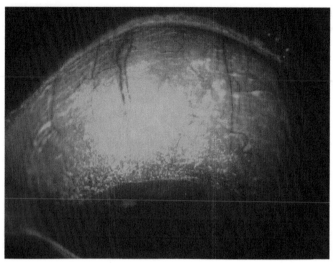

FIG. 12.9 Superior bulbar conjunctival fluorescein staining in a patient with superior limbic keratoconjunctivitis (SLK). Typical findings of diffuse fluorescein-staining dots, together with the irregular superior bulbar conjunctival surface, can be observed.

lid massage, lid spa, and Lipiflow treatment are available to affordable patients as well. Despite the wide range of treatment options, 80% of the prescription is influenced by the reimbursement market. Patients will only get reimbursement if the drugs are on the national list of essential drugs; if not, they are expected to contribute some form of copayment.

OVERVIEW OF DRY EYE IN VIETNAM

Although the prevalence of DED has been thoroughly studied worldwide, there is lack of data on DED in Vietnam. However, according to some experienced ophthalmologists, the prevalence of DED is noticeably high.

Science has come a long way in understanding the underlying etiology of this disease and the concept of DED has changed greatly. In Vietnam, the misconceptions about DED are still very common such as (1) DED is the condition that occurs due to lack of tears so the main treatment is providing lubricants for patients, (2) MGD is synonymous with anterior blepharitis and prescribing antibiotic ointment to apply to the lid margin is a common practice, (3) DED is simply a part of old age, (4) the main cause of DE is vitamin A deficiency in some remote regions. These misconceptions hamper clinical management of DED and need to be reconsidered.

There are many challenges when it comes to management of DED. Many ophthalmologists feel that the diagnosis of DE is time consuming and many do not stain the cornea or use DE questionnaires which makes it difficult to diagnose DED in everyday clinical practice. Although the awareness of DED in Vietnam has been increasing recently, DED is not in the top 10 priorities of the eye diseases listed as important. DED treatment is basically out-of-pocket and patients often tolerate their condition until it is severe and disabling.

The diagnostic tests for identify DED are very simple and limited. Fluorescein impregnated strips are the only tool that is accessible for most ophthalmologists. Schirmer test is far and few between. Recently Keratograph 5M with more advanced testing is available at the two largest eye centers in Vietnam (Hanoi and Ho Chi Minh city). Even with the current tools, there is no consensus on which diagnostic criteria should be used or which approach should be utilized to access the disease. That has made DED an undiagnosed and underattended problem. Some clinicians inappropriately diagnose different conditions as DED, while others rarely make a diagnosis of DED and, thus, underdiagnose it. Given this situation, a simple yet effective diagnostic tool is required. The DED classification system proposed by Asia Dry Eye Society 2017 (ADES)[22] seems to be an appropriate choice that meets all the needs. Only through use of fluorescein, DE classification based on tear film break-up patterns can be determined and that assists the ophthalmologist in selecting the choices of treatment for DED patients. The ADES diagnostic criteria and classification systems are straightforward tools and practical, therefore, it is employed by more and more ophthalmologists, especially corneal specialists in Vietnam.

The mainstay first-line therapy for DED is lubricants or artificial tears. Attitude toward treatment is usually not to identify the underlying etiology of DED but giving patients several brands of lubricants and having patients choose their favorite. There has been an increasing amount of commercially available artificial tear options, both in preserved and preservative-free formulations. The most common agents are hyaluronic acid (0.1%−0.4%) and carboxy methylcellulose. Secretagogue eye drops (diquafosol sodium) is possible to prescribe. Other therapeutic options for treating DED such as punctual plugs, topical cyclosporine A (0.05%), autologous serum are not common in major cities, let alone rural areas.

DED management is an area that is gaining more attention from both ophthalmologists and patients in recent years in Vietnam. Given the high prevalence of the disease and the effects it might have on patient's quality of life, a consensual approach to DED among Vietnamese ophthalmologists is needed in order to reach a correct diagnosis and proper treatment of DED.

CONCLUSIONS

Previous reports of epidemiological studies in Asian countries have clearly shown that the prevalence of DE is high in Asian countries, but the cause of the high prevalence has not been clarified. It has been suggested that air pollution is associated with the prevalence of DE in some countries.[139,140] Whether the high prevalence of DE is due to ethnicity, long VDT work hours, or environmental factors such as climate or air pollution should be clarified in future multicenter studies that include not only Asian countries but also Western countries.

At a meeting of the Asia Dry Eye Society, it was agreed that tear film stability is a core mechanism, and diagnostic criteria for DE were reported in 2017.[22] This was followed by agreement on the classification of DE in 2020, along with a treatment strategy that includes TFOT.[45] At the time of writing this chapter (April 2021), more than 3 years have passed since the Asia Dry Eye Society reported the diagnostic criteria for DE, and the concept of diagnosing DE mainly by focusing on the tear film stability seems to have penetrated into Asian countries. On the other hand, the treatment strategies, types of ophthalmic drugs, and the status of TFOT implementation may vary from country to country due to the influence of the regulatory approval status in each country. In some countries, the choice of drugs to be prescribed is also greatly influenced by the medical administration, such as the medical insurance reimbursement system.

The introduction of diagnostic equipment for DED differs greatly from country to country. For this reason, the amount of information available for TFOD varies greatly from country to country. However, fluorescein staining strips are available in all countries, and it is possible to diagnose abnormalities in the tear film by using tear film break-up patterns. The use of fluorescein staining strips and tear film break-up pattern analysis should continue to be educated and disseminated to non-DE specialists because they are simple, provide a lot of information about tear film abnormalities, and are economically efficient.

Artificial tear eye drops, sodium diquafosol ophthalmic solution, rebamipide ophthalmic solution, and cyclosporine ophthalmic solution are used to treat DEs. In some countries, artificial tear eye drop is the mainstay of DE treatment, and treatment is not sufficiently based on the concept of TFOD. The secretagogue eye drops play a very important role in TFOT. Therefore, in countries where secretagogue is not yet approved by the regulatory authorities, it may be difficult to perform TFOT strategy. If secretagogue eye drops become available in many countries in the future, the concept of TFOT will become more widespread.

In recent years, research groups in Japan have proposed the idea that DE is a lifestyle disease, and have begun to attempt to prevent the onset of the disease by improving lifestyle rather than after the disease has developed.[141] In a study of office workers, it was found that those who exercised more showed greater tear secretion, suggesting that exercise is an effective intervention for DE.[142] In the DE animal model, reduction of oxidative stress has been shown to be effective in preventing the onset of DE,[143] and it is expected that more research will be conducted in the future to intervene in DE through the intake of antioxidants in humans. Since Asian countries have similar lifestyles, it is possible that this idea will spread widely in Asian countries in the future.

ACKNOWLEDGMENTS

The authors express our sincere thanks to Ms. Catherine Oshima for administrative support and editing of the manuscript.

Conflicts of Interest

Vilavun Puangsricharern, Louis Tong, and Chi Hoang Viet Vu report no conflicts of interest.

Murat Dogru reports grants from Icom, Kobayashi Pharmaceuticals and Otsuka Pharmaceutical.

Takashi Kojima reports personal fees from Staar Surgical, personal fees from Santen Pharmaceutical, personal fees from Otsuka Pharmaceutical, personal fees from Johnson & Johnson, personal fees from Alcon, outside the submitted work.

Zuguo Liu reports his consultancy and research funding received from Santen, Xingqi, Haoshili, and Shengyuan. Personal fees from Alcon, Johnson & Johnson, Narvites, and Zhuhaiyisheng.

Chi Chin Sun—to be confirmed.

Kazuo Tsubota reports his position as CEO of Tsubota Laboratory, Inc., Tokyo, Japan, a company working on treatment, prevention, and medical devices for dry eye. Also, consultancy and research funding received from Santen Pharmaceutical Co., Ltd., and Otsuka Pharmaceutical Co., Ltd. Research funding from Jins, Inc., Wakasa Seikatsu Corp, Wakamoto Pharmaceutical Co., Ltd., AMO Japan K.K., Pfizer, R-Tech Ueno, Ophtecs, Alcon Japan, and Rohto Pharmaceutical Co., Ltd. Investment or patent with Tear Solutions, Tissue Tech, Inc. and Kowa Company.

Norihiko Yokoi has received personal fees from Santen Pharmaceutical Co., Ltd., Otsuka Pharmaceutical Co., Ltd., and consultancies from Rohto Co., Ltd. and Alcon Japan Co., Ltd., and patents for the ophthalmologic apparatus with Kowa Co., Ltd.

REFERENCES

1. Uchino M, Uchino Y, Dogru M, et al. Dry eye disease and work productivity loss in visual display users: the Osaka study. *Am J Ophthalmol.* 2014;157(2):294–300.
2. Grzybowski A, Kanclerz P, Tsubota K, Lanca C, Saw SM. A review on the epidemiology of myopia in school children worldwide. *BMC Ophthalmol.* 2020;20(1):27.
3. Choi JH, Li Y, Kim SH, et al. The influences of smartphone use on the status of the tear film and ocular surface. *PLoS One.* 2018;13(10):e0206541.
4. Ayaki M, Kawashima M, Negishi K, Tsubota K. High prevalence of sleep and mood disorders in dry eye patients: survey of 1,000 eye clinic visitors. *Neuropsychiatric Dis Treat.* 2015;11:889–894.
5. Kojima T, Dogru M, Kawashima M, Nakamura S, Tsubota K. Advances in the diagnosis and treatment of dry eye. *Prog Retin Eye Res.* 2020;78:100842.
6. Sano K, Kawashima M, Takechi S, Mimura M, Tsubota K. Exercise program improved subjective dry eye symptoms for office workers. *Clin Ophthalmol.* 2018;12:307–311.
7. Yoon SY, Bae SH, Shin YJ, et al. Low serum 25-hydroxyvitamin D levels are associated with dry eye syndrome. *PLoS One.* 2016;11(1):e0147847.
8. Ayaki M, Kawashima M, Uchino M, Tsubota K, Negishi K. Gender differences in adolescent dry eye disease: a health problem in girls. *Int J Ophthalmol.* 2018;11(2):301–307.
9. Yotsukura E, Torii H, Inokuchi M, et al. Current prevalence of myopia and association of myopia with environmental factors among schoolchildren in Japan. *JAMA Ophthalmol.* 2019;137(11):1233–1239.
10. Uchino M, Nishiwaki Y, Michikawa T, et al. Prevalence and risk factors of dry eye disease in Japan: Koumi study. *Ophthalmology.* 2011;118(12):2361–2367.
11. Zhang Y, Chen H, Wu X. Prevalence and risk factors associated with dry eye syndrome among senior high school students in a county of Shandong Province, China. *Ophthalmic Epidemiol.* 2012;19(4):226–230.
12. Ahn JM, Lee SH, Rim THT, et al. Prevalence of and risk factors associated with dry eye: the Korea National Health And Nutrition Examination Survey 2010–2011. *Am J Ophthalmol.* 2014;158(6):1205–1214.e7.
13. Um S-B, Kim NH, Lee HK, Song JS, Kim HC. Spatial epidemiology of dry eye disease: findings from South Korea. *Int J Health Geogr.* 2014;13:31.
14. Uchino M, Dogru M, Uchino Y, et al. Japan ministry of health study on prevalence of dry eye disease among Japanese high school students. *Am J Ophthalmol.* 2008;146(6):925–929.
15. Lu P, Chen X, Liu X, et al. Dry eye syndrome in elderly Tibetans at high altitude: a population-based study in China. *Cornea.* 2008;27(5).
16. Jie Y, Xu L, Wu YY, Jonas JB. Prevalence of dry eye among adult Chinese in the Beijing Eye Study. *Eye.* 2009;23(3):688–693.
17. Guo B, Lu P, Chen X, Zhang W, Chen R. Prevalence of dry eye disease in Mongolians at high altitude in China: the Henan Eye Study. *Ophthalmic Epidemiol.* 2010;17(4):234–241.
18. Han SB, Hyon JY, Woo SJ, Lee JJ, Kim TH, Kim KW. Prevalence of dry eye disease in an elderly Korean population. *Arch Ophthalmol.* 2011;129(5):633–638.
19. Tong L, Saw S-M, Lamoureux EL, et al. A questionnaire-based assessment of symptoms associated with tear film dysfunction and lid margin disease in an Asian population. *Ophthalmic Epidemiol.* 2009;16(1):31–37.
20. Tan LL, Morgan P, Cai ZQ, Straughan RA. Prevalence of and risk factors for symptomatic dry eye disease in Singapore. *Clin Exp Optom.* 2015;98(1):45–53.
21. Na K-S, Han K, Park Y-G, Na C, Joo C-K. Depression, stress, quality of life, and dry eye disease in Korean women: a population-based study. *Cornea.* 2015;34(7).
22. Tsubota K, Yokoi N, Shimazaki J, et al. New perspectives on dry eye definition and diagnosis: a consensus report by the Asia Dry Eye Society. *Ocul Surf.* 2017;15(1):65–76.
23. Wei Z, Liu H, Liang Q. Advances on the epidemiology of the dry eye. *Chin J Ophthalmol Med.* 2020;1:46–50.
24. Zhang X, Qu Y, et al. Dry eye management: targeting the ocular surface microenvironment. *Int J Mol Sci.* 2017;18(7):1398.
25. Asia Dry Eye Association China Branch, Ocular Surface and Tear Film diseases Group of Ophthalmology Committee of Cross-Straits Medicine Exchange Association, Ocular Surface and Dry Eye Group of Chinese Ophthalmologist Association. Chinese expert consensus on the definition and classification of dry eye (2020). *Chin J Ophthalmol.* 2020;57(10):734–742.

26. Zuguo L, Hua W. Focusing on the management of chronic dry eye disease. *Chin J Ophthalmol.* 2018;2:81–83.

27. Zhang Y, Gong L. Recent advances in P2Y2 receptor agonist for the treatment of dry eye. *Chin Ophthalmic Res.* 2014;9:856–859.

28. Xiao X, He H, Lin Z, et al. Therapeutic effects of epidermal growth factor on benzalkonium chloride–induced dry eye in a mouse model. *Invest Ophthalmol Visual Sci.* 2012;53(1):191–197.

29. Dong F, Liu C-Y, Yuan Y, et al. Perturbed meibomian gland and tarsal plate morphogenesis by excess TGFα in eyelid stroma. *Dev Biol.* 2015;406(2):147–157.

30. Keratology Group of Ophthalmology Branch of Chinese Medical Association. Chinese expert consensus on the treatment of corneal and ocular surface diseases with autologous serum eye drops. *Chin J Ophthalmol.* 2020; 56(10):735–740.

31. Zhang Z, Yang W-Z, Zhu Z-Z, et al. Therapeutic effects of topical doxycycline in a benzalkonium chloride–induced mouse dry eye model. *Invest Ophthalmol Visual Sci.* 2014;55(5):2963–2974.

32. Zhou Y. Study on the therapeutic effect of Melaleuca oil on mites in patients with dry eye. *Adv Clin Med.* 2020; 10(8).

33. Ma K, Li Q, Zhang Z, Xiang M, Zhao Y. Research progress in physical therapy for dry eye. *Int Eye Sci.* 2018;4: 71–74.

34. Zhao H, Liu Z, Xiao X, et al. The clinical effects of non-heating moisture chamber glasses in the treatment of dry eye. *Chin J Optometry Ophthalmol.* 2014;50:517–521.

35. Liu Z, Hong J. Strengthen Chinese translational medicine research in ocular surface. *[Zhonghua yan ke za zhi] Chin J Ophthamol.* 2014;9:646–649.

36. Liu Z, Jin M, Li Y, et al. Efficacy and safety of houttuynia eye drops atomization treatment for meibomian gland dysfunction-related dry eye disease: a randomized, double-blinded, placebo-controlled clinical trial. *J Clin Med.* 2020;9(12):4022.

37. Dhaliwal DK, Zhou S, Samudre SS, Lo NJ, Rhee MK. Acupuncture and dry eye: current perspectives. A double-blinded randomized controlled trial and review of the literature. *Clin Ophthalmol.* 2019;13:731–740.

38. Uchino M. What we know about the epidemiology of dry eye disease in Japan. *Invest Ophthalmol Visual Sci.* 2018; 59(14):DES1–DES6.

39. Bron AJ, de Paiva CS, Chauhan SK, et al. TFOS DEWS II pathophysiology report. *Ocul Surf.* 2017;15(3):438–510.

40. Yokoi N, Georgiev GA. Tear film–oriented diagnosis and tear film–oriented therapy for dry eye based on tear film dynamics. *Invest Ophthalmol Visual Sci.* 2018;59(14): DES13–DES22.

41. The definition and classification of dry eye disease: report of the definition and classification subcommittee of the international Dry Eye WorkShop (2007). *Ocul Surf.* 2007;5(2):75–92.

42. Yokoi N, Uchino M, Uchino Y, et al. Importance of tear film instability in dry eye disease in office workers using visual display terminals: the Osaka study. *Am J Ophthalmol.* 2015;159(4):748–754.

43. Craig JP, Nichols KK, Akpek EK, et al. TFOS DEWS II definition and classification report. *Ocul Surf.* 2017;15(3): 276–283.

44. Tsubota K, Pflugfelder SC, Liu Z, et al. Defining dry eye from a clinical perspective. *Int J Mol Sci.* 2020;21(23).

45. Tsubota K, Yokoi N, Watanabe H, et al. A new perspective on dry eye classification: proposal by the Asia Dry Eye Society. *Eye Contact Lens.* 2020;46.

46. Watanabe H. Medical treatment for dry eye in Japan. *Invest Ophthalmol Visual Sci.* 2018;59(14):DES116–DES120.

47. Yokoi N, Georgiev GA. Tear-film-oriented diagnosis and therapy for dry eye. In: Yokoi N, ed. *Dry Eye Syndrome: Basic and Clinical Perspectives.* London: Future Medicine; 2013:96–108.

48. Yokoi N, Georgiev GA. Tear-film-oriented diagnosis for dry eye. *Jpn J Ophthalmol.* 2019;63(2):127–136.

49. Yokoi N. *TFOD and TFOT Expert Lecture. Paradigm Shift in the Clinical Practice for Dry Eye.* Medical Review Co., Ltd.; 2020:1–48.

50. Toda I, Shimazaki J, Tsubota K. Dry eye with only decreased tear break-up time is sometimes associated with allergic conjunctivitis. *Ophthalmology.* 1995;102(2): 302–309.

51. Deleted in review.

52. Kase S, Shinohara T, Kase M, Ishida S. Effect of topical rebamipide on goblet cells in the lid wiper of human conjunctiva. *Exp Ther Med.* 2017;13(6):3516–3522.

53. Itakura H, Kashima T, Itakura M, Akiyama H, Kishi S. Topical rebamipide improves lid wiper epitheliopathy. *Clin Ophthalmol.* 2013;7:2137–2141.

54. Aoki T, Yokoi N, Kato H, et al. Mechanism and current state of treatment for filamentary keratitis with dry eye [in Japanese]. *Nippon Ganka Gakkai Zasshi (J Jpn Ophthalmol Soc).* 2019;123:1065–1070.

55. Takahashi Y, Ichinose A, Kakizaki H. Topical rebamipide treatment for superior limbic keratoconjunctivitis in patients with thyroid eye disease. *Am J Ophthalmol.* 2014; 157(4):807–812.e2.

56. Kinoshita S, Oshiden K, Awamura S, Suzuki H, Nakamichi N, Yokoi N. A randomized, multicenter phase 3 study comparing 2% rebamipide (OPC-12759) with 0.1% sodium hyaluronate in the treatment of dry eye. *Ophthalmology.* 2013;120(6):1158–1165.

57. Hyon JY, Kim HM, Lee D, et al. Korean guidelines for the diagnosis and management of dry eye: development and validation of clinical efficacy. *Kor J Ophthalmol.* 2014; 28(3):197–206.

58. Bron AJ, Evans VE, Smith JA. Grading of corneal and conjunctival staining in the context of other dry eye tests. *Cornea.* 2003;22(7).

59. Jee D, Park M, Lee HJ, Kim MS, Kim EC. Comparison of treatment with preservative-free versus preserved sodium hyaluronate 0.1% and fluorometholone 0.1% eyedrops after cataract surgery in patients with preexisting dry-eye syndrome. *J Cataract Refract Surg.* 2015;41(4).

60. Jee D, Park SH, Kim MS, Kim EC. Antioxidant and inflammatory cytokine in tears of patients with dry eye syndrome treated with preservative-free versus preserved eye drops. *Invest Ophthalmol Vis Sci.* 2014;55(8):5081–5089.

61. Park Y, Song JS, Choi CY, Yoon KC, Lee HK, Kim HS. A randomized multicenter study comparing 0.1%, 0.15%, and 0.3% sodium hyaluronate with 0.05% cyclosporine in the treatment of dry eye. *J Ocul Pharmacol Therapeut.* 2016;33(2):66–72.

62. You IC, Li Y, Jin R, Ahn M, Choi W, Yoon KC. Comparison of 0.1%, 0.18%, and 0.3% hyaluronic acid eye drops in the treatment of experimental dry eye. *J Ocul Pharmacol Therapeut.* 2018;34(8):557–564.

63. Oh HJ, Li Z, Park S-H, Yoon KC. Effect of hypotonic 0.18% sodium hyaluronate eyedrops on inflammation of the ocular surface in experimental dry eye. *J Ocul Pharmacol Therapeut.* 2014;30(7):533–542.

64. Lee HS, Ji YS, Yoon KC. Efficacy of hypotonic 0.18% sodium hyaluronate eye drops in patients with dry eye disease. *Cornea.* 2014;33(9).

65. Li Y, Cui L, Lee HS, Kang YS, Choi W, Yoon KC. Comparison of 0.3% hypotonic and isotonic sodium hyaluronate eye drops in the treatment of experimental dry eye. *Curr Eye Res.* 2017;42(8):1108–1114.

66. Byun Y-S, Rho CR, Cho K, Choi JA, Na KS, Joo C-K. Cyclosporine 0.05% ophthalmic emulsion for dry eye in Korea: a prospective, multicenter, open-label, surveillance study. *Kor J Ophthalmol.* 2011;25(6):369–374.

67. Kang D-H, Lee Y-W, Hwang K-Y, et al. Changes of tear film lipid layer thickness by 3% diquafosol ophthalmic solutions in patients with dry eye syndrome. *Int J Ophthalmol.* 2019;12(10):1555–1560.

68. Park DH, Chung JK, Seo DR, Lee SJ. Clinical effects and safety of 3% diquafosol ophthalmic solution for patients with dry eye after cataract surgery: a randomized controlled trial. *Am J Ophthalmol.* 2016;163:122–131.e2.

69. Jun I, Choi S, Lee GY, et al. Effects of preservative-free 3% diquafosol in patients with pre-existing dry eye disease after cataract surgery: a randomized clinical trial. *Sci Rep.* 2019;9(1):12659.

70. Yang JM, Choi W, Kim N, Yoon KC. Comparison of topical cyclosporine and diquafosol treatment in dry eye. *Optom Vis Sci.* 2015;92(9).

71. Lee JH, Song IS, Kim KL, Yoon SY. Effectiveness and optical quality of topical 3.0% diquafosol versus 0.05% cyclosporine A in dry eye patients following cataract surgery. *Journal of Ophthalmol.* 2016;2016:8150757.

72. Yoon K-C, Im S-K, Park Y-G, Jung Y-D, Yang S-Y, Choi J. Application of umbilical cord serum eyedrops for the treatment of dry eye syndrome. *Cornea.* 2006;25(3).

73. Yoon KC, Jeong IY, Im SK, Park YG, Kim HJ, Choi J. Therapeutic effect of umbilical cord serum eyedrops for the treatment of dry eye associated with graft-versus-host disease. *Bone Marrow Transplant.* 2007;39(4):231–235.

74. Yoon K-C, Heo H, Im S-K, You I-C, Kim Y-H, Park Y-G. Comparison of autologous serum and umbilical cord serum eye drops for dry eye syndrome. *Am J Ophthalmol.* 2007;144(1):86–92.e2.

75. Yoon KC. Use of umbilical cord serum in ophthalmology. *Chonnam Med J.* 2014;50(3):82–85.

76. Kim JH, Kim HY, Ryu YH, et al. The effect of an antioxidative and anti-inflammatory functional dietary supplement in dry eye syndrome. *J Korean Ophthalmol Soc.* 2008;49(9):1397–1405.

77. Choi W, Lee JB, Cui L, et al. Therapeutic efficacy of topically applied antioxidant medicinal plant extracts in a mouse model of experimental dry eye. *Oxid Med Cell Longev.* 2016;2016:4727415.

78. Choi W, Kim JC, Kim WS, et al. Clinical effect of antioxidant glasses containing extracts of medicinal plants in patients with dry eye disease: a multi-center, prospective, randomized, double-blind, placebo-controlled trial. *PLoS One.* 2015;10(10):e0139761.

79. Yang JM, Li F, Liu Q, et al. A novel TRPM8 agonist relieves dry eye discomfort. *BMC Ophthalmol.* 2017;17(1):101.

80. Teo CHY, Ong HS, Liu Y-C, Tong L. Meibomian gland dysfunction is the primary determinant of dry eye symptoms: analysis of 2346 patients. *Ocul Surf.* 2020;18(4):604–612.

81. Tong L, Chaurasia SS, Mehta JS, Beuerman RW. Screening for meibomian gland disease: its relation to dry eye subtypes and symptoms in a tertiary referral clinic in Singapore. *Invest Ophthalmol Visual Sci.* 2010;51(7):3449–3454.

82. Man REK, Veerappan AR, Tan S-P, et al. Incidence and risk factors of symptomatic dry eye disease in Asian Malays from the Singapore Malay Eye Study. *Ocul Surf.* 2017;15(4):742–748.

83. Waduthantri S, Yong SS, Tan CH, Htoon HM, Tong L. Lubricant with gelling agent in treating dry eye in adult Chinese patients. *Optom Vis Sci.* 2012;89(11).

84. Waduthantri S, Tan CH, Fong YW, Tong L. Specialized moisture retention eyewear for evaporative dry eye. *Curr Eye Res.* 2015;40(5):490–495.

85. Tong L, Beuerman R, Simonyi S, Hollander DA, Stern ME. Effects of punctal occlusion on clinical signs and symptoms and on tear cytokine levels in patients with dry eye. *Ocul Surf.* 2016;14(2):233–241.

86. Tong L, Zhou L, Beuerman R, Simonyi S, Hollander DA, Stern ME. Effects of punctal occlusion on global tear proteins in patients with dry eye. *Ocul Surf.* 2017;15(4):736–741.

87. Teo ZL, Chu C, Tong L. Severe dysfunctional tear syndrome patients and resolution of central corneal staining: retrospective cohort study. *Br J Ophthalmol.* 2020;104(12):1669.

88. Petznick A, Tong L, Chung R, et al. Autologous plasma eyedrops prepared in a closed system: a treatment for dry eye. *Eye.* 2013;27(9):1102.

89. Chong PQY, Yeo S, Too CL, Boo C, Tong L. Effects of wearing a daily disposable lens on tear film: a randomised controlled trial. *Clin Exp Optom.* 2016;99(3):241–247.

90. Garrigue J-S, Amrane M, Faure M-O, Holopainen JM, Tong L. Relevance of lipid-based products in the management of dry eye disease. *J Ocul Pharmacol Therapeut.* 2017; 33(9):647−661.

91. Lim P, Han TA, Tong L. Short-term changes in tear lipid layer thickness after instillation of lipid containing eye drops. *Transl Vis Sci Technol.* 2020;9(8):29.

92. Jerkins G GJ, Tong L, Tan J, Tauber J, Mearza A, Srinivasan S. A comparison of efficacy and safety of two lipid-based lubricant eye drops for the management of evaporative dry eye disease. *Clin Ophthalmol.* 2020;14: 1665−1673.

93. Tong L, Sun CC, Yoon KC, Lim Bon Siong R, Puangsricharern V, Baudouin C. Cyclosporine anionic and cationic ophthalmic emulsions in dry eye disease: a literature review. *Ocul Immunol Inflamm.* 2020:1−10.

94. Sim HS, Petznick A, Barbier S, et al. A randomized, controlled treatment trial of eyelid-warming therapies in meibomian gland dysfunction. *Ophthalmol Ther.* 2014;3(1):37−48.

95. Zhao Y, Veerappan A, Yeo S, et al. Clinical trial of thermal pulsation (LipiFlow) in meibomian gland dysfunction with preteatment meibography. *Eye Contact Lens.* 2016; 42(6).

96. Yang Wei K, Turgay C, Hwee Kuan L, Andrea P, Louis HT. Detection of meibomian glands and classification of meibography images. *J Biomed Opt.* 2012;17(8):1−8.

97. Zhao Y, Tan CLS, Tong L. Intra-observer and inter-observer repeatability of ocular surface interferometer in measuring lipid layer thickness. *BMC Ophthalmol.* 2015;15(1):53.

98. Yeo S, Tan JH, Acharya UR, Sudarshan VK, Tong L. Longitudinal changes in tear evaporation rates after eyelid warming therapies in meibomian gland dysfunction. *Invest Ophthalmol Visual Sci.* 2016;57(4):1974−1981.

99. Han SB, Liu Y-C, Mohamed-Noriega K, Tong L, Mehta JS. Objective imaging diagnostics for dry eye disease. *J Ophthalmol.* 2020;2020:3509064.

100. Tong L, Teo CHY, Lee RKJ. Spatial distribution of noninvasive break up times and clinical relevance in healthy participants and mild dry eye. *Transl Vis Sci Technol.* 2019;8(5):30.

101. Lee R,YS, Aung HT, Tong L. Agreement of noninvasive tear break-up time measurement between tomey RT-7000 auto refractor-keratometer and Oculus Keratograph 5M. *Clin Ophthalmol.* 2016;10:1785−1790.

102. Qiu TY, Tong L. Satisfaction and convenience of using terpenoid-impregnated eyelid wipes and teaching method in people without blepharitis. *Clin Ophthalmol.* 2018;12:91−98.

103. Gong L, Sun X, Ma Z, et al. A randomised, parallel-group comparison study of diquafosol ophthalmic solution in patients with dry eye in China and Singapore. *Br J Ophthalmol.* 2015;99(7):903.

104. Tong L, Teng LS. Review of literature on measurements of non-invasive break up times, lipid morphology and tear meniscal height using commercially available hand-held instruments. *Curr Eye Res.* 2018;43(5):567−575.

105. Rashid MAKM, Thia ZZ, Teo CH, Mamun S, Ong HS, Tong L. Evaluation of strip meniscometry and association with clinical and demographic variables in a community eye study (in Bangladesh). *J Clin Med.* 2020;9(10).

106. Ng S-J, Ong HS, Tong L. A practical framework for telemedicine in dry eye disease. *Ocul Surf.* 2020;S1542-0124(20):30165−30168.

107. Tong L, Htoon HM, Hou A, et al. Acupuncture and herbal formulation compared with artificial tears alone: evaluation of dry eye symptoms and associated tests in randomised clinical trial. *BMJ Open Ophthalmol.* 2018;3(1): e000150.

108. Lim EWL, Chee ML, Sabanayagam C, et al. Relationship between sleep and symptoms of tear dysfunction in Singapore Malays and Indians. *Invest Ophthalmol Visual Sci.* 2019;60(6):1889−1897.

109. Liyue H, Chiang PP-C, Sung SC, Tong L. Dry eye-related visual blurring and irritative symptoms and their association with depression and anxiety in eye clinic patients. *Curr Eye Res.* 2016;41(5):590−599.

110. Yeo S, Tong L. Coping with dry eyes: a qualitative approach. *BMC Ophthalmol.* 2018;18(1):8.

111. Tong L, Petznick A, Lee S, Tan J. Choice of artificial tear formulation for patients with dry eye: where do we start? *Cornea.* 2012;31.

112. Poh S, Lee R, Gao J, et al. Factors that influence tear meniscus area and conjunctivochalasis: the Singapore Indian eye study. *Ophthalmic Epidemiol.* 2018;25(1):70−78.

113. Lee SY, Wong TT, Chua J, Boo C, Soh YF, Tong L. Effect of chronic anti-glaucoma medications and trabeculectomy on tear osmolarity. *Eye.* 2013;27(10):1142−1150.

114. Wong TT, Zhou L, Li J, et al. Proteomic profiling of inflammatory signaling molecules in the tears of patients on chronic glaucoma medication. *Invest Ophthalmol Visual Sci.* 2011;52(10):7385−7391.

115. Chao C, Tong L. Tear lactoferrin and features of ocular allergy in different severities of meibomian gland dysfunction. *Optom Vis Sci.* 2018;95(10).

116. Bose T, Hou A, Lee R, Tong L, Chandy KG. A non-invasive way to isolate and phenotype cells from the conjunctiva. *J Vis Exp.* 2017;(125):55591.

117. Stapleton F, Alves M, Bunya VY, et al. TFOS DEWS II epidemiology report. *Ocul Surf.* 2017;15(3):334−365.

118. Dana R, Bradley JL, Guerin A, et al. Estimated prevalence and incidence of dry eye disease based on coding analysis of a large, all-age United States health care system. *Am J Ophthalmol.* 2019;202:47−54.

119. Inomata T, Iwagami M, Nakamura M, et al. Characteristics and risk factors associated with diagnosed and undiagnosed symptomatic dry eye using a smartphone application. *JAMA Ophthalmol.* 2019;138(1):58−68.

120. Lin P-Y, Cheng C-Y, Hsu W-M, et al. Association between symptoms and signs of dry eye among an elderly Chinese population in Taiwan: the Shihpai eye study. *Invest Ophthalmol Visual Sci.* 2005;46(5):1593−1598.

121. Kuo Y-K, Lin IC, Chien L-N, et al. Dry eye disease: a review of epidemiology in taiwan, and its clinical treatment and merits. *J Clin Med.* 2019;8(8):1227.

122. Hung N, Kang E-Y, Lee T-W, Chen T-S, Shyu Y-C, Sun C-C. The risks of corneal surface damage in aqueous deficient dry eye disease: a 17-year population-based study in Taiwan. *Am J Ophthalmol.* 2021;227(7):231−239.

123. Thulasi P, Djalilian AR. Update in current diagnostics and therapeutics of dry eye disease. *Ophthalmology.* 2017; 124(11S):S27−S33.

124. Shimazaki J. Definition and diagnostic criteria of dry eye disease: historical overview and future directions. *Invest Ophthalmol Visual Sci.* 2018;59(14):DES7−DES12.

125. Milner MS, Beckman KA, Luchs JI, et al. Dysfunctional tear syndrome: dry eye disease and associated tear film disorders - new strategies for diagnosis and treatment. *Curr Opin Ophthalmol.* 2017;27(Suppl 1):3−47.

126. Vehof J, Sillevis Smitt-Kamminga N, Nibourg SA, Hammond CJ. Predictors of discordance between symptoms and signs in dry eye disease. *Ophthalmology.* 2017; 124(3):280−286.

127. Wang MTM, Xue AL, Craig JP. Screening utility of a rapid non-invasive dry eye assessment algorithm. *Contact Lens Anterior Eye.* 2019;42(5):497−501.

128. Jones SM, Nischal KK. The non-invasive tear film break-up time in normal children. *Br J Ophthalmol.* 2013; 97(9):1129.

129. Jones L, Downie LE, Korb D, et al. TFOS DEWS II management and therapy report. *Ocul Surf.* 2017;15(3): 575−628.

130. O'Neil EC, Henderson M, Massaro-Giordano M, Bunya VY. Advances in dry eye disease treatment. *Curr Opin Ophthalmol.* 2019;30(3):166−178.

131. Management and therapy of dry eye disease: report of the management and therapy subcommittee of the international dry eye workshop (2007). *Ocul Surf.* 2007;5(2): 163−178.

132. Boboridis KG, Konstas AGP. Evaluating the novel application of cyclosporine 0.1% in ocular surface disease. *Expet Opin Pharmacother.* 2018;19(9):1027−1039.

133. Kim YJ, Ryu JS, Park SY, et al. Comparison of topical application of TSG-6, cyclosporine, and prednisolone for treating dry eye. *Cornea.* 2016;35(4).

134. Lekhanont K, Rojanaporn D, Chuck RS, Vongthongsri A. Prevalence of dry eye in Bangkok, Thailand. *Cornea.* 2006;25(10).

135. Lee AJ, Lee J, Saw SM, et al. Prevalence and risk factors associated with dry eye symptoms: a population based study in Indonesia. *Br J Ophthalmol.* 2002;86(12):1347−1351.

136. Wu SZZ, Chong JK, Tracer N, Wu M, Raju L. Prevalence of dry eye symptoms and relationship to screen time in a New York City pediatric population. *Invest Ophthalmol Visual Sci.* 2020;61(7):340.

137. The Cornea and Refractive Surgery Society of Thailand (CRST). *Dry Eye or Not? [Mobile App].* https://play. google.com/store/apps/details?id=th.co.progaming.drye yeornot&hl=en_US&gl=US, (Retrieved on March 10, 2021).

138. Topcon Company. *SL-D Series Digital Slit-Lamp.* https:// www.topcon.co.jp/en/eyecare/products/product/diagno stic/sl/SL-Dseries_E.html, (Retrieved on March 10, 2021).

139. Zhong J-Y, Lee Y-C, Hsieh C-J, Tseng C-C, Yiin L-M. Association between dry eye disease, air pollution and weather changes in taiwan. *Int J Environ Res Publ Health.* 2018;15(10):2269.

140. Youn J-S, Seo J-W, Park W, Park S, Jeon K-J. Prediction model for dry eye syndrome incidence rate using air pollutants and meteorological factors in South Korea: analysis of sub-region deviations. *Int J Environ Res Publ Health.* 2020;17(14).

141. Kawashima M, Sano K, Takechi S, Tsubota K. Impact of lifestyle intervention on dry eye disease in office workers: a randomized controlled trial. *J Occup Health.* 2018; 60(4):281−288.

142. Kawashima M, Uchino M, Yokoi N, et al. The association between dry eye disease and physical activity as well as sedentary behavior: results from the Osaka study. *J Ophthalmol.* 2014;2014:943786.

143. Kojima T, Simsek C, Igarashi A, et al. The role of 2% rebamipide eye drops related to conjunctival differentiation in superoxide dismutase-1 (Sod1) knockout mice. *Invest Ophthalmol Visual Sci.* 2018;59(3):1675−1681.

CHAPTER 13

Treatment of Dry Eye Disease in Europe

ELISABETH M. MESSMER, MD, FEBO • JOSE BENITEZ-DEL-CASTILLO, MD •
CHRISTOPHE BAUDOUIN, MD, PHD

EUROPEAN DRY EYE SOCIETY

The European Dry Eye Society (EuDES) was founded in 2020. Its goal is to support European researchers and clinicians to expand our knowledge in the area of Dry Eye and other ocular surface diseases. Close collaborations with the existing TFOS and Asian Dry Eye Society are desired. Sharing cutting-edge scientific knowledge and practical skills on dry eye disease (DED) with other European experts, as well as anyone interested in DED and optimizing ocular surface treatment for patients is important to EuDES. EuDES hopes to fill the gap between basic science research in the ivory towers and the practitioners in the trenches, attending to the needs of real people in disabling pain with very poor quality of life. The website of EuDES was just released and is accessible under https://www.dryeye-society.com. An educational program with life talks and other webinars as well as an annual congress (EuDEC) are planned. The authors of this chapter are closely involved in the foundation of this new society and are part of the current Executive Committee.

DEFINITION OF DED IN EUROPE

The definition of the DEWS II report from 2017 is typically also used in Europe; however, there is some containment. The term "homeostasis" is perceived as very theoretical, the loss of visual symptoms in this definition is deeply regret, and the problem to analyze hyperosmolarity in dry eye patients in Europe—although being a definition criterion—is seen critical. Recently a group of dry eye researchers from Europe, Asia, and United States published a revised definition seemingly more relevant to the clinician: "Dry eye is a multifactorial disease characterized by a persistently unstable and/or deficient tear film (TF) causing discomfort and/or visual impairment, accompanied by variable degrees of ocular surface epitheliopathy, inflammation and neurosensory abnormalities."[1]

CLASSIFICATION OF DED IN EUROPE

Barabino et al. recently suggested an update of DED classification defining three types of disease to improve grading of severity[2]: Type I is a transient and reversible form with subclinical inflammation, possible epithelial alterations, and occasional alterations in vision. Type II is a recurrent form characterized by a reduced ability to reequilibrate the ocular surface, frequent symptoms and alterations in vision with clinically evident inflammation, and clear evidence of epithelial alterations. Type III is a chronic form with inability to reequilibrate the ocular surface and accompanied by clinically evident and chronic inflammation, persistent epithelial alterations, and frequent alterations in quality of vision. They state that the vast majority of patients with DED can be easily classified into one of these three forms. Rolando and coworkers support this concept and propose in addition to include the frequency of symptoms (sporadic, intermittent, persistent, or permanent) into the classification of DED.[3]

EPIDEMIOLOGY OF DED IN EUROPE

Epidemiological data are available for a number of European countries including United Kingdom, France, Spain, Italy, Germany, Norway, and Denmark.[4–8] Dry Eye prevalences are reported between 10% and 34% depending on the age and sex of the examined population as well as the definition used. Asymptomatic Meibomian Gland Dysfunction (MGD) occurred in 21.9% and symptomatic MGD in 8.6% in a study from Spain.[9] An Italian study on VDT users found a prevalence of definite DED in 23.4% and suspected DED in 44.4% of persons.[10] The German Register for Glaucoma patients documented a high prevalence of DED in glaucoma patients (56.9% in females, 45.7% in males).[11] Moreover, also in European DED patients, allergy, cataract surgery, rheumatoid arthritis, migraine and stroke, other pain syndromes, and depressive symptoms are confounding factors.[12–14] The economic burden and

Dry Eye Disease. https://doi.org/10.1016/B978-0-323-82753-9.00010-2

reduction of quality of life due to DED is as high as in other areas of the world.[15–19]

DRY EYE DIAGNOSIS IN EUROPE

In its Diagnostic Methodology Report, The Dry Eye Workshop II established a valuable diagnostic flow including triage questions, risk factor analysis, diagnostic tests including questionnaires for symptomology, and analysis of homeostasis markers such as noninvasive break-up time, osmolarity, and ocular surface staining followed by subtype classification with tear meniscus measurements to diagnose aqueous tear deficiency, and meibomian gland evaluation for the diagnosis of MGD. For the European clinician this diagnostic flow, however, seems to be complicated and recommended tests are not available to the general ophthalmologists. In specific dry eye clinics, the recommended diagnostic steps are typically followed with site- and country-specific alterations.

SUBJECTIVE SYMPTOMS OF DED

A multitude of subjective symptoms is reported in dry eye, and the spontaneous terms to express symptoms vary between European countries. Whereas "itchiness," for example, is reported in 38% of the Spanish DED population, it is only prevalent in 16% of French DED patients. "Burning" on the other hand is common in France, Germany, and Italy with over 30%, but not in Spain with only 3% of the reported symptoms.[20] Moreover, DED is perceived differently in various European countries. Whereas it is felt to be a "discomfort" in 77% of patients in United Kingdom (compared 56% of patients in Spain), it is thought to be a "disease" in 34% of DED patients in Spain (compared to 8% in United Kingdom) and a "handicap" in 21% of French DED patients (compared to 2% in Italy).[20] Dry eye symptoms are typically judged as being useful by European Ophthalmologists in the diagnosis of DED; however, symptom questionnaires are rarely used in daily general practice.[21] Questionnaires are usually reserved for specific dry eye clinics. The OSDI questionnaire is well known and commonly used. The standard patient evaluation of eye dryness (SPEED) questionnaire with less questions and an easy interpretation has recently been reported to be suitable for the detection of DED, especially MGD, and replaces the OSDI questionnaire in some countries in Europe as the standard questionnaire.[22]

CLINICAL SIGNS OF DED IN EUROPE

The analysis of homeostasis markers is recommended by the DEWS II. However, there are problems in European Ophthalmology practices to follow this diagnostic algorithm. Noninvasive tear film break-up time is only available in some specific dry eye clinics. Tear film break-up testing is mainly performed invasively with fluorescein. Tear film osmolarity has been shown to be helpful in the diagnosis of moderate to severe DED in German cohorts[23,24]; however, it was not able to diagnose DED in a large Norwegian cohort regardless of cut-off value and intereye difference analysis.[25] Independent of this, tear film osmolarity is rarely measured in Europe due to reimbursement issues. Ocular surface staining is relevant for European Ophthalmologists to grade severity of DED. Baudouin et al. published a clear and practical algorithm of diagnosing severe dry eye with a combination of symptoms (OSDI >33) and fluorescein ocular surface staining using the Oxford Scale of ≥ 3[26]

Lissamine green is rarely used outside of studies to evaluate ocular surface staining. The recommendation of DEWS II to measure tear film quantity by OCT is typically not followed in Europe as anterior segment OCTs are not available in every practice and the calculation of the tear meniscus is still cumbersome. Many clinicians only judge fluorescein tear meniscus at the slit-lamp. Schirmer testing is still in vogue in Europe to diagnose aqueous deficient DED,[21,27,28] although not recommended in the DEWS II workflow. Schirmer testing together with fluorescein BUT were the tests mainly performed by Spanish practitioners[27] and UK ophthalmologists.[21] Schirmer testing was only rarely performed by UK optometrists.[21] Also, in the Netherlands, the use of diagnostic tests between optometrists and ophthalmologists was significantly different[29] Matrix-Metalloproteinase-9-Testing was not recommended by DEWS II; however, it seems to be helpful to diagnose relevant ocular surface inflammation in DED, and institute antiinflammatory treatment.[30] MMP-9 testing is performed rarely by general ophthalmologists but becomes increasingly important for specific dry eye clinics. It is not reimbursed by health insurances.

In addition, the evaluation of lid-parallel conjunctival folds is commonly used by general ophthalmologists in Europe to support the diagnosis of DED.[31]

TREATMENT OF DED IN EUROPE
General Treatment Principles

Treatment of DED in Europe is not uniform. Treatment algorithms are similar but differ in detail between countries. Treatment options may vary profoundly due to the different availability of drugs. In addition, the reimbursement of specific therapies in one country and not in the other influences DED management. Evaporative DED is often overlooked by the general ophthalmologist and may go untreated.

For mild DED, patients usually first see their general practitioner (GP) or their pharmacist. GPs typically are hardly aware of the symptoms and signs of DED and typically diagnose either bacterial conjunctivitis or allergy. Accordingly, in most cases either antibiotics or antiallergics are prescribed by GPs. Also, in pharmacies, DED diagnosis is often missed. This was demonstrated elegantly by a study in the United Kingdom where a mystery shopper with simulated dry eye visited 50 pharmacies in major towns. All pharmacy staff gave a diagnosis with only 42% correctly identifying dry eye.[32] Eight percent of the pharmacists referred directly to a GP or optometrist. Dry eye treatment recommended included topical ocular lubrication and lipid sprays with administration and/or dosage advice in only 10%.[32] Patients with moderate to severe DED are usually seen by ophthalmologists or optometrists (mainly UK) where the diagnosis of DED is established, and treatment for DED is instituted.

ARTIFICIAL TEARS

The mainstay in the treatment for all forms and all severities of DED are artificial tears. They come with many different ingredients and additives. Different options are available in various European countries. However, hyaluronic acid (HA) with different chain lengths, concentrations, qualities, and preparations is the most often used artificial tear in Europe. Artificial tears are typically prescribed with a fixed treatment plan. Patients are instructed to use their artificial tears before symptoms reappear. Applications can range from twice a day to every half hour. Patients may use artificial tears with different mode of actions concomitantly. Patients are informed that special visual tasks such as PC work, reading, or driving may afford increased artificial tear application. For the treatment of MGD, a number of artificial tears with variable lipid components is available. Gels and ointments are added in more severe disease or complaints especially at nighttime. In Europe, artificial tears without preservatives, especially without epitheliotoxic benzalkonium chloride are preferred. Patients are very much aware of the toxicity of benzalkonium chloride and ask for preservative-free or at least benzalkonium-free preparations. Artificial tears with "better preservatives" with less or no toxicity such as polyquad, sodium perborate, and oxychloro-complex are available. An increasing number of artificial tears without preservatives, however, is now on the European market either as unidoses or as preservative-free multidose containers.

Only view studies with appropriate evidence level document the efficacy of artificial tears in the management of DED.

Hyaluronic Acids

HA is a glycosaminoglycan component of the extracellular matrix.

The principal receptor for HA belongs to a family of cell membrane glycoproteins termed CD44 and is involved in a wide range of biological functions including cell adhesion, cell motility, extracellular matrix binding, and lymphocyte homing. CD44 receptors are present in the corneal epithelium and might be responsible for long-lasting adhesion of HA eye drops to the ocular surface.[33] HAs are available in eye drops, gels, and ointments in Europe. Concentration in drops ranges from 0.18% to 0.4%. HA drops alone are often used as basic treatment for aqueous deficient dry eye. Together with lipid-containing artificial tears either as HA–lipid–preparations or together with lipid-containing artificial tears they are used in MGD. Baeyens et al. recently documented the efficacy of 0.18% hypotonic sodium hyaluronate ophthalmic solution in the treatment of symptoms and signs of DED. It was as efficient as 0.3% carbomer with less blur of vision.[34] In a prospective, multicenter, randomized, single-masked phase IIIb, noninferiority study of nonpreserved HA 0.2% versus nonpreserved HA 0.18% both treatments reduced ocular surface staining, tear film BUT, and ocular comfort index values. On treatment day 35 0.2% HA achieved a 47% reduction in staining scores which further increased to 64% on day 84.[35] A preservative-free combination of carboxymethylcellulose (CMC) with HA was compared to CMC alone in a multicenter study in mild to moderate DED. The combined CMC + HA formulation achieved a significant better reduction of overall ocular pain and discomfort compared to CMC alone.[36] HA is also available in combination with Trehalose, a natural bioprotectant in Europe. In a phase III, randomized, active-controlled, investigator masked multicenter study comparing HA alone with HA plus trehalose, both treatments reduced ocular surface staining significantly. HA plus trehalose was able to significantly alleviate symptoms such as stinging, itching, and blurred vision compared to HA alone, and its global performance was judged superior by investigators and patients.[37]

Carboxymethylcellulose

CMC is a component in many lubricants used in the treatment of DED in Europe. It is used in combination or as substitute for HA. CMC has been shown to bind to human corneal epithelial cells (HCECs) probably through interaction of its glucopyranose subunits with glucose transporters. In cell culture studies, CMC binding to matrix proteins stimulated HCEC attachment, migration, and reepithelialization of corneal wounds.[38] In a randomized, controlled, multicenter study comparing CMC alone to CMC with HA, CMC alone was able to significantly reduce subjective symptoms, tear film BUT, and ocular surface staining.[39] CMC is also available together with osmoprotective levocarnithine and erythritol. Moreover, a CMC-lipid preparation with castor oil is frequently used in the care of MGD.

Hydroxypropyl Guar

The mucomimetic agent hydroxypropyl guar (HPG) with tensioactive, gelificaton, and lubrication properties is formulated in eye drops with polyethylene glycol (PEG) and propylene glycol (PG), borate and sorbitol, which compete in the eye drop bottle to reduce borate-mediated cross-linking of HPG. When the low-viscosity formulation is applied to the ocular surface, the sorbitol is diluted by tears, allowing the borate and divalent ions present in the tear film to interact with HPG. This promotes HPG cross-linking to create a structured polymeric network with bioadhesive properties on the ocular surface that prolongs retention of PEG and PG to increase tear film stability, provide sustained lubrication, and protect the ocular surface.[40] In a randomized, double-masked crossover study of patients with dry eye, HPG/PEG/PG maintained visual acuity for a longer duration between blinks 90 min after instillation compared with a CMC-based eye drop.[41] In a multicenter, randomized, observer-masked parallel-group study, ocular surface staining and symptoms were reduced significantly by both HPG/PEG/PG and an osmoprotective CMC product.[40] An improvement in conjunctival impression cytologies in patients with severe DED has been documented in a study from Romania.[42]

ARTIFICIAL TEARS WITH SPECIFIC ADDITIVES

In Europe, a number of artificial tears with very useful additives are on the market and regularly used in the management of DED patients. These additives include **trehalose** (anhydrobiotic, osmoprotective, and antiinflammatory), **erythritol** and **L-carnitine** (antioxidative), **dexpanthenol** (supports wound healing), **Coenzyme Q 10** (antiapoptotic, antioxidative), and topical **Omega fatty acids**.

ARTIFICIAL TEARS WITH LIPIDS

Lipid-containing artificial tears are typically used in the care of MGD patients. Often, they are recommended to be used with either HA, CMC, or HPG in combination. Combination products are also on the European market. Lipid-containing artificial tears support the tear film lipid layer and increase TF-BUT. Lipids used in European preparations include castor oil, paraffin oil, triglycerides, phospholipids, and perfluorohexyloctane. Semifluorinated alkane eye drops, for example, have been shown to increase tear film thickness and lipid layer thickness over time thus stabilizing the tear film and reducing evaporation.[43] Semifluorinated alkane eye drops have also resulted in improved signs and symptoms in MGD patients[44] and improved symptoms of patients with severe ocular graft-versus-host disease[45]

LID HYGIENE

Lid hygiene is recommended as a basic treatment in patients with MGD. There are many different ways to perform lid hygiene, and this has to be adjusted to the patient's possibilities and needs. In general, hot compresses are recommended for approximately 5 min followed by lid massage toward the lid margin with either the clean finger tip or a cotton tip. Many options exist to improve eye lid warming including warming masks, electric eye lid warming devices, and red light.[46] A little plastic massage tool is available for the patient to improve massaging. Multiple lid cleaners either as solution, wipes, or gels are available to support cleaning of the lid margin. The patients are instructed to use these cleaners after lid warming and lid massage, not instead.

In patients presenting with collarettes and broken eye lashes, a hyperinfestation with demodex mites is suspected, and tea tree oil either as wipes or foam recommended to be applied 2×/day after lid hygiene.

In specific dry eye clinics, **microblepharoexfoliation** is offered to reduce lid margin biofilm, debris, and meibomian gland capping. Dry eye specialists typically perform lid warming and **meibomian gland expression** with, e.g., the Tearse forceps. In patients not willing or not able to perform lid hygiene, **automated thermodynamic therapy** is provided again only in specific dry eye clinics. All these additional treatments for MGD are commonly not reimbursed by health insurance companies.

INTENSE PULSED LIGHT TREATMENT

Intense pulsed light (IPL) treatment is a relatively new and approved therapeutic option for MGD. It is typically offered when basic treatment with lipid-containing artificial tears and lid hygiene are not sufficient. The treatment consists of two to four sessions where light impulses are applied to the lower lid and temporal lid margin. The IPL technique is a safe form of treatment when the required safety precautions are followed. Current studies document an improvement of patients' subjective symptoms and objectively measured clinical parameters.[47] In Europe several different IPL devices are on the market equipped with or without additional Low Level Light Therapy. IPL treatment is only offered in specific dry eye centers and is usually not paid by the patient's health insurance.

PRESERVATION OF TEAR FILM
Punctum Plugs
Punctum plugs are a good therapeutic option for patients with low Schirmer test (<5 mm in 5 min) and ocular surface damage. However, ocular surface inflammation has to be controlled concomitantly with topical antiinflammatory medication. Punctum plugs are typically installed into the lower punctum. Their effect may be tested with resorbable collagen plugs; however, silicone plugs or intracanalicular plugs are superior for long-term treatment. Extrusion and loss is the main problem. Very rarely pyogenic granuloma develops around the plug in the punctual area and requires removal of the punctum plug.

Moisture Goggles
Moisture goggles help to preserve the available tear fluid at the ocular surface and prevent evaporation. They are often recommended by the treating physician, but are rarely used by patients due to their unfavorable looks.

ANTIINFLAMMATORY TREATMENT IN DED IN EUROPE
Topical Corticosteroids
Inflammation is an important pathogenetic factor in DED. This knowledge is slowly spreading throughout the ophthalmology community in Europe, however, still is not uniformly present. Nonpreserved topical corticosteroids as a short-term tapering treatment for 2–4 weeks are prescribed when basic treatment with artificial tears and lid hygiene does not improve signs and symptoms of DED. They may be used as a proof of concept whether a longstanding antiinflammatory treatment is reasonable. So called "soft corticosteroids" are preferred. A topical low dose 0.335% preservative-free hydrocortisone is available on the European market

and is used quite frequently in DED management. In a recent study, hydrocortisone 0.3% for 28 days in a tapering dosing scheme has been shown to reduce ocular surface inflammation and decrease subjective symptoms of DED without changes in IOP.[48] In some European countries HA is available in combination with hydrocortisone 0.001%, where the antiinflammatory properties are minor. This product is mainly used as artificial tear promoting homeostasis of the tear film.

Topical Cyclosporine A
Until 2015, pharmacy-formulated cyclosporine A (CSA) in concentrations from 0.5% to 2.0% were used in the care of DED, as anionic CSA 0.05% was never released in Europe. Thereafter, a nonpreserved cationic oil-in-water emulsion of CSA 0.1 was approved for the European market for the treatment of DED. However, the indication is limited to "Treatment of severe keratitis in adult patients with dry eye disease, which has not improved despite treatment with tear substitutes." This indication is based on the so-called SANSIKA study, a multicenter, randomized, double-masked, 2-parallel arms, 6 months phase III study with a 6-month open label treatment safety follow-up of CSA 0.1% vs. Vehicle. This study included patients with severe DED with corneal fluorescein staining grade 4 on the modified Oxford scale. In this study, CSA 0.1% significantly improved corneal fluorescein staining, reduced the ocular surface inflammatory marker HLA-DR, and improved tear film osmolarity compared to vehicle.[49−52]

Discussions in the ophthalmology community concern the term "severe keratitis" in the indication of the drug. Many treating physicians would start treatment with CSA 0.1% in DED with obvious corneal staining of ≥2 in the Oxford Grading Scheme and would not wait for grade 4 staining as done in the study. If corneal staining was already reduced by topical corticosteroids with good effect, CSA 0.1% is also instituted with even lower ocular surface staining scores.[53]

The recommended dose of CSA 0.1% is one drop at bedtime. Patients are instructed to continue their artificial tears. They are also informed that it may take 6−8 weeks until CSA drops take effect and that a typical side effect is burning/stinging on instillation which will improve with time.

Very often, topical corticosteroids are used before or in the first 4 weeks concomitantly with CSA to improve tolerability and to accelerate treatment success. In our own CSA 0.1% patients (E.M.), topical corticosteroids as bridging therapy reduced symptoms significantly earlier as seen in the Sansika study. Patients are typically followed up every 3 months. Treatment with CSA 0.1% should at least be continued for 6 months. The Sansika extension data, however, suggest that CSA 0.1% therapy for 1 year might be superior with less recurrences back to severe ocular surface damage.[54] Although CSA 0.1% is approved for the treatment of DED with ocular surface damage, a number of European countries are still using compounded formulations due to cost and reimbursement issues.[55] Also in countries where CSA 0.1% is approved and reimbursed, general ophthalmologists are sometimes reluctant to prescribe it due to missing knowledge on its properties, fear of side effects, and budget issues.

Hind et al. report on their real-world experience at a Scottish university teaching hospital regarding the tolerability and persistence with topical CSA 0.1% treatment in patients with DED. Mean duration of treatment was 11 months (median 8.5; range 2–30). Sixty three percent of patients (33/52) were also treated with a tapering dose of topical steroids for the first month during the initiation phase of CSA 0.1% use. All patients remained on long-term topical lubrication treatment at least 4 times per day. At last case note CSA 0.1% was well tolerated and treatment persisted successfully in 88% (46/52) of patients. Only six patients discontinued CSA 0.1% due to intolerance in the time period identified, although two were able to restart and persist (intolerant of treatment 4/52; 7.7%). The reason stated for lack of persistence was local irritation, burning, or stinging.[56]

ANTIBIOTIC TREATMENT IN DED
Topical and systemic antibiotics with antiinflammatory properties are used in the management of MGD. Although these treatment options have been in the recommended treatment schedules for quite some time, general ophthalmologists are still reluctant to prescribe oral doxycycline or topical azithromycine in the care of patients with MGD. One reason being the fact that MGD is often not diagnosed in the general ophthalmology practice at all, and treatment for MGD is preferentially initiated in specific dry eye clinics.

Oral Doxycycline
Oral doxycycline treatment is an established therapy in patients with MGD due to rosacea due to its beneficial effect on skin and eye lids. In these cases, a dose of 40–100 mg/day is typically used. However, also in patients with MGD not associated with rosacea, oral doxycycline therapy at a dose of 100 mg/day is instituted as soon as lipid-containing artificial tears and lid hygiene

are not sufficient. A 6-week to 3-month course is typically recommended but can be extended for longer duration.

Topical Azithromycine
Topical azithromycine is available as an oily 1.5% formulation in Europe. Different application protocols exist but seem to be similarly effective. Whereas some physicians apply the typical "Foulks" protocol with azithromycine 2×/day × 2 days followed by 1×/day × 4 weeks, others recommend to apply the oily drop in the conjunctival sac or to the lid margin 2×/day × 1 week for three cycles with 1 week of break in between the cycles.[57] A randomized study in patients with MGD has just demonstrated the equal efficacy of oral doxycycline and topical azithromycine 1.5% in a 4-week study. However, side effects occurred in a much higher rate in the topical azithromycine group (56.3%; eye irritation, blurred vision) compared to the oral doxycycline group (21.1%, gastrointestinal problems). The number of patients discontinuing the treatment due to the side effect was however equal and low with around 5%.[58] Thus, azithromycine is a good option for patients with gastrointestinal disease or pregnant patients. It may also be instituted together with oral doxycycline.

AUTOLOGOUS SERUM
Autologous serum eye drops appear to be the perfect tear substitute containing a number of epitheliotropic factors to support epithelial healing. They are produced at concentrations of 20%–100%. The protocols to prepare and use autologous serum eye drops vary considerably in studies and in Europe.[59] In Germany, the use of autologous serum eye drops has been hampered by regulatory issues. Only institutions with a license to produce blood-derived products are allowed to make and distribute autologous serum eye drops. This massively reduced the number of ophthalmological institutions being able to use and prescribe these drops.[60,61] In Spain, Plasma Rich in Growth factors is preferred.[36]

Albumin eye drops[62] or allogeneic serum eye drops[63] may be an alternative for the treatment of ocular surface disease but have not been established in daily practice. The use of finger prick autologous blood has been advocated but does not appeal to be a good treatment option for most patients.[64]

Taken together, DED treatment in Europe in general follows TFOS DEWS II recommendations. However, diagnostic and treatment options vary between different European countries due to availabilities and reimbursement issues. Pharmacists, optometrists (mainly UK),

GPs, general ophthalmologists, and dry eye specialists are involved in the care of DED patients. Aqueous deficient DED and evaporative DED are often not discriminated by the general ophthalmologist; MGD is frequently overlooked. Specific Dry Eye Clinics are increasingly founded and welcome by DED patients to establish a correct diagnosis and initiate an appropriate treatment in DED.

REFERENCES

1. Tsubota K, Pflugfelder SC, Liu Z, et al. Defining dry eye from a clinical perspective. *Int J Mol Sci.* 2020;21.
2. Barabino S, Aragona P, di Zazzo A, Rolando M. Updated definition and classification of dry eye disease: renewed proposals using the nominal group and Delphi techniques. *Eur J Ophthalmol.* 2020, 1120672120960586.
3. Rolando M, Zierhut M, Barabino S. Should we reconsider the classification of patients with dry eye disease? *Ocul Immunol Inflamm.* 2019:1–3.
4. Bjerrum KB. Keratoconjunctivitis sicca and primary Sjögren's syndrome in a Danish population aged 30-60 years. *Acta Ophthalmologica Scandinavica.* 1997;75: 281–286.
5. Ferrero A, Alassane S, Binquet C, et al. Dry eye disease in the elderly in a French population-based study (the Montrachet study: maculopathy, optic Nerve, nuTRition, neurovAsCular and HEarT diseases): prevalence and associated factors. *Ocul Surf.* 2018;16:112–119.
6. Millán A, Viso E, Gude F, Parafita-Fernández A, Moraña N, Rodríguez-Ares MT. Incidence and risk factors of dry eye in a Spanish adult population: 11-year follow-up from the Salnés eye study. *Cornea.* 2018;37:1527–1534.
7. Reitmeir P, Linkohr B, Heier M, et al. Common eye diseases in older adults of southern Germany: results from the KORA-Age study. *Age Ageing.* 2017;46:481–486.
8. Viso E, Rodriguez-Ares MT, Gude F. Prevalence of and associated factors for dry eye in a Spanish adult population (the Salnes Eye Study). *Ophthalmic Epidemiol.* 2009;16: 15–21.
9. Viso E, Rodríguez-Ares MT, Abelenda D, Oubiña B, Gude F. Prevalence of asymptomatic and symptomatic meibomian gland dysfunction in the general population of Spain. *Investig Ophthalmol Vis Sci.* 2012;53:2601–2606.
10. Rossi GCM, Scudeller L, Bettio F, Pasinetti GM, Bianchi PE. Prevalence of dry eye in video display terminal users: a cross-sectional Caucasian study in Italy. *Int Ophthalmol.* 2019;39:1315–1322.
11. Erb C, Gast U, Schremmer D. German register for glaucoma patients with dry eye. I. Basic outcome with respect to dry eye. *Graefe's Arch Clin Exp Ophthalmol.* 2008;246: 1593–1601.
12. Kaiser T, Janssen B, Schrader S, Geerling G. Depressive symptoms, resilience, and personality traits in dry eye disease. *Graefe's Arch Clin Exp Ophthalmol.* 2019;257: 591–599.
13. Nepp J. [Psychosomatic aspects of dry eye syndrome]. *Der Ophthalmologe: Zeitschrift der Deutschen Ophthalmologischen Gesellschaft.* 2016;113:111–119.
14. Vehof J, Kozareva D, Hysi PG, Hammond CJ. Prevalence and risk factors of dry eye disease in a British female cohort. *Br J Ophthalmol.* 2014;98:1712–1717.
15. Barabino S, Labetoulle M, Rolando M, Messmer EM. Understanding symptoms and quality of life in patients with dry eye syndrome. *Ocul Surf.* 2016;14:365–376.
16. Benítez-Del-Castillo J, Labetoulle M, Baudouin C, et al. Visual acuity and quality of life in dry eye disease: proceedings of the OCEAN group meeting. *Ocul Surf.* 2017;15: 169–178.
17. Clegg JP, Guest JF, Lehman A, Smith AF. The annual cost of dry eye syndrome in France, Germany, Italy, Spain, Sweden and the United Kingdom among patients managed by ophthalmologists. *Ophthalmic Epidemiol.* 2006;13: 263–274.
18. McDonald M, Patel DA, Keith MS, Snedecor SJ. Economic and humanistic burden of dry eye disease in Europe, north America, and Asia: a systematic literature review. *Ocul Surf.* 2016;14:144–167.
19. Messmer E, Chan C, Asbell P, Johnson G, Sloesen B, Cook N. Comparing the needs and preferences of patients with moderate and severe dry eye symptoms across four countries. *BMJ Open Ophthalmol.* 2019;4:e000360.
20. Labetoulle M, Rolando M, Baudouin C, van Setten G. Patients' perception of DED and its relation with time to diagnosis and quality of life: an international and multilingual survey. *Br J Ophthalmol.* 2017;101:1100–1105.
21. Graham JE, McGilligan VE, Berrar D, et al. Attitudes towards diagnostic tests and therapies for dry eye disease. *Ophthalmic Res.* 2010;43:11–17.
22. Finis D, Pischel N, König C, et al. [Comparison of the OSDI and SPEED questionnaires for the evaluation of dry eye disease in clinical routine]. *Der Ophthalmologe: Zeitschrift der Deutschen Ophthalmologischen Gesellschaft.* 2014;111:1050–1056.
23. Jacobi C, Jacobi A, Kruse FE, Cursiefen C. Tear film osmolarity measurements in dry eye disease using electrical impedance technology. *Cornea.* 2011;30:1289–1292.
24. Schargus M, Wolf F, Tony HP, Meyer-Ter-Vehn T, Geerling G. Correlation between tear film osmolarity, dry eye disease, and rheumatoid arthritis. *Cornea.* 2014; 33:1257–1261.
25. Tashbayev B, Utheim TP, Utheim Ø A, et al. Utility of tear osmolarity measurement in diagnosis of dry eye disease. *Sci Rep.* 2020;10:5542.
26. Baudouin C, Aragona P, Van Setten G, et al. Diagnosing the severity of dry eye: a clear and practical algorithm. *Br J Ophthalmol.* 2014;98:1168–1176.
27. Cardona G, Serés C, Quevedo L, Augé M. Knowledge and use of tear film evaluation tests by Spanish practitioners. *Optom Vis Sci.* 2011;88:1106–1111.
28. Yazdani M, Chen X, Tashbayev B, et al. Tear production levels and dry eye disease severity in a large Norwegian cohort. *Curr Eye Res.* 2018;43:1465–1470.

29. van Tilborg MM, Murphy PJ, Evans KS. Agreement in dry eye management between optometrists and general practitioners in primary health care in The Netherlands. *Contact Lens Anter Eye.* 2015;38:283−293.

30. Messmer EM, von Lindenfels V, Garbe A, Kampik A. Matrix metalloproteinase 9 testing in dry eye disease using a commercially available point-of-care immunoassay. *Ophthalmology.* 2016;123:2300−2308.

31. Pult H, Bandlitz S. Lid-parallel conjunctival folds and their ability to predict dry eye. *Eye Contact Lens.* 2018;44(Suppl 2):S113−s119.

32. Bilkhu PS, Wolffsohn JS, Tang GW, Naroo SA. Management of dry eye in UK pharmacies. *Cont Lens Anter Eye.* 2014;37:382−387.

33. Lerner LE, Schwartz DM, Hwang DG, Howes EL, Stern R. Hyaluronan and CD44 in the human cornea and limbal conjunctiva. *Exp Eye Res.* 1998;67:481−484.

34. Baeyens V, Bron A, Baudouin C. Efficacy of 0.18% hypotonic sodium hyaluronate ophthalmic solution in the treatment of signs and symptoms of dry eye disease. *J Fr Ophtalmol.* 2012;35:412−419.

35. Groß D, Childs M, Piaton JM. Comparison of 0.2% and 0.18% hyaluronate eye drops in patients with moderate to severe dry eye with keratitis or keratoconjunctivitis. *Clin Ophthalmol.* 2017;11:631−638.

36. Anitua E, Muruzabal F, de la Fuente M, Merayo J, Durán J, Orive G. Plasma Rich in Growth factors for the treatment of ocular surface diseases. *Curr Eye Res.* 2016;41:875−882.

37. Chiambaretta F, Doan S, Labetoulle M, et al. A randomized, controlled study of the efficacy and safety of a new eyedrop formulation for moderate to severe dry eye syndrome. *Eur J Ophthalmol.* 2017;27:1−9.

38. Garrett Q, Simmons PA, Xu S, et al. Carboxymethylcellulose binds to human corneal epithelial cells and is a modulator of corneal epithelial wound healing. *Investig Ophthalmol Vis Sci.* 2007;48:1559−1567.

39. Aragona P, Benítez-Del-Castillo JM, Coroneo MT, et al. Safety and efficacy of a preservative-free artificial tear containing carboxymethylcellulose and hyaluronic acid for dry eye disease: a randomized, controlled, multicenter 3-month study. *Clin Ophthalmol.* 2020;14:2951−2963.

40. Labetoulle M, Messmer EM, Pisella PJ, Ogundele A, Baudouin C. Safety and efficacy of a hydroxypropyl guar/polyethylene glycol/propylene glycol-based lubricant eye-drop in patients with dry eye. *Br J Ophthalmol.* 2017;101:487−492.

41. Torkildsen G. The effects of lubricant eye drops on visual function as measured by the Inter-blink interval Visual Acuity Decay test. *Clin Ophthalmol.* 2009;3:501−506.

42. Mocanu C, Bărăscu D, Bîrjovanu F, Mănescu R, Iliuşi F. [Assessment of systane in severe dry eye]. *Oftalmologia.* 2008;52:105−110.

43. Schmidl D, Bata AM, Szegedi S, et al. Influence of perfluorohexyloctane eye drops on tear film thickness in patients with mild to moderate dry eye disease: a randomized controlled clinical trial. *J Ocul Pharmacol Therapeut.* 2020;36:154−161.

44. Steven P, Augustin AJ, Geerling G, et al. Semifluorinated alkane eye drops for treatment of dry eye disease due to meibomian gland disease. *J Ocul Pharmacol Therapeut.* 2017;33:678−685.

45. Eberwein P, Krösser S, Steven P. Semifluorinated alkane eye drops in chronic ocular graft-versus-host disease: a prospective, multicenter, noninterventional study. *Ophthalmic Res.* 2020;63:50−58.

46. Doan S, Chiambaretta F, Baudouin C. Evaluation of an eyelid warming device (Blephasteam) for the management of ocular surface diseases in France: the ESPOIR study. *J Fr Ophtalmol.* 2014;37:763−772.

47. Schuh A, Priglinger S, Messmer EM. [Intense pulsed light (IPL) as a therapeutic option for Meibomian gland dysfunction]. *Der Ophthalmologe: Zeitschrift der Deutschen Ophthalmologischen Gesellschaft.* 2019;116:982−988.

48. Kallab M, Szegedi S, Hommer N, et al. Topical low dose preservative-free hydrocortisone reduces signs and symptoms in patients with chronic dry eye: a randomized clinical trial. *Adv Ther.* 2020;37:329−341.

49. Baudouin C, de la Maza MS, Amrane M, et al. One-year efficacy and safety of 0.1% cyclosporine a cationic emulsion in the treatment of severe dry eye disease. *Eur J Ophthalmol.* 2017;27:678−685.

50. Baudouin C, Figueiredo FC, Messmer EM, et al. A randomized study of the efficacy and safety of 0.1% cyclosporine A cationic emulsion in treatment of moderate to severe dry eye. *Eur J Ophthalmol.* 2017;27:520−530.

51. Leonardi A, Messmer EM, Labetoulle M, et al. Efficacy and safety of 0.1% ciclosporin A cationic emulsion in dry eye disease: a pooled analysis of two double-masked, randomised, vehicle-controlled phase III clinical studies. *Br J Ophthalmol.* 2019;103:125−131.

52. Leonardi A, Van Setten G, Amrane M, et al. Efficacy and safety of 0.1% cyclosporine A cationic emulsion in the treatment of severe dry eye disease: a multicenter randomized trial. *Eur J Ophthalmol.* 2016;26:287−296.

53. Pleyer U, Geerling G, Schrader S, Jacobi C, Kimmich F, Messmer E. [If artificial tears aren't enough. The importance of inflammatory processes in dry eye disease. Practical aspects of an anti-inflammatory therapy of dry eye disease]. *Klinische Monatsblatter fur Augenheilkunde.* 2020;237:655−668.

54. Labetoulle M, Leonardi A, Amrane M, et al. Persistence of efficacy of 0.1% cyclosporin A cationic emulsion in subjects with severe keratitis due to dry eye disease: a nonrandomized, open-label extension of the SANSIKA study. *Clin Therapeut.* 2018;40:1894−1906.

55. Labbé A, Baudouin C, Ismail D, et al. Pan-European survey of the topical ocular use of cyclosporine A. *J Fr Ophtalmol.* 2017;40:187−195.

56. Hind J, Macdonald E, Lockington D. Real-world experience at a Scottish university teaching hospital regarding the tolerability and persistence with topical Ciclosporin 0.1% (Ikervis) treatment in patients with dry eye disease. *Eye.* 2019;33:685−686.

57. Foulks GN, Borchman D, Yappert M, Kim SH, McKay JW. Topical azithromycin therapy for meibomian gland

dysfunction: clinical response and lipid alterations. *Cornea.* 2010;29:781−788.

58. Satitpitakul V, Ratanawongphaibul K, Kasetsuwan N, Reinprayoon U. Efficacy of azithromycin 1.5% eyedrops vs oral doxycycline in meibomian gland dysfunction: a randomized trial. *Graefe's Arch Clin Exp Ophthalmol.* 2019;257:1289−1294.

59. Geerling G, Maclennan S, Hartwig D. Autologous serum eye drops for ocular surface disorders. *Br J Ophthalmol.* 2004;88:1467−1474.

60. Geerling G, Unterlauft JD, Kasper K, Schrader S, Opitz A, Hartwig D. [Autologous serum and alternative blood products for the treatment of ocular surface disorders]. *Der Ophthalmologe: Zeitschrift der Deutschen Ophthalmologischen Gesellschaft.* 2008;105:623−631.

61. Kasper K, Godenschweger L, Hartwig D, Unterlauft JD, Seitz B, Geerling G. [On the use of autologous serum eyedrops in Germany: results of a survey among members of the Cornea Section of the German Ophthalmological Society (DOG)]. *Der Ophthalmologe: Zeitschrift der Deutschen Ophthalmologischen Gesellschaft.* 2008;105:644−649.

62. Schargus M, Kohlhaas M, Unterlauft JD. Treatment of severe ocular surface disorders with albumin eye drops. *J Ocul Pharmacol Therapeut.* 2015;31:291−295.

63. van der Meer PF, Seghatchian J, de Korte D. Autologous and allogeneic serum eye drops. The Dutch perspective. *Transfus Apher Sci.* 2015;53:99−100.

64. Than J, Balal S, Wawrzynski J, et al. Fingerprick autologous blood: a novel treatment for dry eye syndrome. *Eye.* 2017;31:1655−1663.

CHAPTER 14

Treatment of Meibomian Gland Disease

JOSEPH TAUBER, MD

The treatment of meibomian gland dysfunction (MGD) first requires both proper diagnosis of the condition and identification of contributory ocular surfaces disorders that may confuse proper attribution of both patient symptoms and signs.[1] Nomenclature remains confusing as many clinicians alternate between diagnosing patients with dry eye, evaporative dry eye, MGD, ocular rosacea, or, more generically, ocular surface disease. While all of these terms are valid descriptors of ocular surface disease, this chapter will focus on treatment of MGD, to be understood as the evaporative dry eye caused by the tear film dysfunction created by stagnant and/or dysfunctional meibum as well as ocular surface inflammation, whether present within occluded glands in the eyelid, conjunctival and corneal epithelium, and the tear film itself. Of course, it is well recognized that most patients with MGD have some degree of concomitant aqueous tear production deficiency,[2-5] conjunctivochalasis,[6,7] and/or allergic eye disease, and these also require their own distinct therapeutic interventions. The value of clinical skills on the part of the eye care provider in differentiating the relative contributions of these overlapping conditions is crucial to success in addressing patient complaints. Clinicians can be loosely divided into categories of lumpers (all ocular surface disease is one pool) and splitters (subgrouping ocular surface disease matters). The clinical management recommendations of this chapter focus on the treatment of MGD in isolation and follow the thinking of a splitter-style clinician, cognizant of the need to also treat all the contributory causes of ocular surface disease. The comprehensive treatment approach for ocular surface disease is beyond the scope of this chapter.

Optimum treatment addresses disease pathophysiology, but our understanding of what truly underlies MGD is incomplete. The etiologies of MGD have been reviewed extensively in the TFOS MGD Workshop Report[8] and other publications[9-11] and will not be repeated here. Of note, significant basic science research[12-16] provides growing evidence that meibomian gland senescence and altered meibocyte differentiation related to PPAR-γ—mediated pathways are critical to the development of clinical MGD. Understanding of the role of meibomian gland periductal fibrosis has also grown in past years.[17] As our understanding of meibocyte physiology and of additional mechanisms of MGD pathogenesis evolve, it is likely that novel treatment strategies will emerge.

At present, most clinicians believe that MGD is a result of hyperkeratinization of ductal epithelium and abnormal thickening of meibum secretions with consequent gland obstruction, atrophy, and dropout as well as variable degrees of secondary inflammation and secondary microbial colonization or superinfection. Optimum treatment, in theory, would prevent or resolve hyperkeratinization (whether on the eyelid margin or within the gland ducts), "normalize" meibum, suppress or eliminate inflammation and superinfection, restore normal meibum output, and prevent functional loss of gland tissue. Some clinicians distinguish between lipid-deficient or hyposecretory MGD (in which a decreased tear lipid layer allows increased evaporation of tears) and oil retentive or obstructive MGD as different conditions based on the presence/degree of meibomian gland obstruction, and possibly in the degree of inflammation in the eyelid margin tissues.[18-21] This may be relevant in constructing a treatment algorithm for MGD patients, depending on whether the main driver of symptoms is tear overevaporation or tissue-based inflammation within the eyelids. Compared with aqueous deficient dry eye, most clinicians underestimate (and undertreat) inflammation as a pathogenic mechanism (and thus target for therapy) in MGD.

Replacement or normalization (restoring homeostasis) of the meibum layer of the tear film represents a significant challenge to clinicians. At present, it must be said that we do not have reproducible methods to either reliably quantitate or characterize meibum in the tear film or even to quantitate gland orifice obstruction. In cases where significant loss of functioning glands precludes restoration of a normal meibum component to the tear, a "substitute" component delivered topically might serve the physiologic role of meibum, that is, to stabilize the tear film and prevent evaporative loss of tears. Perfluorohexyloctanes have been shown to do this in clinical trials and are in development as a treatment for evaporative dry eye.[22,23]

"If you can't measure it, you can't manage it" is a quote (famously incorrectly attributed to economist W. Edward Deming) relevant to the difficulty of assessing treatment efficacy in MGD.[24] There is no standardized methodology to clinically (at the slit lamp) assess the viscosity or the quantity of secreted meibum beyond simple mild—moderate—severe scales. There is debate over whether the patency of gland orifices is best inferred from vigorous compression of the eyelid using a finger, forceps, or various mechanical squeezers versus tools that exert mild or "physiologic blink" force (the Korb MGE).[25,26] Debate also exists as to the irreversibility of gland "dropout" as diagnosed by meibography (defined as nonvisualization of "normal white stripes" thought to represent normally functioning glands).[27,28] Each of these issues has important relevance in determining an appropriate metric (orifice patency vs. meibum consistency) with which to measure efficacy of our treatments for MGD.[29] Further, it may be necessary to treat tissue-based inflammation in addition to restoring the normal meibum component to the tear film.

Currently available treatment options do not address each of the pathogenic processes involved in MGD. Prior to managing the disease, clinicians who treat patients with MGD must be cognizant of the contributory role of medicamentosa (e.g., isotretinoin and others)[30,31] in MGD and the existence of high-risk patient subgroups (atopy, OCP, prostate cancer, etc.).[32,33] While it may not be possible to improve the function of meibomian glands by discontinuing systemic medications such as isotretinoin, the benefits of eliminating preservatives from topical medications is well known. Controlling atopy with appropriate antiallergy medications and controlling the immunologic activity of diseases such as OCP is likewise important, highlighting the benefits of thorough history taking.

Virtually all patients self-treat symptoms of ocular surface disease with topical artificial lubricants as a first step. Despite limited published studies of efficacy,[34] many clinicians recommend lubricants, intended either as general supplementation of tear volume or for a presumed rinsing effect on the ocular surface. The purported benefits of lipid-containing or higher viscosity lubricants[28,35,36] have not yet been confirmed in large, randomized clinical trials. Nonetheless, there is

rationale justification for choosing an artificial lubricant that replaces the deficient component in tears or one that behaves physiologically like tears.

Most clinicians initiate mechanical treatment of MGD with some form of home-based lid hygiene (combinations of heat/warm compress plus massage/expression of meibum). Heating the eyelids usually is perceived as soothing or comforting, but compression or expression of gland contents is the more therapeutic aspect of the procedure. This point needs to be highlighted in instructing patients. Despite published, peer-reviewed studies regarding the required temperature/time needed to melt meibum[37–40] and estimates of the force required to express meibum,[18] no standardization of home eyelid hygiene method exists.[34,41] Even the methods of patient instruction (e.g., written handouts, videos, personal hands-on instruction) and assessment of patient compliance are not standardized and not validated in a statistical sense. Nonetheless, numerous published studies have shown lid hygiene to be effective in relieving both symptoms and signs of MGD and this is generally the first treatment intervention selected by most eye care providers, including corneal specialists.[34,42,43]

Pharmaceutical treatment using orally administered agents is often the next prescribed therapy for patients whose symptoms are uncontrolled with eyelid hygiene.[34,44] Rather than antibiosis (which may be an ancillary side benefit), these agents are primarily prescribed for their antiinflammatory and oil-thinning effects. Tetracycline derivatives, azithromycin and/or omega-3 supplementation, are widely prescribed at varied dosing schedules in hopes of reducing tear film inflammation. Potential side effects are real and can be serious, including tetracycline-induced esophageal erosions, gastric cramping, vaginal yeast infections, and cardiac arrythmias. Omega-3 supplementation can cause anticoagulation issues, particularly in combination with other medications. Patients must be educated about these potential side effects at the time of drug prescription. Published reports support the efficacy of doxycycline or minocycline over other tetracyclines including low doses of these drugs, believed to be antiinflammatory but not antibacterial,[45,46] particularly in patients with rosacea. Azithromycin has been reported to be more efficacious than doxycycline in MGD,[45,47–49] though a variety of dosing regimens have been reported.[45]

Other topical therapies in common use for MGD include antibiotics, steroids, antibiotic-steroid combinations, and even topical hormonal agents.[50] There is no consensus on whether bacterial colonization of the eyelid is causal or secondary to crust accumulation and whether chronic topical antibiotic treatment is appropriate for MGD. Of course, chronic topical antibiotic therapy should be avoided because of the risks of emergence of resistant organisms. Despite their rapid and significant efficacy in controlling acute inflammation or flare ups, topical steroids or steroid/antibiotic combinations generate concerns about ocular hypertension and cataract progression associated with chronic use. While appropriate to treat short-term flares of lid inflammation, these agents should be avoided as chronic therapy.

Thermal pulsation procedures have been widely adopted as a treatment to more completely "express" secretions from stagnated and occluded glands, and numerous published studies have shown the effectiveness and longevity of some of these treatments.[43,51] It is not known if the benefit of such procedures is related to the simultaneous heating and compression or to the vectored nature of the compression. While LipiFlow was the first procedure to gain widespread use based on numerous reports of durable efficacy and symptom improvement,[37] iLux is a handheld heating/compression method that has been shown to provide comparable efficacy.[52] Posttreatment mechanical gland expression[53] and posttreatment topical steroids have been reported to improve outcomes following thermal pulsation procedures.[54] A variety of other, less studied mechanical heating/expression procedures (e.g., Mibo-Flo and TearCare) are also available, with limited published data.[55,56] While heating the MG secretions can melt some enough to make them expressible, it is clinically apparent that not all gland occlusions can be relieved in this way. Meibomian gland duct probing, first reported by Maskin in 2009 (Maskin 2010), is a method designed to reopen clogged duct orifices and central ducts and break adhesions attributed to periductal fibrosis. Probing has been reported as effective for as long as 4−12 months in clearing obstructions, relieving symptoms, and improving TBUT and may be a preferred therapeutic intervention in cases where obstruction is advanced or when prior thermal pulsation has been insufficient.[17,57−60] Debridement of the eyelid margin has been reported to have efficacy as a stand-alone procedure[61,62] and may be performed at the same time as duct probing.

Light-based therapies (including intense pulsed light or IPL) have gained popularity as a treatment for MGD and several studies support their efficacy, though most published studies include MG expression as a cotreatment with IPL, obscuring a clear evaluation of the light-based therapy itself.[63−66] Review of published metaanalyses,[42,67] individual unblinded or open-label reports and reviews suggest potential benefit but a scarcity of RCT evidence for significant improvement in either symptoms, TBUT or corneal staining in MGD patients. Further study is certainly warranted and multiple trials are said to be in progress. The purported mechanisms by which IPL improves symptoms and signs in MGD remain speculative but may include eyelid warming, vascular thrombosis, decreased epithelial cell turnover, photomodulation (at a genetic or protein level), fibroblast activation, increased collagen synthesis, and MMP suppression or impact on inflammatory cytokines or reactive oxygen species.[64]

Topical pharmaceuticals approved for dry eye (cyclosporin and lifitegrast) may have efficacy in the treatment of MGD independent from their efficacy in treating the frequently coexistent aqueous tear deficiency. The presence of inflammation within meibomian glands and within eyelid tissue is difficult to demonstrate but is likely an important cause of eyelid redness, swelling, and induration. Published studies of treatment with topical immunomodulators in MGD populations (small series) have shown efficacy for both cyclosporine[68,69] and lifitegrast[52] in these subgroups of dry eye. Large, randomized trials of treatment in MGD have not been reported. However, given the frequent presence of aqueous deficiency in patients with MGD, the use of immunomodulatory eyedrops in these patients often is reasonable.

Hypochlorous acid is increasingly included in treatment plans for patients with eyelid inflammation and has efficacy as an antimicrobial (bacteria, fungi, and viruses) and possibly as an antiinflammatory agent.[70−73] There is a paucity of data related to the use of these agents for MGD, but because the treatment is well tolerated, even with direct spray onto the ocular surface, hypochlorous acid is used by increasing numbers of patients.

Demodex has been discussed as a pathogenic commensal organism that is present in many patients with MGD, though there is uncertainty and debate regarding how frequently this is the actual cause of patient symptoms.[74] Treatment for *Demodex blepharitis* includes a stepladder style escalation of therapy from topical agents (tea tree oil, terpinol-9) prepared as disposable wipes followed (for incomplete eradication) by an in-office tea tree oil cream for a more intense treatment. Soolantra cream is sometimes prescribed for recalcitrant cases and oral ivermectin has been reported as effective in resistant cases.[75,76]

A number of algorithms have been published[77−79] for the treatment of dry eye disease, with significant similarities between them as well as one for MGD[34] that includes broader recommendations including treatment of aqueous deficiency. No published data are available comparing patient outcomes between these treatment approaches, leaving many clinicians uncertain of how to tailor their sequencing of treatments in patients with uncontrolled symptoms (or signs). Providing yet another algorithm for the treatment of MGD is unlikely to bring consensus, but this author's thirty-plus years of experience treating ocular surface disease in a corneal specialty/clinical research practice yielding very high patient satisfaction has led to a "step-ladder" approach that may help others. This sequence of treatments is recommended for addressing the MGD component that is only one (significant) part of ocular surface disease, and other contributory factors need to be addressed as well.

1. Diagnosis before treatment! Begin with an accurate diagnosis of MGD and intercurrent ocular surface disease using risk factor assessment, patient history, meibography, and tear measurements (aqueous production and lipid layer thickness).
2. Identify patient risk factors and other pathogenic processes (exposure, allergy, conjunctivochalasis, epithelial dystrophy, corneal anesthesia, significant Demodex infestation, etc.) that may be contributory. Treat each as appropriate and as necessary.
3. Exclude medicamentosa contribution from both topical and systemic agents whenever possible.
4. Rehabilitate the tear film using preservative-free lubricants (escalating toward thicker or lipid-containing products including ointment) and effective and regular eyelid hygiene/expression BID. Develop a specific hygiene regimen for your patients based on the results you observe from the method you provide.
5. Address thickened meibum pharmaceutically (omega-3 supplements, doxycycline, azithromycin) especially in cases where meibum appears thickened, viscous, or waxy.
6. Use topical antiinflammatory agents (steroids, azithromycin) judiciously, avoiding long-term therapy. Consider serum tear administration and/or amniotic membrane treatment in resistant cases and for flare-ups of chronic disease.
7. If orifices are patent, thermal pulsation procedures (e.g., LipiFlow or iLux) can augment patient home lid compression, but are not a replacement for home therapy.
8. If orifices are closed or if clinical responses to thermal pulsation procedures are insufficient, consider meibomian gland probing to restore orifice patency.

Management and treatment of MGD requires a full set of clinician skills, including thorough history taking, differential diagnosis, proper diagnosis including coexistent/contributory conditions and knowledge of the many therapeutic options available today. Delivering effective care for each patient requires balancing issues such as choosing between treatments covered by insurance versus self-pay procedures, addressing compliance in an effective way and maintaining patient engagement in plans of ongoing treatment for this chronic and progressive condition. Patient dissatisfaction with inadequate symptom improvement following self-pay procedures can interfere with ongoing care, and clinicians need to properly set patient expectations and explain the need for continued treatment of MGD.

Ongoing research is likely to bring new tools to clinicians, including topical agents that provide the same antievaporative effect that meibum does,[80] agents that reverse abnormal keratinization within the MG and hormonal therapies that maintain the function of meibocytes even as we age.

REFERENCES

1. Ngo W, Situ P, Keir N, et al. Psychometric properties and validation of the standard patient evaluation of eye dryness questionnaire. *Cornea*. 2013;32(9):1204–1210.
2. Nelson JD, Shimazaki J, Benitez-del-Castillo JM, et al. The international workshop on meibomian gland dysfunction: report of the definition and classification subcommittee. *Invest Ophthalmol Vis Sci*. 2011;52(4):1930–1937.
3. Tong L, Chaurasia SS, Mehta JS, et al. Screening for meibomian gland disease: its relation to dry eye subtypes and symptoms in a tertiary referral clinic in Singapore. *Invest Ophthalmol Vis Sci*. 2010;51:3449–3454.
4. Viso E, Gude F, Rodriguez-Ares MT. The association of meibomian gland dysfunction and other common ocular diseases with dry eye:A population-based study in Spain. *Cornea*. 2011;30(1):1–6.
5. Yamaguchi M, Kutsuna M, Uno T, et al. Marx line:fluorescein staining line on the inner lid as indicator of meibomian gland function. *Am J Ophthalmol*. 2006;141:669–675.
6. Chhadva P, Alexander A, McClellan AL, McManus KT, Seiden B, Galor A. The impact of conjunctivochalasis on dry eye symptoms and signs. *Invest Ophthalmol Vis Sci*. 2015;56(5):2867–2871. https://doi.org/10.1167/iovs.14-16337.
7. Marmalidou A, Palioura S, Dana R, Kheirkhah A. Medical and surgical management of conjunctivochalasis. *Ocul Surf*. 2019;17(3):393–399.
8. Knop E, Knop N, Millar T, et al. The international workshop on meibomian gland dysfunction: report of the subcommittee on anatomy, physiology, and pathophysiology of the meibomian gland. *Invest Ophthalmol Vis Sci*. 2011;52:1938–1978.

9. Amano S. Meibomian gland dysfunction: recent progress worldwide and in Japan. *Invest Ophthalmol Vis Sci.* 2018; 59(14):DES87–DES93. https://doi.org/10.1167/iovs.17-23553.

10. Baudouin C, Messmer EM, Aragona P, et al. Revisiting the vicious circle of dry eye disease: a focus on revisiting the pathophysiology of meibomian gland dysfunction. *Br J Ophthalmol.* 2016;100(3):300–306.

11. Suzuki T. Inflamed obstructive meibomian gland dysfunction causes ocular surface inflammation. *Invest Ophthalmol Vis Sci.* 2018;59(14):DES94–DES101. https://doi.org/10.1167/iovs.17-23345.

12. Hwang HS, Parfitt GJ, Brown DJ, Jester JV. Meibocyte differentiation and renewal: insights into novel mechanisms of meibomian gland dysfunction (MGD). *Exp Eye Res.* 2017;163:37–45.

13. Jester JV, Brown DJ. Wakayama symposium: peroxisome proliferator-activated receptor-gamma (PPARgamma) and meibomian gland dysfunction. *Ocul Surf.* 2012; 10(4):224–229. https://doi.org/10.1016/j.jtos.2012.07.001. Epub 2012 Jul 25.

14. Jester JV, Potma E, Brown DJ. PPARγ regulates mouse meibocyte differentiation and lipid synthesis. *Ocul Surf.* 2016; 14(4):484–494.

15. Kim SW, Xie Y, Nguyen PQ, et al. PPARγ regulates meibocyte differentiation and lipid synthesis of cultured human meibomian gland epithelial cells (hMGEC). *Ocul Surf.* 2018;16(4):463–469.

16. Kim SW, Rho CR, Kim J, et al. Eicosapentaenoic acid (EPA) activates PPARγ signaling leading to cell cycle exit, lipid accumulation, and autophagy in human meibomian gland epithelial cells (hMGEC). *Ocul Surf.* 2020;18(3): 427–437.

17. Maskin SL, Testa WR. Growth of meibomian gland tissue after intraductal meibomian gland probing in patients with obstructive meibomian gland dysfunction. *Br J Ophthalmol.* 2018;102:59–68.

18. Blackie CA, Korb DR, Knop E, Bedi R, Knop N, Holland EJ. Nonobvious obstructive meibomian gland dysfunction. *Cornea.* 2010;29(12):1333–1345. https://doi.org/10.1097/ICO.0b013e3181d4f366.

19. Daniel NJ, Jun S, Benitez-Del-Castillo JM, et al. The international workshop on meibomian gland dysfunction: report of the definition and classification subcommittee meibomian gland dysfunction. *Investig Ophthalmol Vis Sci.* 2011;52(4):1930.

20. Eom Y, Na KS, Cho KJ, et al. Distribution and characteristics of meibomian gland dysfunction subtypes: a multicenter study in South Korea. *Kor J Ophthalmol.* 2019; 33(3):205–213. https://doi.org/10.3341/kjo.2018.0104.

21. Li B, Fu H, Liu T, Xu M. Comparison of the therapeutic effect of Meibomian Thermal Pulsation LipiFlow on obstructive and hyposecretory meibomian gland dysfunction patients. *Int Ophthalmol.* 2020;40(12):3469–3479. https://doi.org/10.1007/s10792-020-01533-y. Epub 2020 Aug 1.PMID: 32740882.

22. Agarwal P, Khun D, Krösser S, et al. Preclinical studies evaluating the effect of semifluorinated alkanes on ocular surface and tear fluid dynamics. *Ocul Surf.* 2019;17(2): 241–249.

23. Steven P, Augustin AJ, Geerling G, et al. Semifluorinated alkane eye drops for treatment of dry eye disease due to meibomian gland disease. *J Ocul Pharmacol Therapeut.* 2017;33:678–685.

24. https://deming.org/myth-if-ypu-cant-measure-it-you-cant-manage-it/.

25. Korb DR, Blackie CA. Meibomian gland diagnostic expressibility: correlation with dry eye symptoms and gland location. *Cornea.* 2008;27(10):1142–1147. https://doi.org/10.1097/ICO.0b013e3181814cff.

26. Korb DR, Blackie CA. Meibomian gland therapeutic expression: quantifying the applied pressure and the limitation of resulting pain. *Eye Contact Lens.* 2011;37(5):298–301. https://doi.org/10.1097/ICL.0b013e31821bc7c5.

27. Adil MY, Xiao J, Olafsson J, et al. Meibomian gland morphology is a sensitive early indicator of meibomian gland dysfunction. *Am J Ophthalmol.* 2019;200:16–25. https://doi.org/10.1016/j.ajo.2018.12.006. Epub 2018 Dec 20.

28. Lee SY, Lee K, Park CK, et al. Meibomian gland dropout rate as a method to assess meibomian gland morphologic changes during use of preservative-containing or preservative-free topical prostaglandin analogues. *PLoS One.* 2019;14(6):e0218886. https://doi.org/10.1371/journal.pone.0218886.

29. Asbell PA, Stapleton FJ, Wickström K, et al. The international workshop on meibomian gland dysfunction: report of the clinical trials subcommittee. *Invest Ophthalmol Vis Sci.* 2011;52(4):2065–2085.

30. Fortes BH, Liou H, Dalvin LA. Ophthalmic adverse effects of taxanes: the Mayo Clinic experience. *Eur J Ophthalmol.* 2020. https://doi.org/10.1177/1120672120969045.

31. Moy A, McNamara NA, Lin MC. Effects of isotretinoin on meibomian glands. *Optom Vis Sci.* 2015;92(9):925–930. https://doi.org/10.1097/OPX.0000000000000656.

32. Choi W, Ha JY, Li Y, Choi JH, Ji YS, Yoon KC. Comparison of the meibomian gland dysfunction in patients with chronic ocular graft-versus-host disease and Sjögren's syndrome. *Int J Ophthalmol.* 2019;12(3):393–400.

33. Shrestha T, Moon HS, Choi W, et al. Characteristics of meibomian gland dysfunction in patients with Stevens–Johnson syndrome. *Medicine.* 2019;98(26):e16155. https://doi.org/10.1097/MD.0000000000016155.

34. Geerling G, Tauber J, Baudouin C, et al. The international workshop on meibomian gland dysfunction: report of the subcommittee on management and treatment of meibomian gland dysfunction. *Invest Ophthalmol Vis Sci.* 2011; 52:2050–2064.

35. Garrigue JS, Amrane M, Faure MO, Holopainen JM, Tong L. Relevance of lipid-based products in the management of dry eye disease. *J Ocul Pharmacol Therapeut.* 2017; 33(9):647–661.

36. Rashid S, Jin Y, Ecoiffier T, Barabino S, Schaumberg DA, Dana MR. Topical omega-3 and omega-6 fatty acids for treatment of dry eye. *Arch Ophthalmol.* 2008;126(2): 219–225.

37. Blackie CA, Coleman CA, Holland EJ. The sustained effect (12 months) of a single-dose vectored thermal pulsation procedure for meibomian gland dysfunction and evaporative dry eye. *Clin Ophthalmol.* 2016;10:1385–1396.

38. Borchman D. The optimum temperature for the heat therapy for meibomian gland dysfunction. *Ocul Surf.* 2019;17:360–364.

39. Nagymihalyi A, Dikstein S, Tiffany JM, et al. The influence of eyelid temperature on the delivery of meibomian oil. *Exp Eye Res.* 2004;78(3):367–370.

40. Terada O, Chiba K, Senoo T, et al. Ocular surface temperature of meibomian gland dysfunction patients and the melting point of meibomian gland secretions [in Japanese]. *Nippon Ganka Gakkai Zasshi.* 2004;108:690–693.

41. Aketa N, Shinzawa M, Kawashima M, et al. Efficacy of plate expression of meibum on tear function and ocular surface findings in meibomian gland disease. *Eye Contact Lens.* 2019;45(1):19–22.

42. Cote S, Zhang AC, Ahmadzai V, et al. Intense pulsed light (IPL) therapy for the treatment of meibomian gland dysfunction. *Cochrane Database Syst Rev.* 2020;9(3). https://doi.org/10.1002/14651858.CD013559. Art. No.: CD013559.

43. Sabeti S, Kheirkhah A, Yin J, Dana R. Management of Meibomian Gland Dysfunction: A Review. *Surv Ophthalmol.* 2019. https://doi.org/10.1016/j.survophthal.2019.08.007.

44. Wladis EJ, Bradley EA, Bilyk JR, Yen MT, Mawn LA. Oral antibiotics for meibomian gland-related ocular surface disease: a report by the American Academy of Ophthalmology. *Ophthalmology.* 2016;123(3):492–496. https://doi.org/10.1016/j.ophtha.2015.10.062. Epub 2015 Dec 23.PMID: 26707417.

45. Kagkelaris KA, Makri OE, Georgakopoulos CD, Panayiotakopoulos GD. An eye for azithromycin: review of the literature. *Ther Adv Ophthalmol.* 2018;10, 2515841418783622.

46. Kashkouli MB, Fazel AJ, Kiavash V, et al. Oral azithromycin versus doxycycline in meibomian gland dysfunction: a randomised double-masked open-label clinical trial. *Br J Ophthalmol.* 2015;99:199–204.

47. De Benedetti G, Vaiano AS. Oral azithromycin and oral doxycycline for the treatment of Meibomian gland dysfunction: a 9-month comparative case series. *Indian J Ophthalmol.* 2019;67(4):464–471. https://doi.org/10.4103/ijo.IJO_1244_17.

48. Foulks GN, Borchman D, Yappert M, et al. Topical azithromycin therapy for meibomian gland dysfunction: clinical response and lipid alterations. *Cornea.* 2010;29:781–788.

49. Foulks GN, Borchman D, Yappert M, Kakar S. Topical azithromycin and oral doxycycline therapy of meibomian gland dysfunction: a comparative clinical and spectroscopic pilot study. *Cornea.* 2013;32(1):44–53.

50. Beckman K, Katz J, Majmudar P, Rostov A. Loteprednol etabonate for the treatment of dry eye disease. *J Ocul Pharmacol Therapeut.* 2020;36(7):497–511. https://doi.org/10.1089/jop.2020.0014. Epub 2020 May 8.PMID: 32391735.

51. Greiner JV. Long-term (12-month) improvement in meibomian gland function and reduced dry eye symptoms with a single thermal pulsation treatment. *Clin Exp Ophthalmol.* 2013;41(6):524–530.

52. Tauber J, Owen J, Bloomenstein M, Hovanesian J, Bullimore MA. Comparison of the iLux and the LipiFlow for the treatment of meibomian gland dysfunction and symptoms: a randomized clinical trial. *Clin Ophthalmol.* 2020;14:405–418.

53. Kim HM, Eom Y, Song JS. The relationship between morphology and function of the meibomian glands. *Eye Contact Lens.* 2018;44(1):1–5. https://doi.org/10.1097/ICL.0000000000000336.

54. Kheirkhah A, Kobashi H, Girgis J, Jamali A, Ciolino JB, Hamrah P. A randomized, sham-controlled trial of intraductal meibomian gland probing with or without topical antibiotic/steroid for obstructive meibomian gland dysfunction. *Ocul Surf.* 2020;18(4):852–856.

55. Kenrick CJ, Alloo SS. The limitation of applying heat to the external lid surface: a case of recalcitrant meibomian gland dysfunction. *Case Rep Ophthalmol.* 2017;8(1):7–12. https://doi.org/10.1159/000455087.

56. Karpecki P, Wirta D, Osmanovic S, Dhamdhere K. A prospective, post-market, multicenter trial (CHEETAH) suggested TearCare® system as a safe and effective blink-assisted eyelid device for the treatment of dry eye disease. *Clin Ophthalmol.* 2020;14:4551–4559.

57. Incekalan TK, Harbiyeli II , Yagmur M, et al. Effectiveness of intraductal meibomian gland probing in addition to the conventional treatment in patients with obstructive meibomian gland dysfunction. *Ocul Immunol Inflamm.* 2019;27:1345–1351.

58. Ma X, Lu Y. Efficacy of intraductal meibomian gland probing on tear function in patients with obstructive meibomian gland dysfunction. *Cornea.* 2016;35:725–730.

59. Maskin SL. Intraductal meibomian gland probing relieves symptoms of obstructive meibomian gland dysfunction. *Cornea.* 2010;29(10):1145–1152.

60. Sik Sarman Z, Cucen B, Yuksel N, et al. Effectiveness of intraductal meibomian gland probing for obstructive meibomian gland dysfunction. *Cornea.* 2016;35:721–724.

61. Korb DR, Blackie CA. Debridement-scaling: a new procedure that increases meibomian gland function and reduces dry eye symptoms. *Cornea.* 2013;32(12):1554–1557.

62. Ngo W, Caffery B, Srinivasan S, Jones LW. Effect of lid debridement-scaling in Sjogren syndrome dry eye. *Optom Vis Sci.* 2015;92(9):e316–320.

63. Arita R, Fukuoka S. *Non-pharmaceutical Treatment Options for Meibomian Gland Dysfunction Clinical and Experimental Optometry.* 2020:1–14.

64. Dell S. Intense pulsed light for evaporative dry eye disease. *Clin Ophthalmol.* 2017;11:1167–1173.

65. Meija LF, Gil JC, Jaramillo M. Intense pulsed light therapy: a promising complementary treatment for dry eye disease. *Arch Soc Esp Oftalmol.* 2019;94(7):331–336.

66. Vigo L, Giannaccare G, Sebastiani S, Pellegrini M, Carones F. Intense pulsed light for the treatment of dry

eye owing to meibomian gland dysfunction. *J Vis Exp.* 2019:146. https://doi.org/10.3791/57811.

67. Rennick S, Adcock L. *Intense Pulsed Light Therapy for Meibomian Gland Dysfunction: A Review of Clinical Effectiveness and Guidelines.* Ottawa (ON): Canadian Agency for Drugs and Technologies in Health; 2018. CADTH Rapid Response Reports. PMID: 3030772.

68. Perry HD, Doshi-Carnevale S, Donnenfeld ED, Solomon R, Biser SA, Bloom AH. Efficacy of commercially available topical cyclosporine A 0.05% in the treatment of meibomian gland dysfunction. *Cornea.* 2006;25(2):171–175.

69. Prabhasawat P, Tesavibul N, Mahawong W. A randomized double-masked study of 0.05% cyclosporine ophthalmic emulsion in the treatment of meibomian gland dysfunction. *Cornea.* 2012;31(12):1386–1393.

70. Fukuyama T, Ehling S, Wilzopolski J, Bäumer W. Comparison of topical tofacitinib and 0.1% hypochlorous acid in a murine atopic dermatitis model. *BMC Pharmacol Toxicol.* 2018;19(1):37.

71. Gold MH, Andriessen A, Dayan SH, Fabi SG, Lorenc ZP, Henderson Berg MH. Hypochlorous acid gel technology-its impact on post-procedure treatment and scar prevention. *J Cosmet Dermatol.* 2017;16(2):162–167.

72. Gold MH, Andriessen A, Bhatia AC, et al. Topical stabilized hypochlorous acid: the future gold standard for wound care and scar management in dermatologic and plastic surgery procedures. *J Cosmet Dermatol.* 2020;19(2):270–277.

73. Stroman DW, Mintun K, Epstein AB, et al. Reduction in bacterial load using hypochlorous acid hygiene solution on ocular skin. *Clin Ophthalmol.* 2017;11:707–714. https://doi.org/10.2147/OPTH.S132851.

74. Biernat MM, Rusiecka-Ziółkowska J, Piątkowska E, Helemejko I, Biernat P, Gościniak G. Occurrence of Demodex species in patients with blepharitis and in healthy individuals: a 10-year observational study. *Jpn J Ophthalmol.* 2018;62(6):628–633. https://doi.org/10.1007/s10384-018-0624-3. Epub 2018 Sep 25.PMID: 30255395.

75. Jacob S, VanDaele MA, Brown JN. Treatment of demodex-associated inflammatory skin conditions: a systematic review. *Dermatol Ther.* 2019;32(6):e13103.

76. Sahni DR, Feldman SR, Taylor SL. Ivermectin 1% (CD5024) for the treatment of rosacea. *Expet Opin Pharmacother.* 2018;19(5):511–516.

77. Jones L, Downie LE, Korb D, et al. TFOS DEWS II management and therapy report. *Ocul Surf.* 2017;15(3):575–628.

78. Milner MS, Beckman KA, Luchs JI, et al. Dysfunctional tear syndrome: dry eye disease and associated tear film disorders - new strategies for diagnosis and treatment. *Curr Opin Ophthalmol.* 2017;27(Suppl 1):3–47. https://doi.org/10.1097/01.icu.0000512373.81749.b7. PMID: 28099212.

79. Starr CE, Gupta PK, Farid M, et al. An algorithm for the preoperative diagnosis and treatment of ocular surface disorders. *J Cataract Refract Surg.* 2019;45(5):669–684. https://doi.org/10.1016/j.jcrs.2019.03.023.

80. Tauber J, Wirta DL, Sall K, Majmudar PA, Willen D, Krösser S, SEECASE Study Group. A randomized clinical study (SEECASE) to assess efficacy, safety, and tolerability of NOV03 for treatment of dry eye disease. *Cornea.* 2020. https://doi.org/10.1097/ICO.0000000000002622.

FURTHER READING

1. Ali F, Hala El R, Daoud F, et al. Azithromycin 1.5% ophthalmic solution: efficacy and treatment modalities in chronic blepharitis. *Arq Bras Oftalmol.* 2012;75:178–182.

2. Amparo F, Schaumberg DA, Dana R, et al. Comparison of two questionnaires for dry eye symptom assessment the ocular surface disease index and the symptom assessment in dry eye. *Ophthalmology.* 2015;122(7):1498–1503.

3. Arita R, Morishige N, Shirakawa R, et al. Effects of eyelid warming devices on tear film parameters in normal subjects and patients with meibomian gland dysfunction. *Ocul Surf.* 2015;13:321–330.

4. Badawi D. TearCare system extension study: evaluation of the safety, effectiveness, and durability through 12 months of a second TearCare treatment on subjects with dry eye disease. *Clin Ophthalmol.* 2019;13:189–198.

5. Balci O, Gulkilik G. Assessment of efficacy of topical azithromycin 1.5 percent ophthalmic solution for the treatment of meibomian gland dysfunction. *Clin Exp Optom.* 2018;101:18–22.

6. Blackie CA, Solomon JD, Greiner JV, et al. Inner eyelid surface temperature as a function of warm compress methodology. *Optom Vis Sci.* 2008;85:675–683.

7. Greiner JV. Long-term (3 year) effects of a single thermal pulsation system treatment on meibomian gland function and dry eye symptoms. *Eye Contact Lens.* 2016;42(2):99–107.

8. Hakim H, Thammakarn C, Suguro A, et al. Evaluation of sprayed hypochlorous acid solutions for their virucidal activity against avian influenza virus through in vitro experiments. *J Vet Med Sci.* 2015;77(2):211–215.

9. Hakim H, Thammakarn C, Suguro A, et al. Aerosol disinfection capacity of slightly acidic hypochlorous acid water towards newcastle disease virus in the air: an in vivo experiment. *Avian Dis.* 2015;59(4):486–491.

10. Igami TZ, Holzchuh R, Osaki TH, Santo RM, Kara-Jose N, Hida RY. Oral azithromycin for treatment of posterior blepharitis. *Cornea.* 2011;30:1145–1149.

11. Lam PY, Shih KC, Fong PY, et al. A review on evidence-based treatments for meibomian gland dysfunction. *Eye Contact Lens.* 2020;46:3–16.

12. Lee SY, Tong L. Lipid-containing lubricants for dry eye: a systematic review. *Optom Vis Sci.* 2012;89(11):1654–1661.

13. Liu Y, Kam WR, Fernandes P, et al. The effect of solithromycin, a cationic amphiphilic drug, on the proliferation and differentiation of human meibomian gland epithelial cells. *Curr Eye Res.* 2018;43:683–688.

14. McCulley JP, Shine W. A compositional based model for the tear film lipid layer. *Trans Am Ophthalmol Soc.* 1997; 95:79–88.

15. Mihaltz K, Faschinger EM, Vecsei-Marlovits PV. Effects of lipid- versus sodium hyaluronate-containing eye drops on optical quality and ocular surface parameters as a function of the meibomian gland dropout rate. *Cornea.* 2018; 37:886–892.

16. Navel V, Mulliez A, Benoist d'Azy C, et al. Efficacy of treatments for Demodex blepharitis: a systematic review and meta-analysis. *Ocul Surf.* 2019;17(4):655–669.

17. Opitz DL, Tyler KF. Efficacy of azithromycin 1% ophthalmic solution for treatment of ocular surface disease from posterior blepharitis. *Clin Exp Optom.* 2011;94: 200–206.

18. Savla K, Le JT, Pucker AD. Tea tree oil for Demodex blepharitis. *Cochrane Database Syst Rev.* 2020;6(6): CD013333.

19. Schaumberg DA, Nichols JJ, Papas EB, et al. The international workshop on meibomian gland dysfunction: report of the subcommittee on the epidemiology of, and associated risk factors for, MGD. *Invest Ophthalmol Vis Sci.* 2011;52:1994–2005.

20. Toyos R, McGill W, Briscoe D. Intense pulsed light treatment for dry eye disease due to meibomian gland dysfunction; a 3-year retrospective study. *Photomed Laser Surg.* 2015;33:41–46.

21. Villani E, Marelli L, Dellavalle A, Serafino M, Nucci P. Latest evidence on meibomian gland dysfunction diagnosis and management. *Ocul Surf.* 2020;18:871–892.

22. Leng X, Shi M, Liu X, Cui J, Sun H, Lu X. Intense pulsed light for meibomian gland dysfunction: a systematic review and meta-analysis. *Graefe's Arch Clin Exp Ophthalmol.* 2021. https://doi.org/10.1007/s00417-020-04834-1.

CHAPTER 15

Treatment of Ocular Pain Not Responsive to Traditional Dry Eye Disease Treatments

JERRY KALANGARA, MD • MERIN KURUVILLA, MD • KONSTANTINOS D. SARANTOPOULOS, MD, PHD

INTRODUCTION

Neuropathic ocular pain (NOP) in dry eye disease (DED) has hitherto remained an underdiagnosed and challenging condition to treat. The pathogenesis of NOP includes injury to the corneal nerves, leading to chronic afferent pain signaling driving neural plasticity and peripheral and central neuronal sensitization. The development of neuropathic pain occurs through changes in both peripheral and central neurons leading to allodynia and hyperalgesia.[1] Peripheral sensitization stems mainly from the release of inflammatory cytokines during and after tissue injury and altered responsiveness of peripheral sensory neurons, whereas central sensitization results from the generation of complex genomic, signaling, neuroinflammatory and electrophysiological alterations in the central nervous system that amplify afferent pain signaling.[1] Not infrequently, central pathogenetic processes drive painful symptoms (pain, allodynia, photophobia, neuro-behavioral manifestations), and these may be refractory to treatments targeting the peripheral tissues or nerves.

Given that NOP is complex, that it may coexist with nociceptive mechanisms, yet it includes predominantly neuropathic mechanisms, there is rarely a single treatment that entirely eliminates symptoms. While conventional therapies for DED, such as artificial or autologous serum tears (AST), antiinflammatories, or topical cyclosporine, could affect nociceptive pain by decreasing the release of cytokines and proinflammatory neuropeptides from injured nerves, they have little to no effect on centrally mediated NOP syndromes. Conventional topical treatments also appear to afford limited improvement in the morphologic status or function of corneal nerves. The advent of novel imaging modalities, including in vivo confocal microscopy (IVCM), has made it possible to obtain high resolution, noninvasive, layer by layer imaging of the corneal ultrastructure. The direct visualization of corneal nerves contributes to the evaluation of NOP and possibly to the monitoring of therapeutic response.[2] Furthermore, recent therapeutic strategies have been targeted at reversing neuronal damage through nerve regeneration. However, peripherally targeted approaches do not address those patients with a primary central component to their symptoms. Diagnostic and therapeutic strategies that hinge upon diagnostic criteria, such as the use of specific questionnaires, the lack of response to tears, or the proparacaine challenge test that differentiates between peripheral and centralized NOP in DED have great value in guiding treatments.[3,4] NOP patients who present with persistent pain symptoms despite prior use of tears or the instillation of topical anesthetic drops, such as proparacaine hydrochloride, are more likely to have centrally mediated pain that mandates adjunctive systemic treatments.

In this respect, a multidisciplinary approach consisting of ophthalmologists' and pain specialists' collaboration may be helpful, as well as a multimodal approach to address both peripheral and centralized pain using topical and systemic therapies. NOP also has a significant negative impact on quality-of-life measures with regard to mood, sleep, activity, relationships, and enjoyment, highlighting the importance of adjunctive behavioral therapy, as well.

TOPICAL THERAPIES FOR PERIPHERAL SENSITIZATION

If a primarily peripheral etiology for NOP in DED is suspected, i.e., pain responds to application of topical anesthetic, the treatment goal is to promote healing

Dry Eye Disease. https://doi.org/10.1016/B978-0-323-82753-9.00013-8

and regeneration of damaged nerves, to reduce any further pathological signaling via injured or sensitized nociceptors, and to prevent the development of central sensitization. This can potentially be accomplished through different nerve regenerative therapies. Further, patients with symptoms of hypersensitivity to evaporation may respond to physical shields that can act as barriers to evaporation.

Nerve Regenerative Therapies

AST eye drops are prepared from patient serum. AST contains neurotrophic growth factors including nerve growth factor (NGF) as well as transforming growth factor β (TGF- β), insulin-like growth factor-1, fibronectin, and epidermal growth factors.[5] Several studies have described the successful use of AST in DED that may be attributed to these neuroregenerative properties. Concentrations ranging between 20% and 100% increase nerve density and tortuosity as well as epithelial healing.[6] One recent report evaluating AST in neuropathic corneal pain from various etiologies including DED even correlated the decrease in patient pain scores with an improvement in corneal nerve density based on IVCM assessment.[7]

It must be noted that the inflammatory microenvironment appears to significantly influence peripheral nerve degeneration.[8] Studies using IVCM have demonstrated substantial correlation between increased numbers of dendritic cells and decreased corneal innervation.[9] This signifies a possible corneal neuroimmune crosstalk. Some groups therefore suggest the concomitant use of low dose steroids with AST for successful nerve regeneration,[10] the premise being that steroids would decrease the inflammatory load on the ocular surface, perhaps allowing for uninterrupted neuronal regeneration. Furthermore, steroids may further contribute to analgesia by suppressing any aberrant, ectopic peripheral electrical signaling originating in injured neuronal pathways.[11]

Autologous platelet-rich plasma contains even higher concentrations of therapeutically relevant biological factors including NGF and epidermal growth factors than autologous serum, with reported efficacy in refractory DED. Alio et al. investigated the efficacy of a 6-week course of autologous platelet-rich plasma in 368 patients with refractory DED.[12] 87% of individuals had subjective improvement and 76% had objective increase in corneal fluorescein staining. NOP symptoms were not specifically addressed in this study. However, these blood products are presently not FDA approved, and their use in DED remains investigational.

NGF plays an important role in the regeneration of nerves through the induction of neuronal sprouts and restoration of injured neuron function.[13] NGF also facilitates the growth and differentiation of sensory neurons[14] with improvement of hyperalgesia and allodynia in the animal models of NOP.[13] Oxervate (cenegermin-bkbj) is an ophthalmic solution of human recombinant NGF that has received FDA approval for neurotrophic keratitis and is under investigation for DED treatment in the United States and Europe.[15]

Self-Retained Cryopreserved Amniotic Membrane (CAM) has neurotrophic, antiinflammatory, and antifibrotic effects that facilitates ocular surface rehabilitation.[16] CAM is well tolerated and affords symptom relief as well as improved staining of the ocular surface in DED. Some groups have reported encouraging preliminary results with self-retained CAM specifically in patients with NOP and rapid symptom relief.[3] A small prospective trial of 17 subjects demonstrated the efficacy of CAM in improving corneal sensitivity and increasing corneal nerve density assessed via IVCM in DED.[17]

Contact Lenses (Both Scleral and Silicone-Hydrogel)

When conventional topical therapies fail to afford adequate relief, patients with DED and NOP may derive benefit from trials of extended wear of silicone-hydrogel contact lenses or scleral contact lenses to accelerate corneal restoration. While the mechanisms underlying relief have not been elucidated, protection of corneal nociceptors from environmental stimuli likely plays a role. Several studies have described pain relief with therapeutic soft contact lenses in NOP secondary to ocular surface disease. Wearing soft contact lenses in patients with DED from Sjögren's syndrome improved their OSDI scores to a greater degree than AS.[18]

The lenses that have proven most effective at maintaining the nociceptive barrier are the fluid-filled scleral lenses such as PROSE (Prosthetic replacement of the ocular surface ecosystem, Boston Foundation for Sight).[19] However, the potential infectious risk with prolonged use makes this less feasible as a long-term option. Further, these patients may suffer from concomitant hyperalgesia and contact lens placement on the ocular surface may exacerbate noxious stimuli in this subset. Finally, a recent study indicated that wearing PROSE long term did not promote corneal nerve regeneration when assessed by IVCM.[20]

Investigational Therapies—Topical TRPM8 Agonism

The transient receptor potential melastatin 8 (TRPM8) cation channel is a cold-sensing receptor localized to nerve endings in the cornea and eyelid. Since TRPM8 activation can inhibit other nociceptive inputs, TRPM8 agonism may potentially relieve NOP in DED. In view of its distribution not only in the cornea but also in the eyelid, TRPM8 can be activated by the application of topical agents to the eyelid without the direct instillation of eye drops into the cornea. In a recently published pilot study of 15 patients with NOP secondary to DED who underwent topical application of a selective TRPM8 agonist, cryosim-3, to their eyelids for 1-month, significant reduction in the intensity of eye pain and an increase in quality-of-life measures were noted after 1 week of treatment and sustained at 1 month.[21] The Schirmer and OSDI test scores were similarly improved following 1 month of therapy.

SYSTEMIC THERAPIES FOR CENTRAL AND PERIPHERAL SENSITIZATION

NOP patients who present with persistent pain symptoms despite the instillation of topical anesthetic drops, such as proparacaine hydrochloride, may have a central pain component to their symptoms.[4,22] This in office test is thus crucial for treatment selection. Further, NOP with a prominent central contribution to symptomatology may suffer from concomitant neuropsychiatric conditions such as anxiety and depression[23] as well as neurocognitive abnormalities that further confound therapeutic approaches. While pharmacotherapy may afford significant relief among patients with a prominent central component of NOP, evidence for this is scarce especially in the setting of DED.[24] Further, multiple simultaneous medications may be necessary for symptom control as has been found in other studies for nonocular neuropathic pain.[25] Yet, there is a variety of systemic therapies that may have some benefit for the treatment of NOP which will be discussed below.

Gabapentinoids

Gabapentin and pregabalin bind to the α2 delta subunit of voltage-dependent peripheral and central calcium channels and decrease neuronal calcium influx thus reducing the release of excitatory neurotransmitters and stabilizing central nervous system neurons.[26] Gabapentin is well established as the first-line therapy for diabetic neuropathy and has been investigated for other systemic neuropathic pain conditions. Gabapentin is typically initiated at a daily dose of 300 mg for neuropathic pain disorders with instructions to subsequently titrate to a recommended dose of 1200 mg daily with a maximum daily dose of 3600 mg (1200 mg three times daily or 900 mg four times a day). This gradual dose titration can often offset the most common side effects including dizziness, sedation, and somnolence. Gabapentin as well as pregabalin decrease postoperative pain after eyelid surgery and photorefractive

keratectomy.[27] Both of these agents are labeled for the treatment of postherpetic neuralgia. On the other hand, more recent literature describes potentially limited benefit for pregabalin in NOP and other dry eye symptoms after Laser-Assisted in Situ Keratomileusis (LASIK).[28]

One might conclude that together, there is support for the use of these systemic agents more broadly in neuropathic pain syndromes involving the eye. However, there are limited studies examining its utility in NOP secondary to DED. In a case series of eight patients, six showed complete or partial resolution of NOP on oral gabapentinoids, while the remainder showed no improvement.[29] Ongun et al. evaluated a cohort of 72 patients with ocular pain from DED in whom adjunctive gabapentin was associated with a decrease in pain scores as well as improvements in OSDI score and Schirmer's test results.[30] Notably, the study design incorporated a dosing schedule below the recommended dose of gabapentin 1200 mg daily. Relatively high doses of gabapentinoids have also been used anecdotally with success to treat DED and ocular pain unresponsive to conventional therapies at (gabapentin 900−1200 mg 3 times daily; pregabalin 150 mg twice day).[31] In case higher doses of gabapentinoids have to be used for treating intractable NOP, caution is advised in patients with renal dysfunction, in the elderly, or in those prone to imbalance and falls.

Tricyclic Antidepressants

The International Association for the Study of Pain (IASP) advises secondary amine tricyclic antidepressants (TCAs) such as nortriptyline, desipramine, or amitriptyline for the first-line treatment of neuropathic pain.[32] TCAs bind to serotonin and noradrenaline transporters and inhibit the reuptake of these endogenously analgesic neurotransmitters resulting in their increased levels in the synaptic cleft. Analgesia is thus conferred by enhancement of central endogenous neuroinhibitory circuits. In addition to inhibition of endogenous analgesic neurotransmitter reuptake, TCAs have several other effects that may contribute to their efficacy in neuropathic pain, such as N-methyl-D-aspartate (NMDA) antagonism and sodium channel blockade. TCAs are initially prescribed at a nightly dose of 10−25 mg and titrated by 10−25 mg every week depending on response and tolerance, this can be every 3−7 days up to a maximum of 150 mg nightly. No data are presently available on the off-label use of these agents in DED, but they may be considered for ocular pain concomitant with a more generalized pain syndrome, e.g., fibromyalgia. In a retrospective study of 30 patients with refractory centralized NOP treated with nortriptyline (10–100 mg), 17 (56.7%) of whom had underlying DED, 24 (80%) individuals reported an improvement in pain scores at 4 weeks as compared with baseline. Specifically, >50% improvement was reported in 12 (40%) patients, 30%–49% improvement in 6 (20%) patients, and 1%–29% improvement in 6 (20%) patients.[33] Yet, since these agents possess anticholinergic properties, caution is advised in cases of actual ocular dryness because this may be intensified, as well as in patients with coexisting disease such as glaucoma, urinary retention, cardiac disease, or seizures.

Opioids

Opioids such as tramadol may provide some relief in the management of intractable neuropathic pain, whenever other treatments have failed, but they are often limited by the development of tolerance and their side effects including addiction, dependence, constipation, and potentially respiratory depression and death. Further, these systemic therapies should be utilized in conjunction with a pain specialist who is familiar with their therapeutic effects and drug monitoring. If necessary, tramadol, a weak opioid, might be considered, but should be noted, that it has not been investigated for ocular pain, and therefore its role in management of DED with NOP is unknown. Tramadol acts as a μ-opioid receptor agonist and monoamine reuptake inhibitor. The starting dose of tramadol is 50–100 mg daily in neuropathic pain with gradual titration to a maximal dose 400 mg daily. Once again, caution should be used with this medication class due to its adverse effects profile. Yet, overall, opioids should be rather avoided in this setting due to their propensity for several unwanted effects, including but not limited to the generation of opioid induced hyperalgesia, a state of aberrant enhanced responsiveness to painful stimuli associated with opioid therapy, resulting in exacerbation of pain sensation rather than relief of pain.[34]

Low-Dose Naltrexone (LDN) is a μ- and δ-opioid receptor antagonist, and thereby upregulates opioid signaling and the release of endogenous endorphins. LDN also acts as an antagonist for toll-like receptor 4 (TLR4) that has been linked with neuropathic pain. At low doses (1.5–4.5 mg daily), naltrexone exerts an antineuroinflammatory effect, reducing the effect of proinflammatory cytokines. LDN has been investigated for efficacy in fibromyalgia pain syndrome and refractory neuropathic pain syndromes such as diabetic neuropathy.[35,36] One recently published report demonstrated for the first time that LDN is effective and safe in refractory NOP, based on a nearly 50% improvement in the mean pain score in a cohort of 39 patients of whom 20 (66.7%) had underlying DED.[37] Notably, all patients had a central pain component with incomplete symptom relief after topical anesthetic drops and the improvement in pain was found even in the presence of other concomitant systemic medications.

Anticonvulsants Other than Gabapentinoids

In addition to the above systemic pharmacotherapies, other agents have been used to address chronic neuropathic pain that have not been previously investigated in chronic NOP but may be beneficial in this regard. These include a variety of antiepileptics (e.g., carbamazepine, oxcarbazepine, topiramate) that act via inhibition of sodium channels or other neuroexcitatory suppressant actions.[38] Carbamazepine, for example, is an anticonvulsant that has been used successfully for relief in trigeminal neuralgia, and by extrapolation may have a potential role in managing NOP. The starting daily dose is 200 mg and gradually titrated on a weekly basis. The typical effective dose range is 800–1600 mg divided in two to four daily doses.

Serotonin-Norepinephrine Reuptake Inhibitors

Serotonin-norepinephrine reuptake inhibitors such as duloxetine and venlafaxine have dual mechanisms of action with both central analgesic as well as antidepressant properties. These agents have been extensively studied for systemic neuropathic pain and duloxetine has FDA approval for the management of diabetic neuropathy. A metaanalysis on systemic pharmacotherapy for neuropathic pain in adults included nine studies investigating duloxetine.[39] Seven of these studies showed encouraging results at daily doses of 20–120 mg with the final recommendation showing strong evidence for its use for neuropathic pain.

Combination Therapies

The initial drug selection is guided by several factors, such as prior therapeutic trials, coexisting conditions (fibromyalgia, other painful conditions, depression), and specific side effect profile of each individual agent in the context of coexisting disease (such as renal insufficiency that may impair the clearance of gabapentinoids, or glaucoma, urinary retention, cardiac disease, or seizures, that may prevent the use of TCAs). Each therapeutic trial with a specific agent should be based on careful dose titration up to recommended maximal dose for each drug, and in case of a favorable response, maintenance for a few months and reassessment. In case of lack of response, the drug should be weaned off, and another agent from a different category may be tried. Furthermore, combination therapy is often required in refractory cases of eye pain,[10] involving the combined use of a gabapentinoid with an analgesic antidepressant or LDN, etc.

PROCEDURAL THERAPIES

More aggressive invasive and noninvasive nonpharmacologic and pharmacologic procedural interventions can also be employed for the treatment of NOP. Adjuvant invasive procedures should be reserved for NOP that is refractory to other topical and systemic therapies.

Transcutaneous Electrical Nerve Stimulation

Transcutaneous electrical nerve stimulation (TENS) is a noninvasive form of neuromodulation that has been used to successfully address various chronic pain conditions by delivering electrical current to peripheral nerves through cutaneous electrodes. In a recent report, 9 out of 10 patients with ocular pain reported decreased pain intensity by ∼27.4% with the use of the device for a 3-month period.[40] In another study of 14 patients with chronic NOP secondary to various etiologies, there was a significant reduction in ocular pain scores within 5 min of treatment with a TENS device called RS-4i Plus Sequential Stimulator (RS-4i, RS Medical, Vancouver, WA).[41] Specifically, the intensity of ocular pain measured using the Defense and Veterans Pain Rating Scale (DVPRS, 0−10 scale) decreased by > 2 points in each eye without significant side effects. Another TENS device that may be potentially useful for NOP is called Cefaly (Cefaly US, Inc, Wilton CT). Cefaly is placed centrally in the supraorbital region and externally stimulates branches of the ophthalmic division of the trigeminal nerve (V1). This device has demonstrated efficacy in preventing migraines and it is certainly plausible that its use would benefit any associated NOP.[42] However, investigations are yet to quantify its effect in this setting. TENS is contraindicated in pregnancy, patients with epilepsy, and those with implanted devices such as pacemakers and defibrillators.

Intranasal Electrical Nerve Stimulation

A noninvasive intranasal neurostimulation device called TrueTear (Allergan, San Diego, CA, USA) was recently approved in individuals with DED for augmenting tear production. TrueTear is a handheld device with two prongs applied in the nostrils for 30−60 s of stimulation and activation of the nasolacrimal reflex. A study of 75 patients with DED treated with one session described significantly decreased ocular pain and increased tear volume from baseline.[43] Interestingly, the improvements in ocular pain and tear volume were not directly correlated

and those patients with low to moderate pain scores had the greatest degree of symptom reduction.

Periorbital Nerve Blocks

The analgesic effect of nerve blocks in NOP derives from the targeting of afferent pain signals from sensory nerves innervating the cornea or adjacent tissues such as the fornix or conjunctiva, or from modulating sympathetic and/or parasympathetic autonomic neural pathways that contribute to neuronal sensitization.[44] Not only nerves directly subjected to injury but uninjured nerves, adjacent to the injured ones have been shown to promote neuropathic pain[45−47] and this may apply to NOP, as well.[29] Ocular and periorbital neural pathways (supraorbital, infraorbital, supratrochlear, and infratrochlear nerves) anatomically converge at the spinal trigeminal nucleus and integrated neural input leads to the perception of ocular pain. Thus, the blockade of periorbital nerves adjacent to the injured corneal nerves may suppress ectopic firing and decrease nociceptive signals to the spinal trigeminal level.[29] This would translate into overall decreased perception of NOP. In a case series of 11 patients treated with periorbital nerve blocks for ocular pain from various etiologies, pain relief lasting up to 7 months was reported in 7 cases.[29] Furthermore, sympathetic efferent blockade (by superior cervical ganglion blocks) or parasympathetic blocks (such as sphenopalatine ganglion blocks) depending on unique dichotomous clinical subcategorization of patients[48] may be beneficial in NOP as in other oculo-facial pains.

Botulinum Toxin Type a (BoNT-A/Botox)

Botulinum toxin type A (BoNT-A/Botox) is approved for the treatment of chronic migraines refractory to prophylactic medications. Botox modulates pain through the inhibition of inflammatory mediator release such as calcitonin gene-related peptide (CGRP).[49] In a retrospective study of 91 patients with chronic migraines who received Botox injections, there was significant improvement in not only migraine pain but also dry eye symptoms and photophobia.[50] Symptomatic improvement was independent of an associated improvement in the baseline tear volume, implicating other factors in this effect.[51] This has prompted the use of Botox for suspected NOP alone without chronic migraines.[52] In this preliminary investigation of six patients with severe DED and NOP, periocular Botox injection significantly reduced mean scores for ocular discomfort (0−5 scale) from 4.67 to 2.83 at 1 month. Anti-CGRP agents, such as erenumab, galcanezumab, and fremanezumab, may have a similar application in

NOP via similar mechanisms but there are no available data in this regard.

Intrathecal Targeted Drug Delivery

The placement of a high cervical intrathecal pump for the delivery of bupivacaine and low dose fentanyl has been described for recalcitrant NOP in post-LASIK cases.[53] The invasive nature of the intervention and potential for complications precludes routine application and should be reserved only after exhaustion of all other options.

COMPLEMENTARY THERAPIES

For patients who continue to describe inadequate pain relief despite multimodal treatments with one or more of the above, the use of complementary therapies may afford some relief and/or have a pharmacotherapy sparing effect in many patients.

Omega-3 Fatty Acid Supplementation

Nutritional strategies such as an increased omega-3:omega-6 fatty acid ratio regulates systemic inflammation and is being investigated in chronic pain.[54] While omega-3 fatty acids were effective at decreasing symptoms in a case series of neuropathic pain[55], there was no effect on ocular pain in a randomized controlled study.[56] Omega-3 fatty acid supplementation has further been reported to increase tear film break-up time and improve results of Schirmer's test in clinical trials at doses of 1 g 2 to 3 times a day.[57] This may help to decrease associated NOP in DED.

Vitamin B12 Supplementation

Vitamin B12 supplementation has been used to manage neuropathic and postsurgical pain. *In vivo* studies indicate that vitamin B mediates its analgesic effects either by increasing serotonin levels in the brain or the activation of opioid receptors. It was recently reported that vitamin B12/hyaluronic acid eye drops alleviated DED by attenuating inflammation and oxidative stress.[58] There is also evidence that vitamin B12 improves corneal reinnervation and reepithelization following injury.

Acupuncture

Acupuncture stimulates the production of endogenous opioids as well as the gene expression of various neuropeptides and has been used for the adjunctive treatment of various neuropathic pain conditions. One prospective randomized study recently investigated acupuncture for the treatment of DED.[59] The active treatment group ($n = 24$) demonstrated significant improvements

in the OSDI score from baseline of 34 ± 17 to 19 ± 17 at 1 week ($P < .01$) and 16 ± 12 at 6 months ($P < .01$). The sham group ($n = 25$) also showed improvement although to a lesser degree, with a decrease from baseline OSDI of 36 ± 20 to 24 ± 22 at 1 week, and 25 ± 18 at 6 months.

Cognitive Behavioral Therapy

Cognitive behavioral therapy (CBT) has also been shown to be efficacious in chronic pain syndromes[60] but has not been studied specifically for DED or ocular pain. Patients with chronic ocular pain appear to have underlying dysfunctional coping mechanisms and CBT may therefore be beneficial at enabling them to cope with these psychological sequelae of their chronic pain.[61] While randomized controlled trials are necessary in the context of chronic NOP, this approach may be implemented safely with the goal of mood regulation and improved overall quality of life.

Investigational Therapies—Endocannabinoid System Modulation

The endocannabinoid system is ubiquitous throughout the body including ocular tissues; it is a current target in the treatment of various pathophysiologic processes characterized by ocular pain, inflammation, and nerve damage. The activation of the cannabinoid type 1 receptor contributes to central and peripheral analgesia, whereas modulating the cannabinoid type 2 receptor has immunomodulatory potential. Novel strategies of drug development and even drug delivery such as the topical administration of cannabinoids in the eye are being investigated.[62]

CONCLUSION

Despite progress in elucidating the underlying mechanism of NOP in DED, the management of these patients remains a significant challenge in clinical practice. No single treatment will likely be effective and personalized multimodal therapy will be necessary to address the complex mechanisms underlying this disease.

REFERENCES

1. Rosenthal P, Borsook D. Ocular neuropathic pain. *Br J Ophthalmol.* 2016;100(1):128–134.
2. Alzubaidi R, Sharif MS, Qahwaji R, et al. In vivo confocal microscopic corneal images in health and disease with an emphasis on extracting features and visual signatures for corneal diseases: a review study. *Br J Ophthalmol.* 2016;100(1):41–55.

3. Dieckmann G, Goyal S, Hamrah P. Neuropathic corneal pain: approaches for management. *Ophthalmology.* 2017; 124(11S):S34–S47.

4. Mehra D, Cohen NK, Galor A. Ocular surface pain: a narrative review. *Ophthalmol Ther.* 2020;9(3):1–21.

5. Pan Q, Marrone AA, Stark WJ, Akpek EK. Autologous serum eye drops for dry eye. *Cochrane Database Syst Rev.* 2017;2:CD009327.

6. Aggarwal S, Kheirkhah A, Cavalcanti BM, et al. Autologous serum tears for treatment of photoallodynia in patients with corneal neuropathy: efficacy and evaluation with in vivo confocal microscopy. *Ocul Surf.* 2015;13(3):250–262.

7. Aggarwal S, Colon C, Kheirkhah A, Hamrah P. Efficacy of autologous serum tears for treatment of neuropathic corneal pain. *Ocul Surf.* 2019;17(3):532–539.

8. Benowitz LI, Popovich PG. Inflammation and axon regeneration. *Curr Opin Neurol.* 2011;24(6):577–583.

9. Cruzat A, Witkin D, Baniasadi N, et al. Inflammation and the nervous system: the connection in the cornea in patients with infectious keratitis. *Invest Ophthalmol Vis Sci.* 2011;52(8):5136–5143.

10. Goyal S, Hamrah P. Understanding neuropathic corneal pain–gaps and current therapeutic approaches. *Semin Ophthalmol.* 2016;31(1–2):59–70.

11. Devor M, Govrin-Lippmann R, Raber P. Corticosteroids suppress ectopic neural discharge originating in experimental neuromas. *Pain.* 1985;22(2):127–137.

12. Alio JL, Rodriguez AE, Ferreira-Oliveira R, Wróbel-Dudzińska D, Abdelghany AA. Treatment of dry eye disease with autologous platelet-rich plasma: a prospective, interventional, non-randomized study. *Ophthalmol Ther.* 2017;6(2):285–293.

13. Cirillo G, Cavaliere C, Bianco MR, et al. Intrathecal NGF administration reduces reactive astrocytosis and changes neurotrophin receptors expression pattern in a rat model of neuropathic pain. *Cell Mol Neurobiol.* 2010;30(1):51–62.

14. Takemura Y, Imai S, Kojima H, et al. Brain-derived neurotrophic factor from bone marrow-derived cells promotes post-injury repair of peripheral nerve. *PLoS One.* 2012;7(9):e44592.

15. Aragona P, Giannaccare G, Mencucci R, Rubino P, Cantera E, Rolando M. Modern approach to the treatment of dry eye, a complex multifactorial disease: a P.I.C.A.S.S.O. board review. *Br J Ophthalmol.* 2021;105(4):446–453.

16. Cheng AM, Zhao D, Chen R, et al. Accelerated restoration of ocular surface health in dry eye disease by self-retained cryopreserved amniotic membrane. *Ocul Surf.* 2016;14(1):56–63.

17. John T, Tighe S, Sheha H, et al. Corneal nerve regeneration after self-retained cryopreserved amniotic membrane in dry eye disease. *J Ophthalmol.* 2017;2017:6404918.

18. Li J, Zhang X, Zheng Q, et al. Comparative evaluation of silicone hydrogel contact lenses and autologous serum for management of Sjogren syndrome-associated dry eye. *Cornea.* 2015;34(9):1072–1078.

19. Stason WB, Razavi M, Jacobs DS, et al. Clinical benefits of the Boston ocular surface prosthesis. *Am J Ophthalmol.* 2010;149(1):54–61.

20. Wang Y, Kornberg DL, St Clair RM, et al. Corneal nerve structure and function after long-term wear of fluid-filled scleral lens. *Cornea.* 2015;34(4):427–432.

21. Yoon HJ, Kim J, Yang JM, et al. Topical TRPM8 agonist for relieving neuropathic ocular pain in patients with dry eye: a pilot study. *J Clin Med.* 2021;10(2):250.

22. Crane AM, Feuer W, Felix ER, et al. Evidence of central sensitisation in those with dry eye symptoms and neuropathic-like ocular pain complaints: incomplete response to topical anaesthesia and generalised heightened sensitivity to evoked pain. *Br J Ophthalmol.* 2017; 101(9):1238–1243.

23. Chang VS, Rose TP, Karp CL, et al. Neuropathic-like ocular pain and nonocular comorbidities correlate with dry eye symptoms. *Eye Contact Lens.* 2018;44(Suppl 2):S307–S313.

24. Ebrahimiadib N, Yousefshahi F, Abdi P, Ghahari M, Modjtahedi BS. Ocular neuropathic pain: an overview focusing on ocular surface pains. *Clin Ophthalmol.* 2020; 14:2843–2854.

25. Gilron I, Bailey JM, Tu D, et al. Nortriptyline and gabapentin, alone and in combination for neuropathic pain: a double-blind, randomised controlled crossover trial. *Lancet.* 2009;374(9697):1252–1261.

26. Sarantopoulos C, McCallum B, Kwok WM, et al. Gabapentin decreases membrane calcium currents in injured as well as in control mammalian primary afferent neurons. *Reg Anesth Pain Med.* 2002;27(1):47–57.

27. Pakravan M, Roshani M, Yazdani S, et al. Pregabalin and gabapentin for post-photorefractive keratectomy pain: a randomized controlled trial. *Eur J Ophthalmol.* 2012; 22(Suppl 7):S106–S113.

28. Galor A, Patel S, Small LR, et al. Pregabalin failed to prevent dry eye symptoms after Laser-Assisted In Situ Keratomileusis (LASIK) in a randomized pilot study. *J Clin Med.* 2019;8(9):1355.

29. Small LR, Galor A, Felix ER, et al. Oral gabapentinoids and nerve blocks for the treatment of chronic ocular pain. *Eye Contact Lens.* 2020;46(3):174–181.

30. Ongun N, Ongun GT. Is gabapentin effective in dry eye disease and neuropathic ocular pain? *Acta Neurol Belg.* 2021;121(2):397–401.

31. Andersen HH, Yosipovitch G, Galor A. Neuropathic symptoms of the ocular surface: dryness, pain, and itch. *Curr Opin Allergy Clin Immunol.* 2017;17(5):373–381.

32. Dworkin RH, O'Connor AB, Kent J, et al. Interventional management of neuropathic pain: NeuPSIG recommendations. *Pain.* 2013;154(11):2249–2261.

33. Ozmen MC, Dieckmann G, Cox SM, et al. Efficacy and tolerability of nortriptyline in the management of neuropathic corneal pain. *Ocul Surf.* 2020;18(4):814–820.

34. Mercadante S, Arcuri E, Santoni A. Opioid-induced tolerance and hyperalgesia. *CNS Drugs.* 2019;33(10):943–955.

35. Hota D, Srinivasan A, Dutta P, Bhansali A, Chakrabarti A. Off-label, low-dose naltrexone for refractory painful diabetic neuropathy. *Pain Med.* 2016;17(4):790–791.

36. Patten DK, Schultz BG, Berlau DJ. The safety and efficacy of low-dose naltrexone in the management of chronic pain and inflammation in multiple sclerosis, fibromyalgia, Crohn's disease, and other chronic pain disorders. *Pharmacotherapy.* 2018;38(3):382−389.

37. Dieckmann G, Ozmen MC, Cox SM, Engert RC, Hamrah P. Low-dose naltrexone is effective and well-tolerated for modulating symptoms in patients with neuropathic corneal pain. *Ocul Surf.* 2021;20:33−38.

38. Kobayashi K, Endoh F, Ohmori I, Akiyama T. Action of antiepileptic drugs on neurons. *Brain Dev.* 2020;42(1):2−5.

39. Finnerup NB, Attal N, Haroutounian S, et al. Pharmacotherapy for neuropathic pain in adults: a systematic review and meta-analysis. *Lancet Neurol.* 2015;14(2):162−173.

40. Zayan K, Aggarwal S, Felix E, et al. Transcutaneous electrical nerve stimulation for the long-term treatment of ocular pain. *Neuromodulation.* 2020;23(6):871−877.

41. Sivanesan E, Levitt RC, Sarantopoulos CD, et al. Noninvasive electrical stimulation for the treatment of chronic ocular pain and photophobia. *Neuromodulation.* 2018;21(8):727−734.

42. Tabeeva GR. Neurostimulation of the supraorbital nerve with the Cefaly device - a new method for the treatment of migraine. *Zh Nevrol Psikhiatr Im S S Korsakova.* 2019;119(3):133−140.

43. Farhangi M, Cheng AM, Baksh B, et al. Effect of noninvasive intranasal neurostimulation on tear volume, dryness and ocular pain. *Br J Ophthalmol.* 2020;104(9):1310−1316.

44. Digre KB, Brennan KC. Shedding light on photophobia. *J Neuro Ophthalmol.* 2012;32(1):68−81.

45. Yoon YW, Na HS, Chung JM. Contributions of injured and intact afferents to neuropathic pain in an experimental rat model. *Pain.* 1996;64(1):27−36.

46. Li Y, Dorsi MJ, Meyer RA, Belzberg AJ. Mechanical hyperalgesia after an L5 spinal nerve lesion in the rat is not dependent on input from injured nerve fibers. *Pain.* 2000;85(3):493−502.

47. Tran EL, Crawford LK. Revisiting PNS plasticity: how uninjured sensory afferents promote neuropathic pain. *Front Cell Neurosci.* 2020;14:612982.

48. Chen W, Batawi HI, Alava JR, et al. Bulbar conjunctival microvascular responses in dry eye. *Ocul Surf.* 2017;15(2):193−201.

49. Wheeler A, Smith HS. Botulinum toxins: mechanisms of action, antinociception and clinical applications. *Toxicology.* 2013;306:124−146.

50. Diel RJ, Kroeger ZA, Levitt RC, et al. Botulinum toxin A for the treatment of photophobia and dry eye. *Ophthalmology.* 2018;125(1):139−140.

51. Diel RJ, Hwang J, Kroeger ZA, et al. Photophobia and sensations of dryness in patients with migraine occur independent of baseline tear volume and improve following botulinum toxin A injections. *Br J Ophthalmol.* 2019;103(8):1024−1029.

52. Venkateswaran N, Hwang J, Rong AJ, et al. Periorbital botulinum toxin A improves photophobia and sensations of dryness in patients without migraine: case series of four patients. *Am J Ophthalmol Case Rep.* 2020;19:100809.

53. Hayek SM, Sweet JA, Miller JP, Sayegh RR. Successful management of corneal neuropathic pain with intrathecal targeted drug delivery. *Pain Med.* 2016;17(7):1302−1307.

54. Raphael W, Sordillo LM. Dietary polyunsaturated fatty acids and inflammation: the role of phospholipid biosynthesis. *Int J Mol Sci.* 2013;14(10):21167−21188.

55. Ko GD, Nowacki NB, Arseneau L, Eitel M, Hum A. Omega-3 fatty acids for neuropathic pain: case series. *Clin J Pain.* 2010;26(2):168−172.

56. Dry Eye A, Asbell PA, Maguire MG, et al. n-3 fatty acid supplementation for the treatment of dry eye disease. *N Engl J Med.* 2018;378(18):1681−1690.

57. Liu A, Ji J. Omega-3 essential fatty acids therapy for dry eye syndrome: a meta-analysis of randomized controlled studies. *Med Sci Monit.* 2014;20:1583−1589.

58. Macri A, Scanarotti C, Bassi AM, et al. Evaluation of oxidative stress levels in the conjunctival epithelium of patients with or without dry eye, and dry eye patients treated with preservative-free hyaluronic acid 0.15 % and vitamin B12 eye drops. *Graefes Arch Clin Exp Ophthalmol.* 2015;253(3):425−430.

59. Dhaliwal DK, Zhou S, Samudre SS, Lo NJ, Rhee MK. Acupuncture and dry eye: current perspectives. A double-blinded randomized controlled trial and review of the literature. *Clin Ophthalmol.* 2019;13:731−740.

60. Jacobs DS. Diagnosis and treatment of ocular pain: the ophthalmologist's perspective. *Curr Ophthalmol Rep.* 2017;5(4):271−275.

61. Patel S, Felix ER, Levitt RC, Sarantopoulos CD, Galor A. Dysfunctional coping mechanisms contribute to dry eye symptoms. *J Clin Med.* 2019;8(6).

62. Lafreniere JD, Kelly MEM. Potential for endocannabinoid system modulation in ocular pain and inflammation: filling the gaps in current pharmacological options. *Neuronal Signal.* 2018;2(4):NS20170144.

CHAPTER 16

Pathways and Mechanisms of Ocular Pain and Photophobia in Dry Eye Disease

SNEH PATEL, MS • KONSTANTINOS D. SARANTOPOULOS, MD, PHD

INTRODUCTION

Sensory nerves normally convey signals of pain to the brain. Yet, the overall experience and behavioral manifestations of pain are determined by mechanisms within the peripheral and central nervous system (CNS) that are complex and inadequately understood. The International Association for the Study of Pain defines pain as a *"subjective unpleasant sensory and emotional experience associated with actual or potential tissue damage, or described in terms of such damage."*[1] In this context, pain is not strictly a mechanistic or biological phenomenon, but the experience of pain is influenced by complex emotional, behavioral, and psychosocial processes. The conscious experience of pain and its behavioral manifestations are also driven by environmental, social, and cognitive factors, which dictate the need for a *"holistic"* understanding of painful symptoms and for patient-centered, comprehensive, and multimodal therapies for combating pain.[2]

There is no unique "pain," but rather painful sensory and behavioral manifestations in various forms, driven by variable causes and pathophysiological mechanisms and thus requiring variable therapeutic approaches. Acute pain tends to originate from direct injury, which can be intentional (e.g., secondary to laser-assisted in situ keratomileusis (LASIK) or other ocular surgery) or unintentional (ocular trauma, infections, disease, noxious environmental exposure, actual dryness). Acute pain usually resolves with the healing phase (~3–6 months), but in certain conditions can become recurrent or chronic.[3] In contrast, chronic pain is persistent, by convention extending beyond the expected healing time, and is confounded by a complexity of emotional, behavioral, and psychosocial factors.[3] Peripheral and central sensitizing

mechanisms are one cause of chronic pain, and for most patients, cure is unlikely; this often leads to quality of life being negatively impacted for years on end (self-care and well-being, work, socialization, pleasure, relationships). Chronic pain may originate from prolonged application of noxious (tissue-damaging) stimuli causing persistent activation of specific receptors on nociceptive peripheral sensory fibers, which subsequently wind up the downstream pathways (nociceptive pain). On the other hand, it may originate from dysfunction within sensory nervous system itself, whether due to injury, disease, or other alterations (neuropathic pain). In either case, the pain sensation is amplified by overreactivity of peripheral or central nerves (e.g., peripheral and central sensitization, respectively), leading to persistent symptoms.[4,5]

Anatomically, the sensory pathways that convey signals of pain from the periphery to the CNS consist of a chain of three afferent neurons.[4,5] Pain transmission from the oculofacial region involves afferent trigeminal pathways. The first-order (e.g., primary afferent) neuron responds to noxious stimuli applied to the peripheral oculofacial tissues, which sense noxious stimuli at the periphery (e.g., cornea) and convey the pertinent pain signals to the spinal trigeminal nucleus in the medulla (first-order neuron). The axons of the second-order neurons decussate and reach the thalamus (second-order neuron) via the contralateral trigeminothalamic tracts; at the thalamus, they synapse to third-order neurons, which project to subcortical and cortical centers of the brain (third-order neurons) that form part of the primary somatosensory cortex, where the sensation of pain is perceived.[4,5] Other pathways that are involved in modulation of pain simultaneously deliver inhibitory or excitatory signals from the brain to the periphery

Dry Eye Disease. https://doi.org/10.1016/B978-0-323-82753-9.00005-9

and thus influence how the pain is perceived, representing valuable therapeutic targets as pharmacological or electrical manipulation of the inhibitory circuits may be clinically useful in providing analgesia.[6]

DRY EYE DISEASE

Dry eye disease (DED) constitutes "a multifactorial disease of the ocular surface characterized by a loss of homeostasis of the tear film, and accompanied by ocular symptoms, in which tear film instability and hyperosmolarity, ocular surface inflammation and damage, and neurosensory abnormalities play etiological roles."[7] Its pathogenesis is complex, involving a cycle of tear osmolarity changes, inflammatory damage, and tear film instability.[8] Importantly, there exists heterogeneity in signs and symptoms of DED, thus DED may be understood as an *"umbrella"* term, characterized by multiple phenotypes with different symptoms, signs, and nerve findings.[9] This variability is best exemplified by the lack of consistent relationships between symptoms and signs of disease, by the lack of a *"gold standard"* definition, and the overlap of corneal nerve parameters in individuals who are healthy compared to those with DED.[10,11] Despite this heterogeneity, the most common symptom of DED is ocular pain or discomfort; in fact, ocular surface pain is the leading cause of clinic visits and ophthalmic healthcare costs in patients with DED,[12] and has deleterious effects on quality of life via impaired social functioning and decreased productivity.[13,14] As such, it is a large source of morbidity in the patient population of DED, and an important symptom to work-up when considering a new case of DED.

Ocular pain in DED falls into two categories, as introduced above—nociceptive and neuropathic pain. Nociceptive pain refers to pain that originates from activation of nociceptors secondary to a noxious stimulus at a peripheral nonneural tissue, implying an intact somatosensory nervous system. Conversely, neuropathic pain often arises secondary to a lesion or functional alteration along the somatosensory nerve supply to the cornea that originates from the trigeminal nerve.[4,5] Not infrequently, these two types of pain may coexist. While categorizing the type of pain can be difficult, one can glean this information (which may guide mechanism-specific treatments) by analyzing presenting signs and symptoms. For example, neuropathic-type ocular pain may be spontaneous pain, or may be evoked pain, triggered by wind and/or light (the ocular equivalents of tactile allodynia, and photophobia),[15] and is often described with specific descriptors

(burning, shooting, lancinating, stabbing).[16] Besides this, pain out of proportion to ocular surface findings, persistence of pain despite treatment of potential nociceptive origins, and presence of specific comorbidities (fibromyalgia, irritable bowel syndrome, vulvodynia, interstitial cystitis, atypical facial pain disorders) may suggest a neuropathic cause.[16]

CORNEAL NERVES AND PAIN RECEPTORS

The cornea is the most densely innervated tissue in the body, containing nerves that function in mediating sensation as well as ocular protection and homeostasis. Corneal subbasal nerves originate from the ophthalmic branch of the trigeminal nerve, travel within its nasociliary and long ciliary nerve branches, and branch into nerve fibers that penetrate and innervate the cornea.[17] These nerve fibers form thick bundles that approach the cornea radially to form the limbal plexus.[17] At 1–3 mm away from the limbus, the nerves lose their perineurium and myelin sheath, aiding in corneal transparency. These stromal nerves, encased in only Schwann cells, run at a mean depth of approximately 300 μm from the corneal surface.[17] Within the stroma, they extend laterally and anteriorly, running parallel to the collagen lamellae.[18,19] Branches form the anterior stromal plexus continue anteriorly to form the subepithelial nerve plexus (between Bowman's layer and the anterior stroma), and then penetrate Bowman's layer to form the subbasal nerve plexus, terminating near the corneal epithelium.[18,19] The total surface area of the subbasal nerve system is estimated at 90 mm^2 with 5400–7200 nerve bundles, with each bundle then separating into side branches containing three to seven individual axons each. Overall, this accounts for an estimated 19,000–44,000 total axons. Each nerve fiber houses 10–20 nerve terminals, and thus it is estimated that there are 315,000–630,000 terminals in the cornea, or approximately 7000 per mm.[18,19]

The nerves that make up the subbasal nerve system also function in mediating sensation.[20] The cornea contains several different nociceptive fibers (nociceptors) that are specialized to sense pain due to a variety of stimulus types, including mechanoreceptors (second most prevalent; ∼20% of total corneal sensory nerves), polymodal receptors (most prevalent; ∼70%), and cold receptors (least prevalent; ∼10%).[20–22] Mechanoreceptors transmit sharp pain due to mechanical stimulation (e.g., object contacting the cornea) and are the fastest conductors of the three. Polymodal receptors respond to multiple modalities, including mechanical, thermal, and chemical stimuli, as well as local pH changes. Finally, cold nociceptors sense decreasing temperature and alterations in tear osmolarity.[20-22] Pricking pain is sensed by mechanoreceptors, burning and stinging pain by polymodal receptors, and dryness by cold receptors.[23,24]

ASCENDING PATHWAYS OF PAIN

The somata of corneal nociceptors are located within the trigeminal ganglion, with centrally projecting axons synapsing in the trigeminal subnucleus caudalis/upper cervical transition zone (Vc/C1-2) and the subnucleus interpolaris/subnucleus caudalis (Vi/Vc).[25,26] Second-order axons travel from the spinal trigeminal nuclear complex, decussate, and terminate in the thalamus alongside contralateral spinothalamic fibers.[25,26] It should be emphasized that several neurons in the spinal trigeminal nucleus (mainly within the caudal subnucleus interpolaris, the transition zone between interpolaris and caudalis, and the rostral subnucleus caudalis) receive converging input from the cornea and from adjacent eyelid and facial skin, and can thus be activated by mechanical stimulation from either the ipsilateral cornea or from the periorbital skin. Their receptive fields expand after prolonged noxious stimulation[27,28]; this altered sensory processing manifests as a hyperalgesic state, with enhanced pain to both normally nonnoxious and noxious stimuli across a wide area surrounding the eye and face.[29,30]

This expansion of the receptive field is mediated centrally, and is partly due to attenuation of central inhibitory signals onto activated second-order neurons, to the extent that these neurons can be activated by subliminal inputs from the cornea or periorbital region.[28] Clinically, this sensitization may account for chronic periocular pain that often accompanies corneal pain, as a result of increased excitability of second-order neurons and an expanded periorbital receptive fields with loss of central inhibition. Furthermore, it has been shown that not only nerves directly subjected to injury but uninjured nerves situated adjacent to those that are injured are involved in the pain experience[31-35]; as such, blockade of periorbital nerves may induce analgesia by suppressing ectopic firing and decreasing incoming convergent nociceptive traffic to the spinal trigeminal level.[36] Finally, third-order neurons extend from the thalamus to areas of the primary somatosensory cortex (e.g., trigeminal ganglion, bilateral trigeminal nucleus caudalis, contralateral ventroposteromedial thalamus, anterior cingulate cortex, and middle frontal gyrus), where the sensation of pain is finally processed.[25,26,37]

Central-level processing of pain signals includes interactions between various subcortical and cortical centers involved in the pain response.[4,5] These include the somatosensory SI and SII regions, anterior insula, and anterior cingulate cortex.[4,5,25,26] On the other hand, affective-motivational responses to pain are mediated by the limbic system, including the hypothalamus, which normally regulates autonomic and neuroendocrine responses to pain.[25,26,38] Several other projections involved in autonomic, homeostatic, and behavioral responses after tissue-damaging stimuli have been identified, such as those that extend to the parabrachial nuclei.[39,40] It has even been speculated that pain originating from the peripheral cornea may be preferentially conveyed via a nonthalamic ascending pathway via corneal afferents that activate parabrachial-projecting second-order trigeminal neurons rather than trigeminothalamic ones, although it is also possible that ascending transmission is polysynaptic, with projections at both sites.[41] These polysynaptic pathways may explain why corneal pain is not infrequently poorly localized, and is often referred to adjacent periocular regions, and may also offer some explanation of the strong emotional and aversive dimensions related to corneal pain.[41-43]

Interestingly, these sensory pathways also interact with other pathways involved with processing the sensation of light,[44] explaining why photophobia frequently accompanies ocular pain (Fig. 16.1). These pathways involve projections from intrinsically photosensitive retinal ganglion cells to thalamic neurons, which also receive converging input of pain signals from the trigeminal nucleus caudalis, and subsequently project to the cortex. At this level, the thalamus not only relays signals to the cortex but also dynamically integrates and amplifies all these signals thus constituting a neurophysiological substrate that can both generate pain amplification and also contribute to photophobia.[44,45]

Of note, these denoted pathways of pain are not hardwired signal relays, and are capable of signal modulation.[23] Dynamic plasticity within the periphery, medulla, thalamus, and higher centers of the brain allows for dramatic alterations in the relation between the intensity of the painful stimulus and the responses to this pain. The interplay between incoming signals, excitatory signal modulation, and inhibitory signal modulation eventually determines the intensity of perceived pain, as well as the physiologic response to it.[26,46] Depending on circumstances, the response to the incoming messages may be attenuated or amplified compared to the original signal. Amplification of the

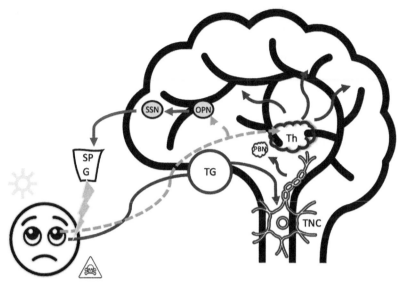

FIG. 16.1 Overlap in ascending pathways of ocular pain (red) and light sensitivity (yellow, green). Ascending ocular pain pathways such as those in inflammatory or neuropathic pain (red) originate either from sensing noxious stimuli or from dysfunction in corneal nerves which send afferents to the trigeminal ganglion (TG), trigeminal nucleus caudalis (TNC), and eventually the posterior thalamus (Th) and primary somatosensory cortex. The overlapping pathway of photophobia begins at retinal ganglion cells (green) that travel to the olivary pretectal nucleus (OPN), superior salivatory nucleus (SSN), and finally the sphenopalatine ganglion (SPG) before driving inflammatory reactions via dilation and extravasation of inflammatory mediators at ocular and dural vessels; there, they can cause parasympathetic-mediated vasodilation of ocular and dural vessels, which are also innervated by trigeminal afferents, providing one pathway of overlap with the ocular pain pathway. A smaller proportion of these ganglion cells (intrinsically photosensitive retinal ganglion cells; green) also process directly to the posterior thalamus, providing a second overlap with the pain pathway. Finally, projections of pain signals to the parabrachial nuclei (PBN) drive emotional and behavioral responses to pain from the eye.

pain signal, or onset of spontaneous pain, often occurs in DED as a result of peripheral or central sensitization of nociceptive neurons.[46]

Ascending nociceptive signals can be modulated by descending inhibition from the CNS, leading to attenuation of the incoming afferent input and thus the perceived intensity of pain. For example, the periaqueductal gray contains opioid peptides and receptors which serve as a mediator for opioid-induced analgesia; their release directly decreases the sensation of incoming pain.[47] On the other hand, other higher centers (e.g., cerebral cortex, limbic system, nucleus raphe magnus, locus coeruleus) also involved in analgesia in response to incoming nociception similarly activate descending pathways that instead lead to analgesia[48] via inhibition of nociceptive processing at the trigeminal/spinal dorsal horn.[37] This inhibition occurs via serotoninergic or noradrenergic fibers that release serotonin and norepinephrine which act as inhibitory neurotransmitters, a process that can be targeted pharmacologically (via tricyclic antidepressants, selective

norepinephrine serotonin reuptake inhibitors, or tramadol). Finally, nociceptive stimuli drive activation of inhibitory interneurons leading to release of encephalin (endorphins), GABA, and glycine, which also work to modulate the incoming signal.[23,49]

Nociceptive Pain

In general, the workup of a new painful case of DED begins with consideration of nociceptive sources of pain,[50] and is usually carried out in the ophthalmologic clinic setting. Nociceptive pain is defined as *"pain that arises from actual or threatened damage to non-neural tissue and is due to the activation of nociceptor,"* and is thus due to direct noxious stimulus to the ocular surface.[1] Implied in this definition is that underlying corneal nerves are healthy and functional, an important distinction from neuropathic ocular pain. The noxious stimuli trigger a nocifensive response which aims to protect the integrity of affected tissues by eliciting withdrawal responses or behavioral modifications. Different noxious stimuli at the level of the cornea will activate specific subsets of nociceptors, leading to discharges of impulses relayed to the CNS to encode the characteristics of the stimulus, to evoke pain sensations referred to the eye, and to mobilize defensive stimulus-avoiding behavioral responses.[25,26]

Several types of noxious triggers to nociceptive pain exist, each corresponding to activation of a particular type of nociceptor as described above. Commonly observed stimuli include direct traumatic or surgical injury, tear film abnormalities (e.g., decreased tear production, high or unstable tear osmolarity, presence of inflammatory mediators), abnormal ocular anatomy of the surrounding eyelid and/or cornea (e.g., pterygium), or direct ocular surface toxicity by an external agent (air pollution, topical glaucoma medications).[51] Importantly, nociceptive ocular pain tends to be acute and self-limited—once the exposure is removed, healing can begin, after which pain tends to subside—in comparison to chronic nociceptive pain, which is more persistent.[52] It is important to note, that under specific circumstances, prolonged exposure to a nociceptive stimulus can manifest as a more chronic type pain via sensitization, explored further below.

Acute Nociceptive Pain

In normal states, noxious stimuli generate an acute nociceptive pain response, characterized by a pain sensation proportional to the severity of the stimulus (although genetic and other factors may result in variability across individuals) and subsequent nocifensive behavioral responses aimed toward withdrawal and protection from the insult. These are "healthy," physiologically adaptive responses, aimed at recognizing harmful stimuli and eliciting reflexive avoidance behaviors in order to avoid further exposure to the stimuli.[20,50,53]

In the cornea, some nerves respond selectively to cold stimuli, while others respond selectively to mechanical forces, but the majority (e.g., the most abundant neurons in the trigeminal system, classified as "polymodal nociceptors") respond to a wide variety of stimuli such as heat, chemical irritants, and presence of heightened inflammatory mediators.[24,54] Pain receptors are specialized receptors coupled to cation channels, the opening of which generates electrical signals in the form of action potentials that successively propagate proximally toward central nerve terminals wherein they elicit neurotransmitter release and synaptic transmission of ascending pain signals.[51,53,55]

Several of such receptors, like transient receptor potential vanilloid 1 (TRPV1) and transient receptor potential melastatin member 8 (TRPM8), which respond to a variety of noxious stimuli, have been identified on both nociceptive fibers in the cornea[54] as well as on nerves of the conjunctiva and eyelid.[56,57] The TRPV1 receptor responds to thermal, acidic, and chemical stimuli, generating nociceptive signals in response to activation that are perceived as burning or sharp painful sensations.[37,38,58,59] Other receptors transduce noxious heat, cold, mechanical, or chemical stimuli' and initiate the signals that will enable the nervous system to distinguish these stimuli as painful.[24] For example, TRPM8 thermoreceptors expressed in both the cornea and the eyelids are coupled to an ion channel which is activated by cold stimuli and/or osmolarity increases, and they mediate reflexive blinking as well as tear production.[38,59–61] TRPV1 coexist with TRPM8 in a high proportion of cold receptors and act to enhance neuronal firing to cold; interestingly, their expression in DED may be upregulated by inflammation, and may contribute to observed cold allodynia seen in certain cases of DED.[62] Because activation of TRPM8 receptors may inhibit other aberrant nociceptive signals, their targeting by specific agonists, such as the topical agonist cryosim-3, has therapeutic potential in DED with related neuropathic pain.[57] Yet, the opposite may also be the case, since TRPM8 antagonists may suppress acute and chronic pain including cold allodynia,[63,64] at the cost of worsening dryness.[61]

The action potentials that are generated in response to noxious stimulation are conveyed to the CNS via synaptic neurotransmission from Aδ fibers and C fibers. Neurotransmitters involved in this synaptic transmission of pain include excitatory amino acids (e.g., glutamate or aspartate) and neuropeptides (e.g., calcitonin gene–related peptide [CGRP] and substance P [sP]).[65] These proteins act on cognate postsynaptic receptors: glutamate mediates signaling by activating cation channels (e.g., α-amino-3-hydroxy-5-methyl-4-isoxazolepropionic acid [AMPA] receptor and N-Methyl-D-aspartate [NMDA] receptor), or by inducing secondary cytosolic messenger signaling (metabotropic receptors). Substance P binds to the neurokinin receptor 1 (NK$_1$) which regulate various mediators of cellular excitability and function.[4,5,58] Acute nociceptive pain is usually signaled via synaptic release of excitatory glutamate acting at AMPA receptors, and minimally via sP acting at the NK1 receptor.[66] CGRP is abundant in trigeminal neurons[67] and secondary sensory neurons in trigeminal nucleus caudalis (TNC),[68] and elicits postsynaptic responses via G protein–coupled receptors that drive multiple processes, including neurogenic inflammation (by recruiting immune cells, and sensitizing sensory neurons) in peripheral tissue,[69] vasodilation, and signaling processes driving central sensitization.[65,70]

Postsynaptic responses lead to brief discharge of action potentials and subsequent activation of discriminative-sensory ascending pathways.[4,5,58] This is also the case in the trigeminal pain transmission, wherein TRPV1 induces release of CGRP and sP from trigeminal nerve terminals. The expression of sP and CGRP in trigeminal nociceptors is rapidly upregulated in response to inflammation, thus CGRP and sP contribute to the development of peripheral hyperalgesia, while CGRP receptor activation promotes activation of AMPA receptors, leading to increased firing of neurons and central sensitization.[71]

Chronic Nociceptive Pain and Sensitization

In some instances, acute nociceptive pain may transition into a chronic pain state. Specifically, prolonged or intense nociceptive stimulation, or loss of normal sensation, may alter the properties of the somatosensory nerve pathways to such an extent that incoming pain signals are amplified to an inappropriate level, leading to spontaneous pain upon nonnoxious stimuli.[52,72] In contrast to acute pain, this occurs because tissue injury or persisting inflammation that is spatially or temporally extensive induces plasticity changes in neural pathways, generating chronic pain.[50] This also applies to the cornea, wherein prolonged noxious stimuli and/or direct injury to corneal nerves may lead to altered nerve morphology and function, which is also associated with chronic pain.[53]

Specific injuries or extensive inflammation can mobilize and activate immune cells, leading to release of numerous inflammatory mediators (e.g., prostaglandins, protons, potassium ions, bradykinin, cytokines, growth factors, purines, and amines; sometimes described as an "inflammatory soup").[50,73,74] This also includes generation of nitric oxide (NO) and proinflammatory cytokines (interleukins, tumor necrosis factor) that induce the enzyme COX2 synthase, which further contribute to the release of prostaglandins, and so-forth.[75] Some of these mediators may function to activate nociceptors directly and evoke chronic pain, while others sensitize the nociceptors, promoting easier activation (by lowering their thresholds of activation) or enhanced responsiveness (by heightened membrane excitability) of receptors.[52,72]

Sensitization refers to the phenomenon of *"increased responsiveness of nociceptive neurons to their normal input, and/or recruitment of a response to normally subthreshold inputs."*[1] Prolonged or extensive tissue injury (due to noxious stimuli, inflammatory damage, hyperosmolarity, environmental exposures, postsurgical changes) can sensitize nociceptors and make them more responsive to

stimuli. The sensitized sensory neural apparatus in turn fosters a hyperresponsive state, generating spontaneous pain and/or pain evoked by normally nonnoxious stimuli (allodynia), or responding with aberrantly excessive pain to a normally painful stimulus (hyperalgesia) which are interestingly shared symptoms of neuropathic ocular pain.[52,72] Some sensitization mechanisms can be rapid, subsequent to posttranslational modification (phosphorylation) of signal effectors such as membrane ion channels, while others are more delayed because they depend on altered transcription, translation, and transport of newly synthesized proteins to either distal or proximal terminals.[5,58,76]

Peripheral sensitization involves release of cytokines, prostaglandins, nerve growth factor, and bradykinin all of which act to increase TRPV1 expression and/or activity within sensory neurons.[74] This is also the case in corneal pain and DED, wherein TRPV1 is upregulated in corneal nerves and within the trigeminal ganglion, in a fashion that correlates with various hyperalgesic responses.[62] Then, ongoing nociceptive input from peripherally sensitized nerves as a result of persistent inflammation provides a sustained input to the second-order neurons and to higher centers. Sensitized C fibers may then release CGRP and sP, which promote prolonged excitatory postsynaptic responses and firing.[77] On the other hand, central sensitization also involves a synergistic activation of both glutamate and sP or CGRP receptors, which if of sufficient magnitude and duration, can excite the NMDA receptor.[78,79] NMDA receptors are linked to Ca^{2+} channels, and their activation results in prolonged release of cytosolic Ca^{2+}, leading to Ca^{2+}-dependent hyperactivity of secondary messenger cascades (e.g., activation of phospholipase A2 and subsequent mediators such as NO, inositol triphosphate (IP_3), diacylglycerol (DAG), activation of protein kinase C (PKC), and phosphorylation of various targets), leading to a series of events that range from genomic alterations to "burst" firing of spinal cord neurons and amplified transmission of nociceptive processing.[23,80,81] Central neurons may then reach a state of heightened neuronal excitability that results in amplified sensation (hyperalgesia, allodynia, photophobia), spontaneous firing, and subsequently spontaneous pain.

Peripheral nociceptor activity at the level of the trigeminal ganglion processes centripetally to the trigeminal nucleus, leading to a sustained input at the central level. Downstream, this heightened traffic of incoming pain signals due to peripherally sensitized corneal nociceptors will in turn significantly enhance the responsiveness of central nociceptive pathways as well, by inducing a series of neuroplastic changes.[82]

Central sensitization often involves permanent changes in the CNS (at the level of neurons, interneurons, ventral horn neurons, thalamus, cortex, and other brain areas), leading to pain that persists after the original injury has healed.[50,76,83] In contrast to physiologically adaptive acute pain, central sensitization is considered a process of maladaptive neuroplasticity, because it facilitates an amplified, exaggerated synaptic response to pain signaling[83] as a result of enhanced excitatory neuronal activity and downregulation of inhibitory neuronal pathways.[84] Pain and other neurobehavioral manifestations of central sensitization do not serve any physiologically adaptive role, but rather contribute to ongoing dysfunction and suffering.[15] This maladaptive pain is commonly seen in DED, specifically when symptoms do not mirror ocular surface findings.[85]

NEUROPATHIC PAIN AND PHOTOPHOBIA

In certain circumstances, eye pain is not a result of nociception from the ocular surface per se, but is rather caused by an injury or alteration to the nerves involved with processing of nociceptive pain, or to adjacent nerves. Several elements can be affected in this manner: nerve terminals, axons of nociceptive sensory neurons, sensory ganglia, and higher-order neurons (e.g., spinal cord, brain stem, thalamus, and cortical structures) involved with processing or responding to nociceptive input.[16] This is termed neuropathic pain, defined as *"pain caused by a lesion or disease of the somatosensory nervous system."*[1] In pure neuropathic pain, there is no association between pain and damage; pain often exists in the absence of any injury or stimulus,[50] yet in other situations neuropathic pain may coexist with nociceptive pain, making it difficult to distinguish one from the other. Various diseases that may lead to lesions encompassing corneal nerves (LASIK or other ocular surgery, trauma, infections such as herpes zoster or acanthamoeba), or to the second- and third-order somatosensory system within the CNS (multiple sclerosis, stroke, tumor) can thus manifest as neuropathic pain.[46,50]

The predominant abnormality that drives neuropathic pain is aberrant electrical hyper-excitability and generation of ectopic firing of sensory neurons after injury to somatosensory nerves, at any region along the nociceptive pain pathway.[86-88] Subsequent alterations in translation and posttranslational modification of neuronal sodium channels[89] and other channels[86,87] secondary to nerve injury have been implicated in the onset of neuropathic pain. Interestingly, given the underlying role of hyperexcitability, drugs that modulate

channels involved in nerve excitation (e.g., sodium channel−blocking drugs) may have roles as analgesics; suppressing the initial afferent barrage by using a local anesthetic, for example, may attenuate the development of subsequent hyperalgesia.[90,91]

Aberrant firing generates action potential that propagate centrally and these elicit spontaneous pain, and/or drive central sensitization, thereby contributing to abnormal pain perception, such as allodynia, hyperalgesia,[42-44] and—additionally in the case of the corneal pain—photophobia.[44] Inflammation or injuries affecting corneal nerves may lead to emergence of neuropathic pain and photophobia as a result of peripheral and central sensitization[92-94] subsequent to persistent ongoing afferent trafficking that induces synaptic reorganization and functional alterations, both of which contribute to chronicity of pain. These alterations include neuroinflammation, astrocyte and microglial activation, and enhancement of excitatory synaptic transmission, resulting in sensitization of ocular-responsive neurons of the caudal trigeminal brainstem and also those in higher centers.[95] This may explain several manifestations of central sensitization and centralized pain states, such as photophobia, migraines, fibromyalgia, and accompanying neurocognitive and emotional disorders.[94] Deficient supraspinal or descending mechanisms may also be involved, such that excitatory input predominates over descending inhibitory pathways because pain-modulating tracts become weak.[50,96] Finally, other mechanisms have been also implicated, including neuroma formation at the sites of damaged peripheral nerves, which exhibit abnormal responsiveness and spontaneous discharges (ectopic firing) and thus driving neuropathic pain and sensitization.[97-101] Activation of satellite glial cells that surround trigeminal ganglia may be another contributor to neuropathic ocular pain and hyperalgesia,[102-104] as well as glial activation in the brain[105-107] which is upregulated by CGRP-dependent mechanisms.[108]

As brought up above, a common symptom of corneal neuropathic pain is the presence of light sensitivity, e.g., photoallodynia and photophobia.[44,50] The thalamic nuclei mediate the transmission of nociceptive pain from the periphery to the CNS as aforementioned, but some of these same areas overlap with areas that mediate the sensory processing of light.[85] Specifically, incoming light is sensed by rods and cones within the retina, which synapse upon retinal ganglion cells that feed into the optic nerve; branches of this nerve stretch to the parabrachial nuclei, and from there the information eventually is relayed into the thalamic geniculate nucleus and the occipital cortex where the information is processed.[109] Yet, some of these afferent fibers instead project to the lateral geniculate nucleus and eventually to the olivary pretectal nucleus, which activates the superior salivatory nucleus and sphenopalatine ganglion located downstream. This parasympathetic overdrive causes activation and sensitization of trigeminal afferents from the eye (via uveal vessel dilation as well as release of neuroinflammatory mediators (e.g., CGRP, vasoactive intestinal peptide, and NO)) which sensitize the corneal trigeminal afferents and higher-order neurons within the nucleus caudalis, thalamus, and higher brain centers, thus generating pain out or proportion.[109] This overlap of light and pain pathways in sensory processing areas of the brain explains how light sensation may lead to increased pain signals, resulting in the manifestation of photophobia and photoallodynia.[85] This would also explain noted observations that patients with DED and photophobia who protect their eyes with sun glasses and avoid intense light and wind tend to report less painful symptoms.[85,109]

DISTINGUISHING NOCICEPTIVE AND NEUROPATHIC PAIN

As suggested, mechanisms of neuropathic pain have shared features with nociceptive pain; though these disorders manifest by vastly differently processes, they are tied to one-another by a common pathophysiology involving sensitization.[50,83] Central sensitization has been implicated in both nociceptive pain and neuropathic pain, directly leading to the presence of evoked pain over the initial site of injury and around the surrounding area (e.g., expansion of the receptive field).[110] Despite the similarities, it is important to distinguish neuropathic from nociceptive pain in a case of DED, as their therapeutic ladders differ greatly. Several clinical features can be used to distinguish neuropathic from nociceptive pain. First, if ocular pain persists after nociceptive sources have been evaluated and treated, neuropathic pain should be considered.[50] Besides this, if individuals display specific symptoms gleaned through the use of validated questionnaires[111-114] (e.g., burning, tingling, wind and light sensitivity) and/or have comorbidities suggestive of corneal nerve damage (migraine, fibromyalgia, recent refractive surgery), neuropathic pain should also be considered.[50] Finally, hyperalgesia (augmented pain response) and allodynia (pain due to a nonnoxious stimuli, e.g., to light [*photoallodynia and photophobia*], to cutaneous touch [*cutaneous allodynia*], to wind) are features also generally seen in individuals with neuropathic pain,[16,50] and directly occur

as a result of central sensitization leading to pain from innocuous stimuli.[58]

CONCLUSION

The ascending pathways of ocular pain are complex, consisting of multiple circuits of nerves stretching from the periphery (cornea) to the CNS (spinal cord and higher cortical centers of the brain), and back. The processing and eventual perception of ocular pain is equally as complex, being influenced by external (environment, cognition, mood) and internal (modulation by higher cortical centers) factors. Nevertheless, ocular pain is an important part of the DED experience, and clinicians should take great care in understanding the differences in pathophysiology and presentation of the types of pain seen in DED (e.g., nociceptive, neuropathic, or both) and how these types of pain may change over time (e.g., sensitization). This is especially important as these factors have implications on how one should therapeutically approach ocular pain in DED.

REFERENCES

1. *IASP Terminology;* 2020. https://www.iasp-pain.org/Education/Content.aspx?ItemNumber=1698.
2. Bushnell MC, Case LK, Ceko M, et al. Effect of environment on the long-term consequences of chronic pain. *Pain.* 2015;156(Suppl 1(0 1)):S42–S49.
3. Grichnik KP, Ferrante FM. The difference between acute and chronic pain. *Mt Sinai J Med.* 1991;58(3):217–220.
4. Stucky CL, Gold MS, Zhang XJPNAS. Mechanisms of pain. *Proc Natl Acad Sci U S A.* 2001;98(21):11845–11846.
5. Basbaum AI, Bautista DM, Scherrer G, Julius DJC. Cellular and molecular mechanisms of pain. *Cell.* 2009;139(2):267–284.
6. Mehra D, Mangwani-Mordani S, Acuna K, Hwang JC, Felix ER, Galor A. Long-term trigeminal nerve stimulation as a treatment for ocular pain. *Neuromodulation: Technology at the Neural Interface.* 2021;24:1107–1114. https://doi.org/10.1111/ner.13402.
7. Craig JP, Nichols KK, Akpek EK, et al. TFOS DEWS II definition and classification report. *Ocul Surf.* 2017;15(3):276–283.
8. Ganesalingam K, Ismail S, Sherwin T, Craig JP. Molecular evidence for the role of inflammation in dry eye disease. *Clin Exp Optom.* 2019;102(5):446–454.
9. Bron AJ, Yokoi N, Gaffney E, Tiffany JM. Predicted phenotypes of dry eye: proposed consequences of its natural history. *Ocul Surf.* 2009;7(2):78–92.
10. Villani E, Bonsignore F, Cantalamessa E, Serafino M, Nucci P. Imaging biomarkers for dry eye disease. *Eye Contact Lens.* 2020;46(Suppl 2):S141–s145.

11. Galor A, Felix ER, Feuer W, Levitt RC, Sarantopoulos CD. Corneal nerve pathway function in individuals with dry eye symptoms. *Ophthalmology*. 2021;128(4):619–621.
12. Yu J, Asche CV, Fairchild CJ. The economic burden of dry eye disease in the United States: a decision tree analysis. *Cornea*. 2011;30(4):379–387.
13. Goyal S, Hamrah P. Understanding neuropathic corneal pain—gaps and current therapeutic approaches. *Semin Ophthalmol*. 2016;31(1–2):59–70.
14. Patel S, Felix ER, Levitt RC, Sarantopoulos CD, Galor A. Dysfunctional coping mechanisms contribute to dry eye symptoms. *J Clin Med*. 2019;8(6):901.
15. Galor A, Zlotcavitch L, Walter SD, et al. Dry eye symptom severity and persistence are associated with symptoms of neuropathic pain. *Br J Ophthalmol*. 2015;99(5):665–668.
16. Galor A, Moein HR, Lee C, et al. Neuropathic pain and dry eye. *Ocul Surf*. 2018;16(1):31–44.
17. Yang AY, Chow J, Liu J. Corneal innervation and sensation: the eye and beyond. *Yale J Biol Med*. 2018;91(1):13–21.
18. Müller LJ, Marfurt CF, Kruse F, Tervo TMT. Corneal nerves: structure, contents and function. *Exp Eye Res*. 2003;76(5):521–542.
19. Müller LJ, Pels L, Vrensen GF. Ultrastructural organization of human corneal nerves. *Invest Ophthalmol Vis Sci*. 1996;37(4):476–488.
20. Shaheen BS, Bakir M, Jain S. Corneal nerves in health and disease. *Surv Ophthalmol*. 2014;59(3):263–285.
21. Belmonte C, Gallar J, Lopez-Briones LG, Pozo MA. Polymodality in nociceptive neurons: experimental models of chemotransduction. In: *Paper Presented at: Cellular Mechanisms of Sensory Processing*. 1994 (Berlin, Heidelberg).
22. Bessou P, Perl ER. Response of cutaneous sensory units with unmyelinated fibers to noxious stimuli. *J Neurophysiol*. 1969;32(6):1025–1043.
23. Belmonte C, Acosta MC, Merayo-Lloves J, Gallar J. What causes eye pain? *Curr Ophthalmol Rep*. 2015;3(2):111–121.
24. Belmonte C, Acosta MC, Gallar J. Neural basis of sensation in intact and injured corneas. *Exp Eye Res*. 2004;78(3):513–525.
25. Rosenthal P, Borsook D. The corneal pain system. Part I: the missing piece of the dry eye puzzle. *Ocul Surf*. 2012;10(1):2–14.
26. Moulton EA, Becerra L, Rosenthal P, Borsook D. An approach to localizing corneal pain representation in human primary somatosensory cortex. *PLoS One*. 2012;7(9):e44643.
27. Hu J, Sessle B, Raboisson P, Dallel R, Woda A. Stimulation of craniofacial muscle afferents induces prolonged facilitatory effects in trigeminal nociceptive brain-stem neurones. *Pain*. 1992;48(1):53–60.
28. Pozo MA, Cervero F. Neurons in the rat spinal trigeminal complex driven by corneal nociceptors: receptive-field properties and effects of noxious stimulation of the cornea. *J Neurophysiol*. 1993;70(6):2370–2378.
29. Dubner R, Bennett G. Spinal and trigeminal mechanisms of nociception. *Annu Rev Neurosci*. 1983;6(1):381–418.
30. Dubner R. Hyperalgesia and expanded receptive fields. *Pain*. 1992;48(1):3–4.
31. Yoon YW, Na HS, Chung JM. Contributions of injured and intact afferents to neuropathic pain in an experimental rat model. *Pain*. 1996;64(1):27–36.
32. Li Y, Dorsi MJ, Meyer RA, Belzberg A. Mechanical hyperalgesia after an L5 spinal nerve lesion in the rat is not dependent on input from injured nerve fibers. *Pain*. 2000;85(3):493–502.
33. Gold MS. Spinal nerve ligation: what to blame for the pain and why. *Pain*. 2000;84(2):117–120.
34. Ringkamp M, Meyer RA. Injured versus uninjured afferents: who is to blame for neuropathic pain? *Anesthesiology*. 2005;103(2):221–223.
35. Tran EL, Crawford LK. Revisiting PNS plasticity: how uninjured sensory afferents promote neuropathic pain. *Front Cell Neurosci*. 2020;14.
36. Small LR, Galor A, Felix ER, Horn DB, Levitt RC, Sarantopoulos CD. Oral gabapentinoids and nerve blocks for the treatment of chronic ocular pain. *Eye Contact Lens*. 2020;46(3).
37. Dieckmann G, Borsook D, Moulton E. Neuropathic corneal pain and dry eye: a continuum of nociception. *Br J Ophthalmol*. 2021.
38. Belmonte C, Nichols JJ, Cox SM, et al. TFOS DEWS II pain and sensation report. *Ocul Surf*. 2017;15(3):404–437.
39. Hermanson O, Blomqvist A. Subnuclear localization of FOS-like immunoreactivity in the rat parabrachial nucleus after nociceptive stimulation. *J Comp Neurol*. 1996;368(1):45–56.
40. Uddin O, Anderson M, Smith J, Masri R, Keller A. Parabrachial complex processes dura inputs through a direct trigeminal ganglion-to-parabrachial connection. *Neurobiol Pain*. 2021;9:100060.
41. Aicher SA, Hermes SM, Hegarty DM. Corneal afferents differentially target thalamic-and parabrachial-projecting neurons in spinal trigeminal nucleus caudalis. *Neuroscience*. 2013;232:182–193.
42. Gauriau C, Bernard JF. Pain pathways and parabrachial circuits in the rat. *Exp Physiol*. 2002;87(2):251–258.
43. Katagiri A, Kato TJ. Multi-dimensional role of the parabrachial nucleus in regulating pain-related affective disturbances in trigeminal neuropathic pain. *J Oral Sci*. 2020;62(2):160–164.
44. Digre KB, Brennan KC. Shedding light on photophobia. *J Neuroophthalmol*. 2012;32(1):68.
45. Hirata A, Aguilar J, Castro-Alamancos MA. Noradrenergic activation amplifies bottom-up and top-down signal-to-noise ratios in sensory thalamus. *J Neurosci*. 2006;26(16):4426–4436.
46. Galor A, Levitt RC, Felix E, Martin ER, Sarantopoulos CJ. Neuropathic ocular pain: an important yet underevaluated feature of dry eye. *Eye*. 2015;29(3):301–312.
47. Xie Y-f, Huo F-q, Tang J-s. Cerebral cortex modulation of pain. *Acta Pharmacol Sin*. 2009;30(1):31–41.
48. Tang J-S, Qu C-L, Huo F-Q. The thalamic nucleus submedius and ventrolateral orbital cortex are involved in

nociceptive modulation: a novel pain modulation pathway. *Prog Neurobiol.* 2009;89(4):383−389.

49. Sivilotti L, Woolf CJ. The contribution of GABAA and glycine receptors to central sensitization: disinhibition and touch-evoked allodynia in the spinal cord. *J Neurophysiol.* 1994;72(1):169−179.

50. Mehra D, Cohen NK, Galor A. Ocular surface pain: a narrative review. *Ophthalmol Ther.* 2020;9(3):1−21.

51. Parra A, Gonzalez-Gonzalez O, Gallar J, Belmonte C. Tear fluid hyperosmolality increases nerve impulse activity of cold thermoreceptor endings of the cornea. *Pain.* 2014; 155(8):1481−1491.

52. Pergolizzi J, Ahlbeck K, Aldington D, et al. The development of chronic pain: physiological CHANGE necessitates a multidisciplinary approach to treatment. *Curr Med Res Opin.* 2013;29(9):1127−1135.

53. Hegarty DM, Hermes SM, Yang K, Aicher SA. Select noxious stimuli induce changes on corneal nerve morphology. *J Comp Neurol.* 2017;525(8):2019−2031.

54. Moulton EA, Borsook D. C-fiber assays in the cornea vs. skin. *Brain Sci.* 2019;9(11):320.

55. Alamri A, Bron R, Brock JA, Ivanusic JJ. Transient receptor potential cation channel subfamily V member 1 expressing corneal sensory neurons can be subdivided into at least three subpopulations. *Front Neuroanat.* 2015;9:71.

56. Yang JM, Wei ET, Kim SJ, Yoon KC. TRPM8 channels and dry eye. *Pain.* 2018;11(4):125.

57. Yoon HJ, Kim J, Yang JM, Wei ET, Kim SJ, Yoon KC. Topical TRPM8 agonist for relieving neuropathic ocular pain in patients with dry eye: a pilot study. *J Clin Med.* 2021;10(2):250.

58. Scholz J, Woolf CJ. Can we conquer pain? *Nat Neurosci.* 2002;5(11):1062−1067.

59. Schecterson LC, Pazevic AA, Yang R, Matulef K, Gordon SE. TRPV1, TRPA1, and TRPM8 are expressed in axon terminals in the cornea: TRPV1 axons contain CGRP and secretogranin II; TRPA1 axons contain secretogranin 3. *Mol Vis.* 2020;26:576.

60. Piña R, Ugarte G, Campos M, et al. Role of TRPM8 channels in altered cold sensitivity of corneal primary sensory neurons induced by axonal damage. *J Neurosci.* 2019; 39(41):8177−8192.

61. Parra A, Madrid R, Echevarria D, et al. Ocular surface wetness is regulated by TRPM8-dependent cold thermoreceptors of the cornea. *Nat Med.* 2010;16(12): 1396−1399.

62. Li F, Yang W, Jiang H, et al. TRPV1 activity and substance P release are required for corneal cold nociception. *Nat Commun.* 2019;10(1):1−13.

63. De Caro C, Russo R, Avagliano C, et al. Antinociceptive effect of two novel transient receptor potential melastatin 8 antagonists in acute and chronic pain models in rat. *Br J Pharmacol.* 2018;175(10):1691−1706.

64. Fakih D, Baudouin C, Goazigo R-L, Mélik Parsadaniantz SJ. TRPM8: a therapeutic target for neuroinflammatory symptoms induced by severe dry eye disease. *Int J Mol Sci.* 2020;21(22):8756.

65. Chatchaisak D, Srikiatkhachorn A, Maneesri-le Grand S, Govitrapong P, Chetsawang BJ. The role of calcitonin gene-related peptide on the increase in transient receptor potential vanilloid-1 levels in trigeminal ganglion and trigeminal nucleus caudalis activation of rat. *J Chem Neuroanat.* 2013;47:50−56.

66. Fernández-Montoya J, Avendaño C, Negredo PJ. The glutamatergic system in primary somatosensory neurons and its involvement in sensory input-dependent plasticity. *Int J Mol Sci.* 2018;19(1):69.

67. Lazarov NE. Comparative analysis of the chemical neuroanatomy of the mammalian trigeminal ganglion and mesencephalic trigeminal nucleus. *Prog Neurobiol.* 2002; 66(1):19−59.

68. Lennerz JK, Rühle V, Ceppa EP, et al. Calcitonin receptor-like receptor (CLR), receptor activity modifying protein 1 (RAMP1), and calcitonin gene-related peptide (CGRP) immunoreactivity in the rat trigeminovascular system: differences between peripheral and central CGRP receptor distribution. *J Comp Neurol.* 2008;507(3):1277−1299.

69. Cady RJ, Glenn JR, Smith KM, Durham PL. Calcitonin gene-related peptide promotes cellular changes in trigeminal neurons and glia implicated in peripheral and central sensitization. *Mol Pain.* 2011;7:94.

70. Sun R-Q, Tu Y-J, Lawand NB, Yan J-Y, Lin Q, Willis WDJJ. Calcitonin gene-related peptide receptor activation produces PKA-and PKC-dependent mechanical hyperalgesia and central sensitization. *J Neurophysiol.* 2004;92(5): 2859−2866.

71. Martins D, Santos F, Britto L, Lemos J, Chacur MJ. Neurochemical effects of photobiostimulation in the trigeminal ganglion after inferior alveolar nerve injury. *J Biol Regul Homeost Agents.* 2017;31(1):147−152.

72. Costigan M, Scholz J, Woolf CJ. Neuropathic pain: a maladaptive response of the nervous system to damage. *Annu Rev Neurosci.* 2009;32:1−32.

73. Coutaux A, Adam F, Willer J-C, Le Bars DJ. Hyperalgesia and allodynia: peripheral mechanisms. *Joint Bone Spine.* 2005;72(5):359−371.

74. Pinho-Ribeiro FA, Verri Jr WA, Chiu IM. Nociceptor sensory neuron−immune interactions in pain and inflammation. *Trends Immunol.* 2017;38(1):5−19.

75. Jakubowski M, Levy D, Goor-Aryeh I, et al. Terminating migraine with allodynia and ongoing central sensitization using parenteral administration of COX1/COX2 inhibitors. *Headache.* 2005;45(7):850−861.

76. Latremoliere A, Woolf CJ. Central sensitization: a generator of pain hypersensitivity by central neural plasticity. *J Pain.* 2009;10(9):895−926.

77. Iyengar S, Ossipov MH, Johnson KW. The role of calcitonin gene−related peptide in peripheral and central pain mechanisms including migraine. *J Pain.* 2017; 158(4):543.

78. Ren K, Dubner RJ. Central nervous system plasticity and persistent pain. *J Pain.* 1999;13(3):155−163.

79. Sessle BJ. Neural mechanisms and pathways in craniofacial pain. *Can J Neurol Sci.* 1999;26(3):7−11.

80. Taylor BK, Sinha GP, Donahue RR, Grachen CM, Morón JA, Doolen S. Opioid receptors inhibit the spinal ampa receptor Ca^{2+} permeability that mediates latent pain sensitization. *Exp Neurol.* 2019;314:58−66.

81. Cull-Candy S, Kelly L, Farrant M. Regulation of Ca^{2+}-permeable AMPA receptors: synaptic plasticity and beyond. *Curr Opin Neurobiol.* 2006;16(3):288−297.

82. Kalangara JP, Galor A, Levitt RC, Felix ER, Alegret R, Sarantopoulos CD. Burning eye syndrome: do neuropathic pain mechanisms underlie chronic dry eye? *Pain Med.* 2016;17(4):746−755.

83. Ebrahimiadib N, Yousefshahi F, Abdi P, Ghahari M, Modjtahedi BS. Ocular neuropathic pain: an overview focusing on ocular surface pains. *Clin Ophthalmol.* 2020; 14:2843.

84. Kurose M, Meng ID. Dry eye modifies the thermal and menthol responses in rat corneal primary afferent cool cells. *J Neurophysiol.* 2013;110(2):495−504.

85. Diel RJ, Mehra D, Kardon R, Buse DC, Moulton E, Galor A. Photophobia: shared pathophysiology underlying dry eye disease, migraine and traumatic brain injury leading to central neuroplasticity of the trigeminothalamic pathway. *Br J Ophthalmol.* 2020.

86. Woolf CJ, Mannion RJ. Neuropathic pain: aetiology, symptoms, mechanisms, and management. *Lancet.* 1999;353(9168):1959−1964.

87. Bridges D, Thompson S, Rice AS. Mechanisms of neuropathic pain. *Br J Anaesth.* 2001;87(1):12−26.

88. Baron R. Neuropathic pain: a clinical perspective. *Handb Exp Pharmacol.* 2009:3−30.

89. Devor M. Sodium channels and mechanisms of neuropathic pain. *J Pain.* 2006;7(1):S3−S12.

90. Kalso E. Sodium channel blockers in neuropathic pain. *Curr Pharm Des.* 2005;11(23):3005−3011.

91. Bhattacharya A, Wickenden AD, Chaplan SR. Sodium channel blockers for the treatment of neuropathic pain. *Neurotherapeutics.* 2009;6(4):663−678.

92. Mcmonnies CW. The potential role of neuropathic mechanisms in dry eye syndromes. *J Optom.* 2017; 10(1):5−13.

93. Masuoka T, Gallar J, Belmonte C. Therapeutics. Inhibitory effect of amitriptyline on the impulse activity of cold thermoreceptor terminals of intact and tear-deficient Guinea pig corneas. *J Ocul Pharmacol Ther.* 2018;34(1−2):195−203.

94. Guerrero-Moreno A, Baudouin C, Melik Parsadaniantz S, Goazigo R-L. Morphological and functional changes of corneal nerves and their contribution to peripheral and central sensory abnormalities. *Front Cell Neurosci.* 2020; 14:436.

95. Rahman M, Okamoto K, Thompson R, Katagiri A, Bereiter DA. Sensitization of trigeminal brainstem pathways in a model for tear deficient dry eye. *Pain.* 2015; 156(5):942.

96. Rosenthal P, Borsook D. Ocular neuropathic pain. *Br J Ophthalmol.* 2016;100(1):128−134.

97. Faweett J, Keynes R. Peripheral nerve regeneration. *Neurosci Res.* 1990;13(1):43−60.

98. Aggarwal S, Colon C, Kheirkhah A, Hamrah P. Efficacy of autologous serum tears for treatment of neuropathic corneal pain. *Ocul Surf.* 2019;17(3):532−539.

99. Bayraktutar BN, Ozmen MC, Muzaaya N, et al. Comparison of clinical characteristics of post-refractive surgery-related and post-herpetic neuropathic corneal pain. *Ocul Surf.* 2020;18(4):641−650.

100. Moein H-R, Akhlaq A, Dieckmann G, et al. Visualization of microneuromas by using in vivo confocal microscopy: an objective biomarker for the diagnosis of neuropathic corneal pain? *Ocul Surf.* 2020;18(4):651−656.

101. Dermer H, Hwang J, Mittal R, Cohen A, Galor A. Corneal sub-basal nerve plexus microneuromas in individuals with and without dry eye. *Br J Ophthalmol.* 2021. https://doi.org/10.1136/bjophthalmol-2020-317891. Published Online First: 04 January.

102. Katagiri A, Shinoda M, Honda K, Toyofuku A, Sessle BJ, Iwata K. Satellite glial cell P2Y12 receptor in the trigeminal ganglion is involved in lingual neuropathic pain mechanisms in rats. *Mol Pain.* 2012;8.

103. Launay P-S, Reboussin E, Liang H, et al. Ocular inflammation induces trigeminal pain, peripheral and central neuroinflammatory mechanisms. *Neurobiol Dis.* 2016;88:16−28.

104. Fakih D, Zhao Z, Nicolle P, et al. Chronic dry eye induced corneal hypersensitivity, neuroinflammatory responses, and synaptic plasticity in the mouse trigeminal brainstem. *J Neuroinflammation.* 2019;16(1):268.

105. Ji R-R, Berta T, Nedergaard M. Glia and pain: is chronic pain a gliopathy? *Pain.* 2013;154:S10−S28.

106. Matsui T, Hitomi S, Hayashi Y, et al. Microglial activation in the trigeminal spinal subnucleus interpolaris/caudalis modulates orofacial incisional mechanical pain hypersensitivity associated with orofacial injury in infancy. *J Oral Sci.* 2021;63(2):170−173.

107. Ceruti S. From astrocytes to satellite glial cells and back: a 25 year-long journey through the purinergic modulation of glial functions in pain and more. *Biochem Pharmacol.* 2021;187:114397.

108. Liang H, Hu H, Shan D, et al. CGRP modulates orofacial pain through mediating neuron-glia crosstalk. *J Dent Res.* 2020;100(1):98−105.

109. Galor A, Levitt RC, Felix ER, Sarantopoulos CD. What can photophobia tell us about dry eye? *Expert Rev Ophthalmol.* 2016;11(5):321−324.

110. Galor A, Patel S, Small LR, et al. Pregabalin failed to prevent dry eye symptoms after laser-assisted in situ keratomileusis (LASIK) in a randomized pilot study. *J Clin Med.* 2019;8(9):1355.

111. Schiffman RM, Christianson MD, Jacobsen G, Hirsch JD, Reis BL. Reliability and validity of the ocular surface disease index. *Arch Ophthalmol.* 2000;118(5):615−621.

112. Chalmers RL, Begley CG, Caffery B. Validation of the 5-item dry eye questionnaire (DEQ-5): discrimination across self-assessed severity and aqueous tear deficient

dry eye diagnoses. *Contact Lens Anterior Eye.* 2010;33(2): 55–60.

113. Farhangi M, Feuer W, Galor A, et al. Modification of the neuropathic pain symptom inventory for use in eye pain (NPSI-eye). *Pain.* 2019;160(7):1541–1550.

114. Qazi Y, Hurwitz S, Khan S, Jurkunas UV, Dana R, Hamrah P. Validity and reliability of a novel ocular pain assessment survey (OPAS) in quantifying and monitoring corneal and ocular surface pain. *Ophthalmology.* 2016;123(7):1458–1468.

Index

Note: Page numbers followed by "f" indicate figures, "t" indicate tables and "b" indicate boxes.

Printed and bound by CPI Group (UK) Ltd, Croydon, CR0 4YY

03/10/2024

01040300-0002